SURGERY IN
AMERICA
SECOND EDITION

SURGERY IN AMERICA

SECOND EDITION

---

*From the Colonial Era to
the Twentieth Century*

---

*EDITED BY
A. SCOTT EARLE*

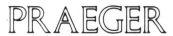

PRAEGER SPECIAL STUDIES • PRAEGER SCIENTIFIC

New York • Philadelphia • Eastbourne, UK
Toronto • Hong Kong • Tokyo • Sydney

Library of Congress Cataloging in Publication Data

Main entry under title:

Surgery in America.

    Bibliography: p.
    Includes index.
    1. Surgery—United States—History—Addresses.
essays, lectures.   I. Earle, A. Scott.
RD27.3.U6S94   1983   617′.0973   83-17808
ISBN 0-03-061999-8 (alk. paper)

Published in 1983 by Praeger Publishers
CBS Educational and Professional Publishing
a Division of CBS Inc.
521 Fifth Avenue, New York, NY 10175 USA

© 1983 by Praeger Publishers

3456789 052 987654321

Printed in the United States of America
on acid-free paper

Introduction

Some years ago, while garnering material for a planned history of American surgery, it became obvious that the story of surgery's growth in this country had been told—and told well—by the men who contributed most to its progress. I attempted, in the first edition of this anthology and again in this one, to present this story in the words of those who practiced in the past and knew the surgery of their times.

Almost twenty years have slipped by since the first edition of this anthology appeared. It has now been out of print for over ten years, including, unfortunately, the bicentennial year when there was revived demand for the book. No matter—it does seem time to revive *Surgery in America* with an enlarged second edition.

Several criteria were used in choosing the selections included in this anthology. Some, of course, demanded inclusion. These are the classics of American surgery: McDowell's papers on ovariotomy and Warren's and Bigelow's account of the first use of ether for surgical anesthesia. Other selections were chosen not because they represented surgical milestones but because they were representative writings of men such as Philip Syng Physick and Nathan Smith, who are important figures in the history of early American surgery, men whose importance derives more from their influence as teachers and outstanding surgeons in their day than from any single contribution.

Some of the selections chosen were taken from texts, lectures, or articles that shaped the practice and philosophy of American surgeons: examples are excerpts from John Syng Dorsey's *Elements of Surgery* (the first American surgical text to attempt to cover the entire field of surgery) and John Jones's "Introductory Lecture to His Course in Surgery." Still others of the writings, such as Samuel White's description of a successful enterotomy performed in 1806, are little known today but are sharp in their portrayal of surgery as it was when the article was written.

A few of the items have been edited by others; they derive much of their interest from this editing. H. H. A. Beach's selections from the early surgical records of the Massachusetts General Hospital and Robert Buck's delightful annotation of a colonial apprentice's diary fall into this group. Others of the selections document great feats of surgery almost forgotten: Valentine Mott's tour de force, the ligation (sadly, not quite successful) of the innominate artery in 1818 is one example; another is Nathan Smith's ovariotomy performed soon after McDowell's. Such operations, performed while European surgery was at its peak, forecast the boldness and ingenuity that brought American surgery to the fore a century later.

In choosing the selections, I have attempted to maintain as high a level of readability as possible. Where there has been a choice between two versions, the informal one is usually more entertaining and easier to read. Thus, Beaumont's account of Alexis St. Martin's wound has been taken from his journal rather than from the more stilted account in *Experiments and Observations,* and Sims's description of his operation for vesicovaginal fistula has been taken from his autobiography rather from his article in the *American Journal of the Medical Sciences.*

This edition has been enlarged considerably over the first. Several items have been added that now seem more important to me than they did before—Thomas Smith's inaugural thesis, for example, describing his 1805 experiments on intestinal repair. Selections have also been added that I simply did not know about at the time the first edition appeared (e.g., the successful suture of multiple intestinal wounds by country doctor Aquila Toland in 1837). Still other items have taken on added meaning because of recent events. I have included, for example, material on the assassination of President Garfield in 1881. This was an event that was important to American surgery at the time that it happened; it is also of interest today, during a time when there is an open season on world leaders. Another article has been added that tells the story of President Cleveland's operations. Garfield's surgical care was poor; Cleveland's was good. American surgery improved during the thirteen years between the two events.

In adding further material, I have tried (as I did in the earlier edition) to choose items that give a feeling both for surgery as it was then practiced and for the time in which the item was written. Two articles are now included that could only have been written on America's western frontier. One is on scalping injuries, the other on arrow wounds; both were treated very much in the manner of their time.

A clinical article by William Stewart Halsted now accompanies his essay on the training of a surgeon (Halsted also figures prominently in another added paper on local anesthesia in surgery by R. J. Hall). The new addition is the paper in which he describes and rationalizes his operation for cancer of the breast. This paper has an importance to surgery far beyond its immediate subject, although it is important for that, also. It would be impossible to overemphasize Halsted's importance to the history of American surgery. He brought scholarship to his profession and the best of European surgery to America, emphasized the importance of meticulous surgical technique, standardized surgical procedures, and taught surgeons who went out from Johns Hopkins as specialists and teachers of the highest order. With Halsted more than any other figure, American surgery came of age.

I have edited some of the articles in this anthology, trying to keep the editorial hand light. In almost every case editing has consisted only of shortening the article to increase readability. In a few of the earlier items—John Jones's "Introductory Lecture" most notably—punctuation has been changed to conform more closely to present-day custom. I believe that in every case the author's meaning and style have remained intact. Surgeons, particularly during the nineteenth century, were wordy and often poorly educated men (I am not aware of any women who practiced surgery during the years covered by this anthology). Today's surgeons, to whom this book is primarily directed, should not have to wade through poorly written, seemingly endless articles—no matter how interesting they may be—in order to get the author's gist. In each introductory note, I have indicated the extent of editing that was carried out for that selection. I suggest that the reader obtain a copy of the original article if the item is of particular interest.

A sense of frustration is inevitable when one reflects on the gems of surgical history that lie waiting to be unearthed in the small mountain of writing turned out prior to the beginning of this century (small only in comparison with the massive bulk that has accumulated since then). I believe that I have mined a few, but I know that there are many more waiting to be found. The knowledgeable reader may detect the absence of certain selections that are often cited as landmarks in the history of American surgery (Bobbs's cholecystostomy, Marks's wound of the heart, and a number of other "firsts"). These and other similar articles have been reviewed and are simply not, in my opinion, of sufficient importance to warrant inclusion. The reader may complain that there were yet other surgical writings that appeared before 1900 that might have been included here. I cannot disagree but offer the excuse that an editor has both a prerogative and a need to be arbitrary in selecting articles for an anthology such as this one.

Footnotes have been used freely and are intended to be read with the selections. With these notes I have tried to establish relationships both among surgeons and between them and the events of their time in the hope that this will be as much a history as an anthology. Pertinent citations have often been included directly in the text in order to reserve the footnotes for background material. In this way I have tried to preserve a flow and readability as uncluttered as possible in a work of this type.

No attempt has been made to glorify the American surgeon of the past. The reader should understand that surgery in America, on the average, did not compare favorably with that practiced in Europe, particularly during the last quarter of the nineteenth century. There are a number of reasons for this—poor preliminary education, inadequate medical training based in large part on an apprentice–preceptor system, proprietary medical schools, an overwhelming tradition to practice as "physician and surgeon" (still with us in more than vestigial form in certain areas of this country), and strong-minded emphasis on the practical rather than the theoretical. (This latter "extreme emphasis on utility" has been cited by R. H. Shryock in his excellent essay "American Indifference to Basic Science During the Nineteenth Century," in *Medicine in America: Historical Essays*.)

There are many surgical writings published during the present century that deserve inclusion in an anthology such as this one; we have debated about using them but have decided that these will have to wait. Aging and improved perspective will help them. The beginning of the twentieth century is a convenient cutoff date and is about the point at which modern surgery began. Further, the development of the subspecialties beginning at that time makes the surgical history of our era so complex that it is difficult to do it justice. Indeed, it has been difficult to ignore the trend toward specialization that occurred during the last years of the nineteenth century, especially at Johns Hopkins with Halsted's encouragement. In any event, there are now a number of collections of histories and anthologies devoted to the various surgical specialties; I have listed a few of these in the Bibliography.

Finally, I am realistic enough to realize that only those with a deep interest in the history of surgery will read this book through page by page. It was not really designed for this. It is a book for browsing, an attempt to present the reader with a time machine that, with the aid of some imagination and reflection, will bring alive the story of the development of our specialty in America.

Acknowledgments

I asked for and received help from many individuals and libraries in preparing both the first, and now this, the second edition of *Surgery in America: Selected Writings*. The following in particular must be mentioned.

The late Henry R. Viets, M.D., Curator of the Boston Medical Library, was especially supportive during the preparation of the first edition of this book and offered invaluable encouragement and help. I believe that his insistence on accuracy—including full dates and middle names—has borne fruit. The 1965 edition of this work was prepared while the editor was living in a part of Idaho where medical library facilities were not available; therefore, the services of the National Library of Medicine were used extensively. This library filled innumerable requests for material, much of it old and obscure. Many of the illustrations in the first edition (carried forward also into this one) were supplied by the library both from their portrait collection and from reproductions made by their photographic services. Without that help there would have been no first edition. I am deeply grateful for that past assistance.

A special note of thanks must go to John B. Blake, Ph.D., at that time the Chief of the History of Medicine Division of the National Library of Medicine, who provided me with data that I was unable to find elsewhere and arranged for the reproduction of many of the illustrations found in the original edition of this book that have been used again in this one.

The New York Academy of Medicine has provided several of the portraits used in this anthology; also, during the preparation of the first edition, Gertrude L. Annan of the New York Academy's library was most helpful in identifying various New York practitioners. Other libraries and librarians were also helpful with the preparation of the original edition. These included Kathleen Worst and the Library of the American College of Surgeons; Joseph I. Waring, M.D., of the Historical Library of the Medical College of South Carolina; W. D. Postell of the Rudolph Matas Medical Library of Tulane University; S. A. G. Kaith; the Boston Medical library; the Library of the Worcester (Massachusetts) Antiquarian Society; and Warren Wheeler of the Massachusetts Historical Society, for his help in obtaining the reproductions of early Boston newspapers.

For the present edition, I am particularly grateful to the librarians of the Brittingham Memorial Library of the Cleveland Metropolitan Hospital for helping me with the many out-of-the-ordinary requests that I made of them. John B. Blake, Ph.D., and Peter Olch, M.D., of the National Library of Medicine kindly provided me with the background material on surgeon J. H. Bill, Jr. Both the Public Library of Nashville and Davidson County (Mary Glenn Hearne) and the Tennessee State Library and Archives (Leslie Pritikin) helped by providing material on James and Felix Robertson. I want also to thank Walter A. Strauss, Chairman of the Department of Comparative Literature at Case Western Reserve University, for the translation of the quotation from Richard Volkmann, quoted by W. S. Halsted in "The Training of the Surgeon."

I owe special thanks to David Dunsmore, Vincent Messina, and Michele Timock, medical photographers of the Cleveland Metropolitan Hospital, for their help in preparing many of the illustrations that have been added to this edition.

I am particularly grateful to Mrs. Glen Jenkins, Rare Book Curator of the Allen Memorial Library of Medicine in Cleveland, for her continuing assistance in helping me find obscure articles and references and in providing a number of useful suggestions that were incorporated into the present edition of this anthology.

I gratefuly acknowledge the permission given to me to reproduce the following articles:

The New England Journal of Medicine and Robert W. Buck, M.D., for the article "Tucker's Wife's Leg."

The American Journal of Surgery for the use of Rudolph Matas's article "Surgery Fifty Years Ago."

The Bulletin of the College of Physicians of Philadelphia for John Jones's "Introductory Lecture to His Course in Surgery."

The C. V. Mosby Company for the use of material from Jesse E. Myer's *Life and Letters of Dr. William Beaumont*.

Lippincott and Harper & Row for use of edited material from *The Surgical Operations on President Cleveland in 1893* by W. W. Keen.

Finally to my wife Barbara and to our children, my thanks and more for their understanding and support during the long hours spent in compiling this material.

Contents

List of Illustrations

SURGERY IN AMERICA
SECOND EDITION

Abigail Eliot's Head Injury

INCREASE MATHER (1639–1723)

The following item is, I believe, the first mention in print of a specific surgical procedure to be performed in an American colony (probably around 1640). The operating surgeon, Mr. Oliver, did not do much of an operation—which probably was all for the best—but he and Mr. Prat (Pratt), who was also called, did provide surgical consultation and care when it was needed. Abigail Eliot's recovery seemed miraculous to the colonists, and for that reason this case report found its way into Increase Mather's book, Remarkable Providences Illustrative of the Earlier Days of American Colonisation, *published in 1684 (the year before he became president of Harvard College).*

Mather was a prolific writer. He also became one of the most influential individuals living in the Massachusetts Bay Colony. He had graduated from Harvard College in 1656 and then studied divinity in Dublin, Ireland, before returning to Massachusetts in 1661 to become a minister in Boston. He is remembered today as an ecclesiastic, writer, and politician. Mather returned to England some years later (in 1688) as an emissary to the crown from the Congregational churches of the Bay Colony. This was very much a political mission, and one result of it was the privilege, given to him by William III, to nominate the colonial governor and other officers. Mather, in spite of his political influence, considered himself above all else a minister. He maintained a healthy interest in science and encouraged scientific study at Har-

vard, which he felt should be more than simply a school for educating ministers.

Who were Mr. Oliver and Mr. Prat (Pratt), who are mentioned in Mather's accounting of Abigail Eliot's accident? Neither man is listed in any of the standard American medical biographies, but Pratt is to be found on the first page of Packard's History of Medicine in the United States as a surgeon hired in England in 1628 to serve the Massachusetts Bay "plantacon" (plantation) in New England. He received "40 lb." (pounds) to pay for his chest and first year's salary. John Pratt fulfilled his three-year contract with the Massachusetts Bay Company and then settled in Cambridge. Nothing is known today of his training or experience. An obituary of sorts is to be found in Governor Winthrop's Journals, where it is mentioned that Pratt, then over 60, perished when the ship on which he was returning to England went down off the coast of Spain in 1645; this information also serves to place Abigail Eliot's accident in the very early years of the colonial era.

Mr. (Thomas) Oliver is also mentioned by Governor Winthrop, who identifies him as a skillful physician and surgeon living in Boston between 1632 and 1644; apparently nothing further is known of him today.

The account of Abigail Eliot's wound included here is to be found on page 54 of the 1890 edition of Increase Mather's Remarkable Providences (London; Reeves and Turner, 1890).

Abigail Eliot's Head Injury

Remarkable was the preservation and restoration which the gracious providence of God vouchsafed to Abigail Eliot, the daughter of elder Eliot, of Boston, in New England; concerning whom, a near and precious relative of hers informs me, that when she was a child under a cart, an iron hinge, being sharp at the lower end, happened to strike her head, between the right ear and the crown of her head and pierced into the skull and brain. The child making an outcry, the mother came, and immediately drew out the iron, and thereupon some of the brains of her child which stuck to the iron, and other bits were scattered on her forehead. Able chyrurgeons were sent for—in special Mr. Oliver and Mr. Prat. The head being uncovered, there appeared just upon the place where the iron pierced the skull, a bunch as big as a small egg. A question arose, whether the skin should not be cut and dilated from the orifice of the wound to the swelling, and so take it away. This Mr. Prat inclined unto, but Mr. Oliver opposed pleading that then the air would

get to the brain, and the child would presently die. Mr. Oliver was desired to undertake the cure; and thus was his operation:—He gently
drove the soft matter of the bunch into the wound, and pressed so
much out as well he could; there came forth about a spoonful; the matter which came forth was brains and blood (some curdles of brain were
white and not stained with blood): so did he apply a plaister. The skull
wasted where it was pierced to the bigness of a half crown piece of silver or more. The skin was exceeding tender, so that a silver plate, like
the skull, was always kept in the place to defend it from any touch or
injury. The brains of the child did swell and swage according to the
tides:— when it was spring-time her brain would heave up the tender
skin, and fill the place sometimes; when it was neap-tide, they would
be sunk and fallen within the skull. This child lived to be the mother of
two children; and (which is marvellous) she was not by this wound
made defective in her memory or understanding.

The First Published Accounts of Elective Surgical Operations in the Colonies

ZABDIEL BOYLSTON (1679–1766)

The two advertisements that follow are the first published accounts of elective surgical operations performed in the North American Colonies. Both appeared in Boston newspapers: both operations were performed by Zabdiel Boylston of that city. Elective surgery had surely been carried out prior to Boylston's time, but we have no earlier record of actual operative procedures.

Zabdiel Boylston was born in Muddy River (Brookline), Massachusetts, on March 9, 1679. He learned his medicine and surgery as an apprentice of one John Cutter of Boston. Boylston is best known today as the physician who introduced smallpox inoculation into the Colonies. His surgical ability—and this must have been considerable —has been ignored. Zabdiel Boylston led a long and useful life as a practitioner of Boston. He died on his farm in Brookline on March 1, 1766.

The first of the two advertisements that follow describes an operation for bladder stone, apparently the third that Boylston performed. It appeared in the Boston News-Letter, no. 327, July 17–24, 1710. The second advertisement is an account of a breast amputation and certainly must have been one of the earliest operations for cancer to have been performed in the Colonies. It appeared in the Boston Gazette, no. 50, November 21–28, 1720.

New-England. Numb. 327.

The Boston News-Letter.

Published by Authority.

From Monday July 17. to Monday July 24. 1710.

Boston, July 19th. 1710.

THE SPEECH of His Excellency *JOSEPH DUDLEY*, Esqr. Captain General and Governour in Chief, in and over Her Majesties Province of the *Massachusetts-Bay* in *New-England*, &c. to the Honourable the Council and Representatives in General Court Assembled.

Gentlemen,

IN Answer to our Repeated Humble Addresses to Her Majesty, Her Majesties Ships of War, Forces and Stores by the good Providence of Almighty GOD, are happily arrived, for our Relief against the Common Enemy in our Neighbourhood. I have no doubt of your ready and chearful Obedience to Her Majesty's Commands for our Quota of the Forces, Transports and other necessary Provisions for the Service.

The Season of the Year is far advanced, and will demand our instant proceeding to every Article that is necessary.

Her Majesty has been pleased to Appoint and Constitute the Honourable Col. Nicholson *to Command the Forces in the present Intended Expedition. And I am glad of his presence with us, That he may be a Witness, that we are as much in Earnest to do our Duty, in Obedience to Her Majesty's Commands, as we are sensible of his great care and solicitude to represent on our behalf the benefit of the present Expedition.*

Gentlemen,

I shall take the good Agreement, and Unanimous Proceeding of the Assembly in their present Session, as an Indication of Success in our Endeavour for the Suppression of an ill Neighbour; In Addition to all the other glorious Articles of Success to Her Majesty's Arms in Europe.

A few days I hope may dispatch the Resolves necessary, that I may have the Service and Assistance of the Officers in the several Counties to which they belong: And there shall be nothing wanting on my part, to make every thing equal and easy for the satisfaction and benefit of all Her Majesty's good Subjects of this Province.

Turin, January 1. N.S. They write from Genoa, that General Mahoni was arrived there from Sicily, accompanied by thirteen French Officers; and it was believed, that all the French Troops had been commanded to quit that Island, as they have already done the Kingdom of Spain, and retire into France. We are also advised, that there hath lately been an Insurrection in Galicia, which was occasioned by a Report received among the People, that the French Merchants were preparing to transport great quantities of Corn into France, which they bought up in that Province, where there is a great Scarcity of that Commodity. Letters from Dauphine & Province confirm the Accounts of the Misery of the Country, and the lamentable Condition of the Soldiers for want of their Pay.

Vienna, January 1. We have Advice that the Prince of Moldavia has been displaced by the Ottoman Court and that another is put into his room, because he gave Intelligence to the Muscovites that several hundred Swedes and Cossacks had left Bender and were passing thro' his Country for Hungary, upon which Intelligence the Muscovites laid wait and cut them off. The said disgraced Prince is put under Confinement, and 300000 Crowns which he profer'd for his Liberty have been refus'd.

Milan, January 1. They talk of a Marriage between the Emperors Daughter and the Duke of Savoys Eldest Son.

Dantzick, January 2. Thanks be to God the Plague, which has swept away so many of our Inhabitants, is entirely ceased and last Week the Burials amounted only to 79 which is something under the usual number, when this City is altogether free from Contagious Diseases. The Burials for the Year past amounted to 31603, whereby it appears that about 14000 Persons dyed of the Plague within that Year. We have been scarce delivered from that terrible Calamity, when we are threatened with another, by the Pretensions of the Saxon Troops quartered in our Neighbourhood. They demand a great Sum of Mony upon account of our having own'd Stanislaus for King of Poland, and paid him in that Quality the Toll and other Duties belonging to the Polish Crown; and our Magistrates having taken that Affair into Consideration, have written to several Princes & States to desire them to interpose their good Offices in our favour.

Plimouth, January 3. This Evening came in the Restoration and Plimouth, with a French Privateer of twenty Guns.

Dartmouth, January 2. This Day came into this Port the Peterborough Galley of Bristol, Capt. Samuel Jacob Commander, for London, who discharged his Cargo, taken in at Newfoundland, at Barcelona, reloaded Wines at Saloe, and came from thence the sixth of December, and stopped at Maiorca the 7th, where he found the Tinpot and Dolphin, two Dutch Privateers, who had taken & brought in with them, as Prize, after a hot Dispute, the Fey-Pink of thirty three Guns, and four hundred and odd Men, a French Privateer, but formerly an English Man of War, taken in the Streights by the French.

Edinburgh, January 3. On the 28th past Mr. Greenshield the Clergyman, who was Imprisoned here for Innovations in Matters of Religion, made a second motion to the Lords of the Session to be set at liberty, in opposition to the Magistrates, but the Lords gave it against him 11 to 4, but the next day he brought an Appeal to the Peers of Great Britain assembled in Parliament, which was allowed in Court.

Venice, January 3. N. S. They write from Naples, that Cardinal Grimani had lately made several Alterations in the Ministry of that Kingdom; that divers rich Prizes had been taken from the Enemy on the Coast of Calabria, and brought into Reggio; that the French Troops in Sicily were preparing to quit that Island; and that General Mahoni, and most of the Principal Officers were already sailed from thence.

Milan, January 4. N. S. The Emperor & the King of Spain have ordered a Council to be assembled in this City, consisting of General Thaun, General Zumjungen, Baron Martini, & two Councellors of the Regency, wherein they are to concert the Measures which are to be taken for the more effectual Prosecution of the War; and also to establish the necessary Funds for the Service of the next Campaign. His Catholick Majesty hath declared, that all the Subjects of this State should make application to his Council, and obtain their assent, before they except of any Benefices that shall be granted them by the Court of Rome; his Majesty being willing that all Persons should be preferred according to the Instances they have given of their Zeal and Fidelity to his Service. Letters from Barcelona of the 9th of December advise, Te Deum had been Sung, and other publick Demonstrations of Joy had been given in that City, on the occasion of the Pope's acknowledging Charles the Third as Catholick King of Spain. Advices from Genoa say, that three English Men of War sailed lately from thence for Barcelona, having on Board great Sums of Mony for the Service of his Catholick Majesty; and that the Enemy who were employed in the Siege of Orbitello, were obliged to retire to Porto Longone, having sustained considerable loss in that Expedition.

Vienna, January 4. N. S. This Court appears very well satisfied with the Measures which have been taken by the High-Allies to carry on the War, and are resolved to exert their utmost Power, to oblige the French King to grant such Terms as may effectually tend to the Security of the Empire, and the Tranquility of Europe. The Emperor hath prolonged the Term within which the Hungarian Malecontents are to return to their Allegiance, and to receive the Benefit of his late gracious Declaration of Pardon; and also ordered the Articles which the last Diet of *Presburg* had resolved to grant the States of *Hungary* to be made publick. The Substance of which is, That the States of *Hungary* shall have the Liberty to proceed to the Election of a new King, if the Line-Male of the late Emperor Leopold shall happen to be extinct. That the *Hungarian* Nation shall be entirely governed by their own Laws. That no Gentleman or Burgher of *Hungary* shall be Arrested before a due Citation, unless in Cases of High Treason; on Conviction of which Crime their Goods shall be Confiscated. That a General Diet shall be Assembled every three Years. That the Treasury of *Hungary* shall be dependant on that of *Vienna*, for the better Administration of the publick Revenue; and therefore be no ways Regulated by the general Diet. That the Emperor shall have the disposal of all Ecclesiastical Preferments. That the Affairs of Religion shall be established on the Resolutions of the Diets of *Presburg* and *Ardemburg*. That an *Hungarian* Counsellor may be elected at the first Diet, who is to have the Charge of the Execution of the Laws. That if Prince Ragotzi and his Adherents do not make their Submission to his Imperial Majesty within the last Term granted for their Pardon, they shall be declared Traitors and Enemies to their Country, & their Goods shall be Confiscated for the Service of the Publick. His Imperial Majesty further promises to restore the Lands taken from the Turks to the lawful Proprietors, if they can prove their Title. It is uncertain whether these Overtures of Accommodation will Reconcile the Differences of that Kingdom; but it is said, that Prince Eugene will mediate with the States of *Hungary* at the next Diet of Presburg, in order to determine that War.

Last

Figure 1. The Boston *News–Letter* for July 17th to July 24th, 1710. The advertisement appeared on the back page and apparently represents the first published account of an elective surgical procedure to be carried out in the North American Colonies (Courtesy Massachusetts Historical Society.)

Advertisement.

For the benefit of any that has or may have Occasion. HEnry Hill Distiller in the Town of Boston New-England, having had a Child grievously afflicted with the Stone, apply'd himself to Mr. Zabdiel Boylstoun of the said Boston, Practitioner in Physick and Chirurgery : who on the 24th of June last, in presence of sundry Gentlemen, Physicians and Chyrurgeons, Cut the said Child, & took out of his Bladder a stone of considerable bigness, and with the blessing of God in less than a months time has perfectly Cured him, and holds his Water : This is his third Operation performed in the Stone on Males and Females, and all with good success : He likewise pretends to all other Operations in Surgery. Which Operation the said Hill could not omit to make Publick.

The Boston News-Letter–July, 1710

ADVERTISEMENT

For the benefit of any that has or may have Occaſion. Henry Hill Diſtiller in the Town of Boſton New-England, having had a Child grievouſly afflicted with the Stone, apply'd himſelf to Mr. Zabdiel Boylſtoun of the ſaid Boſton, Practitioner in Phyſick and Chirurgery; who on the 24th of June laſt, in preſence of ſundry Gentlemen, Phyſicians and Chyrurgeons, Cut the ſaid Child, & took out of his Bladder a ſtone of conſiderable bigneſs, and with the bleſſing of God in leſs than a months time has perfectly Cured him, and holds his Water: This is his third Operation performed in the Stone on Males and Females, and all with good ſucceſs: He likewiſe pretends to all other Operations in Surgery. Which Operation the ſaid Hill could not omit to make Publick.

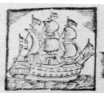
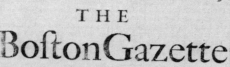

NEW-ENGLAND. No. 50.

THE
Boston Gazette

Publiſhed by Authority.

From MONDAY November 21. to MONDAY November 28. 1720.

A ‖ The Humble Addreſs of the Preſident & Fellows of *Harvard College* in *Cambridge*.

To His Excellency SAMUEL SHUTE Eſq; Captain General and Governour in Chief, in and over His Majeſty's Province of the *Maſſachuſetts-Bay* in *New-England*, and to the Honourable His Majeſty's Council, and Houſe of Repreſentatives in General Court Aſſembled at *Boſton*, *November*, 1720.

WHEREAS it has pleaſed the Great and General Aſſembly of this Province, in anſwer to the Memorials of the Honourable and Reverend the Overſeers of the ſaid College, laid before them at their Seſſions, Novemb. 15th. 1717. and Novemb. 13th. 1718. to Grant and Order an Additional Brick Building to Harvard College, for the Reception and Accommodation of the Tutors and Students there ; and moſt Generouſly from time to time to Allow, Grant and Order to be paid out of the Publick Treaſury to the Committee appointed for the Effecting the ſaid Building, ſuch Sums of Money, as in Your Great Wiſdom and Goodneſs You ſaw neceſſary for ſo great and good a Service.

And whereas it has pleaſed Almighty GOD (to whoſe Honour and Glory our Fathers firſt Founded the ſaid College, and who has made it a ſingular Bleſſing and Honour to the Province unto this day) ſo far to Smile upon Your Pious Expence in this Additional Building, and to proſper the Faithful Cares of the Worthy Gentlemen, the Committee appointed to Overſee the ſame, as that we now ſee with Joy a fine and goodly Houſe Erected and Finiſhed, ſuch as doth every way anſwer the then Views and Propoſals of the Honourable and Reverend the Overſeers Your late Memorialiſts, and will be a laſting Monument, if GOD pleaſe, of the Juſt Regards of the Preſent Government for the Support of Religion and Learning among us in Times to come.

We the Preſident and Fellows of the College do therefore hold Our Selves indiſpenſibly Obliged from the Relation we ſtand in to the College, as well as from the Affection we bear to theſe Churches of our LORD JESUS, firſt of all to give Thanks unto Almighty GOD, who has Inclined and led the Government into, and thro' ſo Great and Noble a Work ; and then alſo to make our Acknowledgments to Your Excellency and Honours for this Great Benefaction to the College, Beſeeching the LORD GOD of our Fathers Graciouſly to Accept of, and abundantly to Reward unto His People this their Offering to His Name.

And as to our Selves, who have the Pleaſure and the Honour, to Addreſs Your Excellency and Honours upon this happy Occaſion, We beg leave to ſay, That we under the Influence and Aſſiſtance of the Divine Grace, in our reſpective Capacities, according to the Truſt repoſed in us, ſhall always Exert our Selves, as we are in Duty bound, to Preſerve and Advance that Society in the Principles and Practice of Piety and Loyalty, and all Vertue, as well as in good Literature, which we know will be the moſt Acceptable Acknowledgment from

May it pleaſe Your Excellency & Honours,

Your moſt Dutiful & Obedient Servant,

John Leverett,

In the Name of the Preſident & Fellows of *Harvard College*.

Madrid, Auguſt 12.

Their Catholick Majeſties, the Prince, and the Infantes, continue at the Eſcurial in perfect Health. The intended Expedition againſt Oran being laid aſide for this Seaſon, the Forces which were order'd for Cadiz to imbark for that Enterprize, are countermanded. The new Levies are continued through the whole Kingdom; the Court intending to augment their Forces to 70000 Foot and 20000 Horſe, but the Veteran Regiments have loſt ſo many Men, that it will be difficult to compleat them, and much more to raiſe new ones. The laſt Convoy which ſail'd from Malaga for Ceuta are ſafely landed, notwithſtanding the great Fire from two Batteries which the Moors had erected to prevent their landing, and from 3000 of their choiceſt Men, which they had placed behind the Rocks for the ſame Purpoſe. The Moors have ſince made an Attack on that Place, but were repulſed with great loſs. Several Projects having been offer'd to this Court to erect Companies of Inſurance in this Kingdom, the ſame have been rejected as Ruinous to Trade, and only calculated to enrich Private Perſons with the Spoils of the Publick.

From

Figure 2. The Boston *Gazette* for November 21st to November 28th. 1720. The advertisement, which appeared on the last page, describes another major operation performed by Zabdiel Boylston. (Courtesy Massachusetts Historical Society.)

FOr the *Publick Good of any that have or may have Cancers*——*Thefe may Certify, That my Wife had been labouring under the dreadful Diſtemper of a Cancer in her Left Breaſt for feveral Years, and altho' the Cure was attempted by fundry Doctors from time to time, to no effect ; And when Life was almoſt defpair'd of by reafon of its repeated bleedings, growth & ſtench, and there feemed immediate hazard of Life, we fend for Doctor* Zabdial Boylſton *of Boſton, who on the 28th. of July* 1718. (*in the prefence of feveral Miniſters & others affembled on that Occaſion*) *Cut her whole Breaſt off ; and by the Bleſſing of* GOD *on his Endeavours, ſhe has obtained a perfect Cure.*

I deferred the Publication of this, leaſt it ſhould have broke out again.   Edward Winſlow.
Rochefter, Octob. 14th. 1720.

The Boston Gazette–November, 1720

ADVERTISEMENT

For the Publick Good of any that have or may have Cancers–Theſe may Certify, That my Wife had been labouring under the dreadful Diſtemper of a Cancer in her Left Breaſt for Several Years, and altho' the Cure was attempted by Sundry Doctors from time to time, to no effect; And when Life was almoſt deſpair'd of by reaſon of its repeated bleedings, growth & ſtench, and there ſeemed immediate hazard of Life, we ſend for Doctor Zabdial Boylſton of Boſton, who on the 28th. of July 1718. (in the preſence of ſeveral Miniſters & others aſſembled on that Ocaſion) Cut her whole Breaſt off; and by the Bleſſing of GOD on his Endeavours, ſhe has obtained a perfect Cure.

I deferred the Publication of this, leaſt it ſhould have broke out again.

Edward Winſlow

Rocheſter, Octob. 14th. 1720

Joseph Baker's Bladder Stone

SILVESTER GARDINER (1707–1786)

The following case report was published as a news item in two Boston newspapers during November of 1741 and obviously represented that day's equivalent of a news release. One suspects that the surgeon, Silvester Gardiner, composed the article, which was (except for typographic differences) the same in the two papers. The operation was unusual; first, because the patient was a young child; and second, because the lithotomy was carried out by the "lateral approach" that had been described by the British surgeon William Cheselden (1688 –1752) only a few years earlier, in 1727 (see Dorsey's description in this anthology, page 75). No operation in surgery arrives de novo; Cheselden's was a modification of one introduced around 1700 by Jacques de Beaulieu (Frere Jacques, 1651–1719), an itinerant French lithotomist. The advantage of the lateral approach, which used a transverse perineal incision extending laterally from the midline, was that there was less chance of damaging the rectum or producing urinary incontinence. This operation was used until it was supplanted by open suprapubic lithotomy and closed transurethral lithotomy in the last century.

Silvester Gardiner was born in Kingston, Rhode Island, in 1707; he received his medical education in England and France. He arrived in London and became Cheselden's pupil at St. Thomas Hospital shortly after the new operation was introduced in 1724. The American

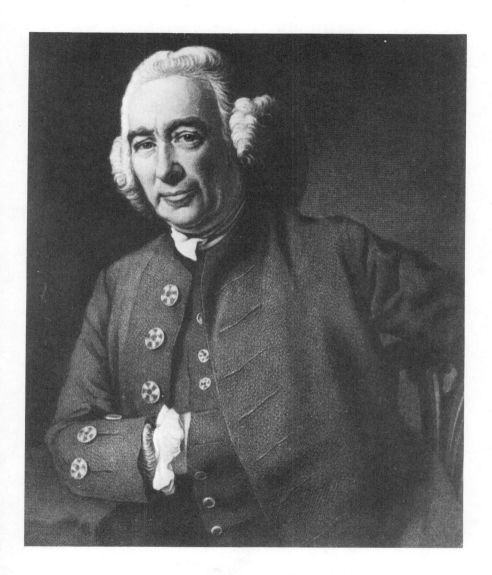

Figure 3. Silvester Gardiner (1707-1786). (Courtesy National Library of Medicine.)

*would have had many opportunities to observe and possibly to help
with lithotomies as well as all of the other procedures performed in that
era; Cheselden was one of Englands best-known and most competent
surgeons (one of his lithotomies was performed in 54 seconds!). Gardiner remained abroad for eight years before returning to America to
settle in Boston (1734). He surely was one of the best-trained physicians
in this country at that time, and presumably delivered a quality of care
equal to that available in England and France at that time.*

*Gardiner practiced in Boston as both a physician and a surgeon.
He was well accepted and was active in organizing a medical society,
probably the one referred to in the following article. He soon branched
out, began to import pharmaceuticals, and established America's first
chain of drugstores with busy apothecary shops in Boston; New Haven;
and Meriden, Connecticut. Gardiner eventually became one of New
England's wealthiest and most successful entrepreneurs (the town of
Gardiner, Maine was named for him). Unfortunately, he was also one
of New England's most ardent loyalists; he lost most of his wealth in
1776 when he fled to Canada and then to England, where he received a
crown pension. Finally, in 1785 Gardiner returned to America, where
in time he regained many of his holdings. He settled and practiced in
Newport, Rhode Island, and died there a respected citizen at the age of
79.*

Joseph Baker's Bladder Stone

A Medical *Society* in Boston *with no quackiſs view, as is the manner of ſome, but for the Comfort and Benefit of the unhappy and miſer-
able Sufferers by the excruciating Pain occaſioned by a Stone in the
Bladder, do publiſh the following Caſe in* Boſton, October 8, 1741. *Joſ-
eph Baker,* Aetat. 6 was cut for the Stone in the Bladder, according to
Mr. *Cheſelden's* late Improvement of the *lateral* Way, by Mr. *Gardiner*
of *Boſton* (who had ſome Part of his Education in the Hoſpitals and In-
firmaries of *London* and *Paris*) in the Preſence of the *Medical Society*
and others, without Reſerve.

This boy by his complaints, ſeems to have had the Rudiments of
this Stone from his Birth, and by Degrees the Paroxiſms of Pain became
ſo violent, that Death or the Operation were unavoidable. This Stone
was extracted in the *Lateral* Method, without Diſtraction or Dilacer-
ation of the Parts, which too frequently kill the Patient in a few days or
Weeks; or if the Patient eſcapes with his Life, the Urine continues to

iſſue involuntarily by the Wound, enduring an uncomfortable Life. Several such miſerabile Inſtances we have had in the Province, for want of Skill and Diſcretion in the Operator.

The Stone when extracted, was of a Lenticular Form, ſomewhat elongated, imitating the converging Part of the Bladder, its Surface *inſtar Lapidus arenosi*[1], but more hard and compact, [its circumference] 4.75 inches; its central Thickneſs .85 inch;[2] the longeſt Diameter 1.5 inch; the ſhorteſt Diameter 1.25 inch.

The Dreſſings were ſoft, eaſy and ſimple, with a Milk Diet to mitigate the ſcalding of the Water in the Wound: The fourth Day the Urine began to trickle the natural Way; the eleventh Day it paſſed the natural Way in a full and ſtrong Stream; 15 Day no more Urine by the Wound, and makes Water only three or four times in twenty four Hours; after the twenty third no more Dreſſings, the Wound being well cicatrized, and the Boy at Play about the Houſe.

Thus in about three Weeks a compleat and eaſy Cure for the Stone in the Bladder, was effected by the *lateral* Way.

---

1. Resembling sand stone.

2. There are two versions of this case; one, in The Boston *Evening Post* for November 9, 1741, was used here. The other announcement, in The Boston *News-Letter*, November 5–13, 1741, is worded almost identically. The measurements of the stone differ, however, between the two versions. The words "circumference" were omitted in the *Post*, and the central thickness is given in the *News-Letter* as 8.5 inches, obviously an incorrect figure.

Tucker's Wife's Leg

ROBERT WILLIAM BUCK, M.D., ed. (1893–   )

John Hartshorn was an apprentice in Boston during the middle of the eighteenth century and learned his medicine and surgery from Silvester Gardiner, the surgeon in the preceding selection. During his apprenticeship, young Hartshorn kept a diary, which is now held by the Countway Medical Library in Boston. This unique document gives an excellent picture of the day-to-day practice of medicine in colonial Boston. The following excerpt represents only a small fraction of the material contained in John Hartshorn's diary, but it gives a good description of a major operation and of pre-operative and post-operative care as it was practiced in that era.

Dr. Robert W. Buck is an internist and graduate of Harvard Medical School (1921) who practiced in Boston for three decades. During that time he taught at Tufts Medical School and authored a book on physical diagnosis. In 1952 he became the secretary of the Massachusetts Medical Society, a position he held for fifteen years. Dr. Buck has written a number of articles on individuals of importance in the history of medicine. He is presently retired in Waban, Massachusetts. The following selection, delightfully edited, is reprinted with his kind permission. "Tucker's Wife's Leg" appeared originally in the New England Journal of Medicine *(246:937, 1952).*

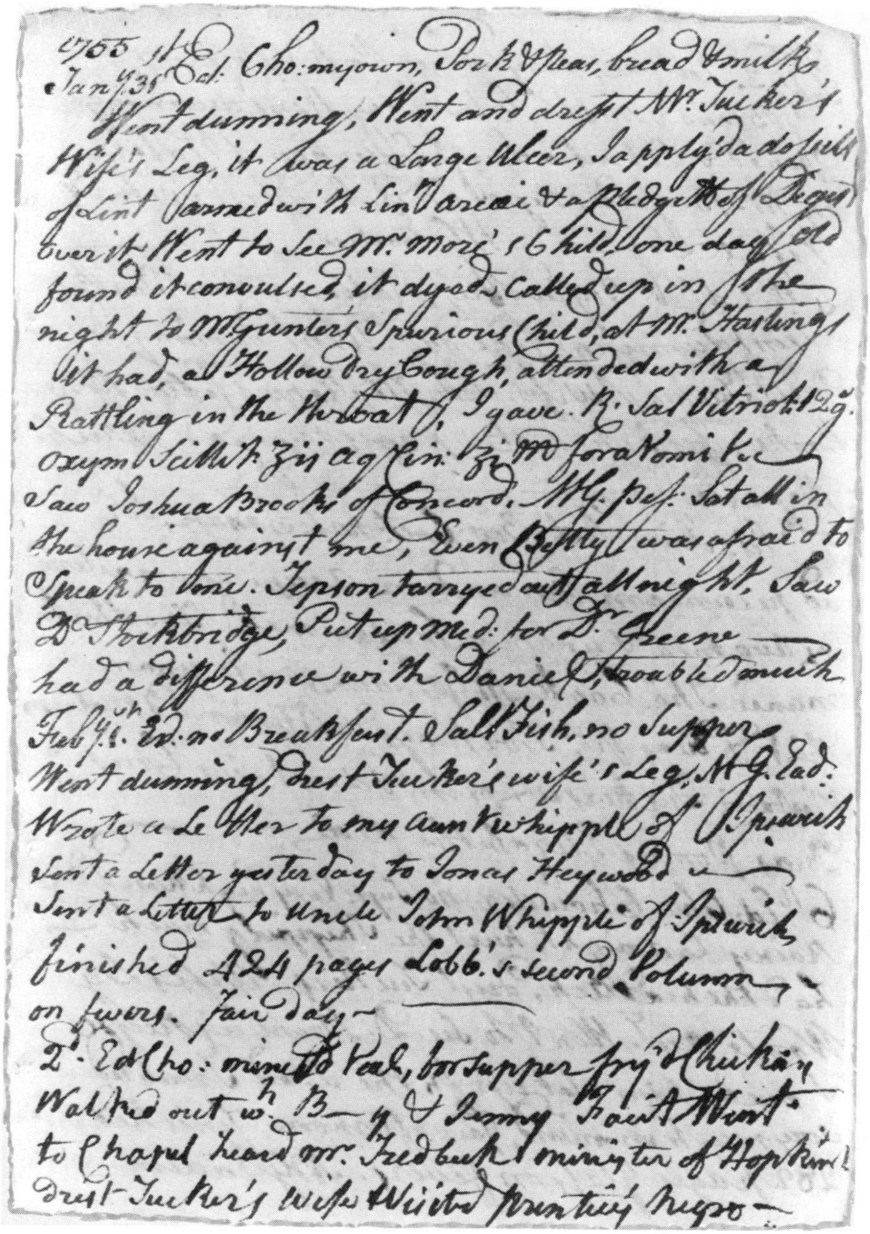

Figure 4. A page from John Hartshorn's manuscript-diary. The entry begins "January 31, Ed. [ate] chocolate: my own, Pork & peas. bread and milk. Went dunning. Went and drest Mr. Tucker's Wife's Leg, it was a Large Ulcer. . . ." (Courtesy Boston Medical Library.)

Tucker's Wife's Leg

In August, 1752, three months before his seventeenth birthday, John Denison Hartshorn of Concord, Massachusetts, came to Boston (population 16,500) to study medicine with Dr. Silvester Gardiner, who was then at the height of his career as a successful surgeon-apothecary. His shop was on Marlborough (now Washington) Street, at the corner of Winter. The boy apprenticed himself to the doctor for five years, and his master undertook to instruct him in Physick, Surgery and the business of an apothecary. Before John's term of service was completed, preparation began for the war against the French, and the young medical student died of typhus fever contracted while tending the victims of an epidemic among the British troops encamped in Boston.

His diary is preserved at the Boston Medical Library. The entries, in script as legible as print, doggedly record each day's events—first, what he had to eat; then a brief account of his professional chores. His artless history of the case of Tucker's wife's leg inspires gratitude that one did not live in Boston two centuries before penicillin.

Hartshorn was in the third year of his studies when, on January 31, 1755, he was called "to dress Mr. Tucker's Wife's Leg; it was a Large Ulcer." He notes that he "apply'd a dossill [a small pledget] of Lint armed with Linimentum Arcaei [rosin and turpentine] and Dig. Praecip. [digestivum praecipitatum, a digestive used to promote ripening of pus and usually containing turpentine, egg yolk and oil of roses or hypericum]." For three weeks the record varies little from day to day:

> Feb. 3. Ed. [edi, I ate] Rice, Boyled Leg Pork & Potatoes, Bread & milk ...Drest Tucker's wife's leg...

> Feb. 4. Ed. Cho. [chocolate], Boyled Rice & Cabbage, Roast Turkey... Drest Tucker's wife...

Occasionally he airs his Latin:

> Feb. 5...visitavi Tucker's uxorem & drest ejus Crus

> Feb. 6. Ed. Cho., Chowder; no Sup...Drest Tucker's Wife's Leg...

> Feb.7. Ed. Ch., Pork & Peas, Bread & milk...Went & drest Tucker's wife's leg. She had worms. I gave her ʒi Bailey's worm powder...

> Feb. 9...Went to dress Tucker's wife...

And so on until:

> Feb. 21. Ed. Cho., Pork & Peas, Bread & milk. . . Drest Tucker's wife.
> Went again at night. She had an exquisite pain acrost her abdomen
> which almost caused convulsions, her body [bowels] regular. I gave her
> 3i Calomel. . .& ordered her to drink plentifuly of Tea made of March-
> mallows, which soon gave her Ease.

On March 2 he discovered "a Sinus running an inch towards her
ancle, out of which issued Ichor." On March 6 Dr. Gardiner "suspected
the Bones was defective" and told his apprentice to fill the sinus with
dossills armed with digest. praecip., which is just what John had inde-
fatigably been doing for more than five weeks. He followed directions
and kept up the daily visits.

In the middle of March, John was sent to Springfield to collect an
old account owing to the Doctor. Having provided himself with a writ
of attachment, he mounted old Ranger and set out, arriving at 10 p.m.
in Worcester, where he lodged with a Mrs. Stearns. He says he had
"harshed Veal & Turnip for Supper, eat for breakfast Tea and Toast"
and paid 16 shillings and sixpence for the accommodation. He stopped
on the following night at Cold Spring, which he found "a very unpleasant place, very poor Huts, the roads uneven & full of Water as the
freshetts were very high, but lodged well, had a drink of bear & supped
on apple pye and Cheese."

In Springfield he searched the records and unfortunately found all
the debtor's lands already made over to another creditor. Completion
of legal formalities and the return trip took several days; he arrived
back in Boston in time for dinner on March 21. On the following day:

> March 22. Ed. Salt Fish, Bread & Milk. . . Went to dress Tucker's wife,
> found her in much pain, the external part of her ancle. Jepson[1] [the senior
> apothecary] had put a caustic on when I was gone, but [it] had not cast
> off. I drest by filling the sinus with Lint & a digest over all. . .

> March 23. Ed. Cho., Boyled Veal & Turnip, apple & minc'd Pye. . . Drest
> Tucker's wife by introducing dossills of Lint into the Sinus to dilate it. . .

---

1. William Jepson (?1733–1783) was a "graduate" of Gardiner's who went
into practice with his preceptor. In 1757 he moved from Boston to Hartford,
Connecticut, where he practiced and managed an apothecary shop in partner-
ship with Gardiner. Later, the two men fell out, and aired their differences in
the newspapers of the day. Jepson's name is also to be found on the rosters of
Revolutionary War surgeons from Connecticut.

apply'd a poultice of Bread & milk & ung. Dialth [unguentum de althaea, a marshmallow ointment]; could discover the head of the Tibia w'h my Probe.

The young medical man persisted in his efforts to help Mistress Tucker day after interminable day. He tried "a sticking plaister w'h a Hole in the middle, applied the Lapd. Infernal [*lapis infernalis*, crude potassium carbonate obtained by evaporating and calcining lye] & then a Slip of plaister over that, and in two hours took it off and put on a small pledget of Digest." He made an eschar with the caustic; he made a small incision with his lancet, and there came forth a large quantity of pus; he drest and drest and drest, all through April. On the first of May, the sore was fetid, which gave him a "suspicion of the Bones being Carious."

> May 6, Ed. Cho., Boyled Beef. No Supper. . . Went to see Mrs. Tucker, a Large Cavity appeared between her Os Calcis & the head of the Tibia. I injected Tinct. myrrh & aloes to deterge it, fomented it, etc., put her under a Diet drink made as follows. Rx. Sarsaparil ℥iis, Sassafras ℥i, Senna, Turpeth, Hermodactyl, Polypod. of the Oak, each half an ounce, Cinamon & Liquorice and ℥is Antim. 1 rad. grosly Pulv. & tied in a Rag. Boyl 24 hours in 5 quarts Water to 3 quarts.

No improvement ensued, however; the patient worsened. She developed a cough, vomiting and weakness. Several new sinuses appeared. On May 17 she was delirious with "a symptomatic fever caused by pain." Finally, on the 26th, Dr. Gardiner himself saw the young woman and concluded that she had a Static. She must have her leg laid open or cut off, or she must die.

> May 29. Ed. Cho., Pork & Peas, no Supper. . . Dr. Gardiner, Doctr. Thos Williams,[2] Doct. Pecker,[3] Jepson & myself, went and amputated Tucker's wife's leg, after much persuasion and many arguments. We sat her in a chair & put a Large Bowl of Sand under her, applyd the Tourniquet with

---

2. "Doctr. Thos. Williams" was probably Thomas Williams (1718-1775) of Deerfield, Massachusetts. Williams was the best known American Army surgeon during the French and Indian Wars. Subsequently he became a prominent practitioner and preceptor in Western Massachusetts. His brother, Ephraim, was the founder of Williams College.

3. "Doc Pecker" apparently refers to James Pecker (? 1741-1794), a practitioner of Boston. He is listed as one of the original members of the Massachusetts Medical Society at the time of its founding in 1781.

a Compress or two upon the arteries, I handed the instruments, Dr. Williams held the tourniquets, after binding a Tape around the Leg about 5 inches below the patella for a Guide to the Knife. D.G. began the Incision & divided quite thro the membrana adiposa, then Pecker drawing the Skin tought, next the muscles were divided, then the Catlin[4] to divide the interosseous muscles, then w'h the Saw the Leg was separated, five vessels were taken up, Lint apply'd & 2 pledgets Digest over them., Two longitudinal compresses, three double headed Bandages, afterwards an onodyne of Batm. drops ʒss. [Balsamum anodynum Bateanum, or anodyne balsam of Bates, made of opium, camphor, saffron and spirits of wine]. Brought the leg home & Pecker dissected it. Fine day...I was sent for to Tucker's in the afternoon they fearing a Hemmorage, but I found it only a serous oozing.

Two days later he reports that he had watched with Tucker's wife all night. He says "she rested but little, was something delirious, was very droughty (thirsty), sweat profusely, urined once no stool." But the patient made an uninterrupted recovery. On June 19, to be sure, she had one or two sloughs on her stump, but the doctor's disciple easily took care of these. He apply'd Dig Praecip, and touched w'h Vitriol Rosmar [copper sulfate]." The visits continued throughout July and August.

July 2. Ed. Cho., my own, Roast Lamb & Baked Pudding. no supper... Drest Tucker's wife &...drank a glass of madeira.

July 3. Ed. Cho., my own, fast day . . . Drest Tucker's wife and drank some punch there.

By this time of course, Tucker's wife and the young apprentice must have become pretty well acquainted.

Toward the end of July there appears one of John's rare reports on current events:

July 23. Ed. Cho., Fry'd Cod & harshed Beef. . . News from the Ohio that Gen'l Braddock was killed & his army defeated, his whole artillery being taken. [This was only ten days after the date of the famous defeat!]

However, Mistress Tucker's steady progress and the regular visits continued without interruption. By the end of September there had been a total of 170 visits over a period of eight months, and at last:

---

4. A catlin was a double edged amputation knife, long and sharp-pointed.

> September 20. Ed. Cho., salt fish, no Supper... Tucker's wife quite well...

Naturally, John continued to drop by from time to time. Tucker's wife had the heartburn December 22; in February, 1756, she hurt her stump; in March he visited "Mr. Tucker's Mother, a woman of about 50"; March 6–14 he had to make four visits to Tucker's wife, as the stump of her leg "had got foul and required several applications of Digest Praecip." It was clean on the occasion of the last visit.

The final notation, written nine months and a day after that July evening when the young surgeon drest Tucker's wife & drank some punch there, may indeed give rise to some sober speculation, but *honi soit qui mal y pense:*

> April 4. Ed. Cho., Boyled mutton, for Sup. fry'd Veal... Went to see Tucker's wife who was yesterday brought to Bed of a girl. Went to Chapel forenoon and to Eliot's meet'g afternoon. Cold day, had the headache much at night...

A Case of
Extra-Uterine Foetus

JOHN BARD, M.D. (1716–1799)

The following description of an abdominal pregnancy was the first scientific paper on a surgical subject to come from the North American Colonies. Its author, John Bard, was born in Burlington, New Jersey, on February 1, 1716. He learned his medicine and surgery as an apprentice to a surgeon of Philadelphia. Bard practiced in Philadelphia a while, but then moved to New York on the advice of his good friend, Benjamin Franklin. John Bard became a prominent practitioner in New York and is said to have dissected an executed criminal in 1750 "for the instruction of the youths then engaged in the study of medicine." This was the first known dissection for this purpose in the Colonies. John Bard was also the father of Samuel Bard (1742–1821), a founder of the medical school of Kings College and one of New York's most illustrious physicians. The elder Bard died in Hyde Park on March 30, 1799.

On the basis of the paper reprinted here, Garrison and others have credited John Bard with carrying out the first successful operation ever performed for ectopic pregnancy. A critical reading reveals that this interpretation is overgenerous; however, the problem was well handled and, most important, the patient survived. "A Case of Extra-Uterine Foetus" appeared in London's Medical Observations and Inquiries *(2:369, 1762).*

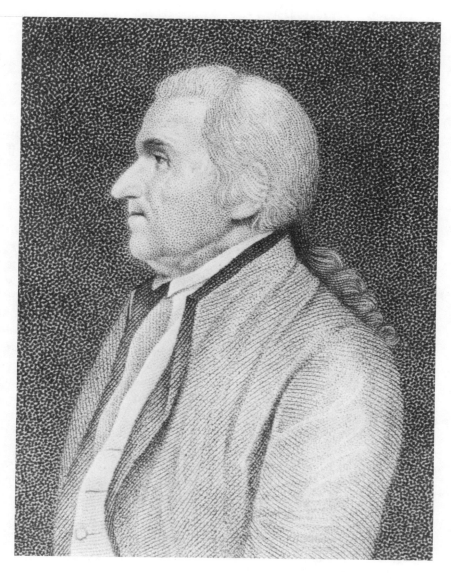

Figure 5. John Bard (1716-1799). (Courtesy National Library of Medicine.)

A case of an extra-uterine foetus, described by Mr. John
Bard, Surgeon at New York; in a letter to Dr. John
Fothergill,[1] and by him communicated to the Society.
Read March, 24, 1760.

Sir,

Dr. Colding,[2] some time ago, shewed me a letter he was favoured with from you; wherein you acquaint him with the design of publishing the London Medical Essays; and invite him to encourage that work, by communicating any useful or curious observations, which might fall under his notice in this part of the world. Encouraged by this invitation to the Doctor, whom I have the honour to be intimate with, I have taken the freedom, though a stranger, to send you the history of a case, which has lately fallen under my care.

Mrs. Stagg, the wife of a mason, about 28 years of age, having had one child without any uncommon symptom, either during her pregnancy or labour, became, as she imagined, a second time pregnant. She was more disordered in this, than in her former pregnancy, frequently feverish, the swelling of her belly not so equal, nor the motion of the child so strong and lively. At the end of nine months, when she expected her delivery, she had some labour pains, but without a flow of waters, or any other discharge. The pains soon went off, and the swelling of her belly grew gradually less; but there still remained a large, hard, indolent, moveable tumour, inclining a little to the right side. She had a return of her menses, continued regular five months, conceived again, and enjoyed better health: the swelling of her belly became more equal and uniform, and, at the end of nine months, after a short and easy labor, she was delivered of a healthy child. The tumour on the right side had again the same appearances as before her last pregnancy. Five days after delivery, she was seized with a violent fever, a purging, suppression of the lochia, pain in the tumour, and profuse

---

1. Dr. John Fothergill (1712-1780) was a noted physician and physician and philanthropist of London. He had a deep interest in Britain's American colonies. He encouraged medical education and contributed both materially and by his advice to the founding of the first medical schools in America.

2. "Dr. Colding" was Cadwalader Colden, M.D. (1688-1776). Colden was born in Scotland and studied medicine at Edinburgh. He came to New York in 1718. Colden was active in politics, wrote several book son medical and scientific subjects, and corresponded with anumber of prominent men of science in the Colonies and in England. Next to Benjamin Franklin, he was the Colonies' leading scientist.

fetid sweats. By careful treatment, these threatening symptoms were, in some measure, removed; but there still remained a loss of appetite, slow hectic fever, night sweats, and a diarrhoea. To the tumour, which continued painful, and gradually increased, were applied fomentations and emollient pultices; and, at the end of nine weeks, I perceived so evident a fluctuation of matter in it, that I desired Dr. Huck,[3] physician to the army, to visit this patient with me, and be present at the opening [of] it. From the whole history we concluded, that we should find an extra-uterine foetus. I made an opening in the most prominent part of the tumour, about the middle of the right rectus muscle, beginning as high as the navel, and carrying it downwards. There issued a vast quantity of extremely fetid matter, together with the third phalanx of a finger of a child. Introducing my finger into the abscess, I found an opening into the cavity of the abdomen by the side of the rectus muscle, through which I felt the child's elbow. I then directed my incision obliquely downwards to the right ilium, and extracted a foetus of the common size, at the ordinary time of delivery. The frontal, parietal, and occipital bones, as also the third phalanges of the fingers of one hand, separated by putrefaction, remained behind; which I also took out. We imagined the placenta and funis umbilicalis were dissolved into pus, of which there was a great quantity. By the use of fomentations and detersive injections, while the discharge was copious, fetid, and offensive; and by the application of proper bandages, and dressing with dry lint only, when the pus became laudable, the cavity contracted, filled up, and was cicatrized in ten weeks. The source of the hectic being removed, with the help of the bark, elix. of vitriol, and a proper diet, whe quickly recovered good health. Her milk, which had left her from the time she was first seized with the fever, returned in great plenty after the abscess was healed; and she now suckles a healthy infant.

I am,
SIR
With great respect,
Your most humble servant,
JOHN BARD

New York
Dec. 25, 1759.

---

3. Richard Huck, M.D. (1720-1785), was a graduate of Marischal College, Aberdeen. He was stationed in New York as a surgeon to the British 33rd Regiment under the Earl of Loudoun until 1762. He later returned to London where he practiced after becoming a licentiate of the Royal College of Physicians.

Introductory Lecture to His Course in Surgery

JOHN JONES, M.D. (1729–1791)

John Jones, who was destined to become the Colonies' foremost surgeon, was born in Jamaica, New York, in 1729. He died sixty-two years later in Philadelphia.

Jones is best known today as the author of the first American medical text, a vade mecum for the military and naval surgeons who served the American cause during the Revolution. Jones was also the first professor of surgery and a co-founder of the Kings College (Columbia) Medical School in New York. The introductory lecture to his course, reproduced here in a somewhat shortened form, is a document of considerable value and interest. It gives the surgical philosophy of an intelligent man who had received his early medical training in the Colonies as an apprentice and then went abroad to learn surgery from Europe's greatest surgeons. Surgery, at the time that this lecture was written, was finally becoming a respectable part of medicine, but Jones was still somewhat defensive about its status. He recognized not only that surgeons should be technically able, but also that they should be acquainted with the entire scope of medicine—good advice even today. And with considerable insight he saw the need for continuing research ("experimental philosophy") and for an appreciation of the scientific method ("observation") if surgery was to advance. Jones's lecture shuold be compared with William Stewart Halsted's "The Training of a Surgeon" (page 352). There is a kinship between the two

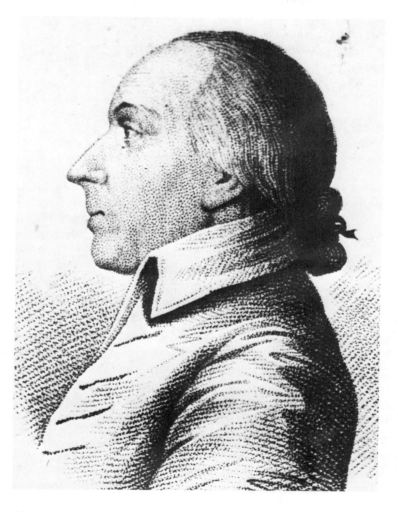

Figure 6. John Jones (1729-1791). (Courtesy National Library of Medicine.

men, and there is a great deal of surgical philosophy in these two lectures that can be appreciated by a thoughtful reader today.

This lecture, printed from Jones's manuscript, was published in the Transactions and Studies of the College of Physicians of Philadelphia *(4th series. 8:180, 1940), with an introduction and notes by W. B. McDaniel, 2d, the librarian of the College of Physicians of Philadelphia. The original punctuation has been somewhat altered here for ease in reading.*

John Jones's Introductory Lecture to His Course in Surgery
Kings College Medical School (1769)[1]

This ancient branch of medicine call'd Surgery, according to the strict grammatical meaning of the word, signifies manual operation; but the science & art of surgery, tho more clear & certain in its objects than that of a Physic, is equally various, extensive, & difficult of attainment. And I have ever been of opinion that young Physicians might lay the truest foundation for medical knowledge by an attentive observation of those disorders which surgery presents to their view.

Surgery may, with great propriety, be divided into medical, & manual. The first comprehends an infinite variety of diseases which require the assistance of both internal, & external applications: the last is confin'd to those cases which admit of relief from the hand alone, or assisted with instruments. Hence it will appear very evident how necessary it is for the student in surgery to make himself thoroughly acquainted with all those branches of medicine, which are requisite to form the most accomplished Physician; to which must be superadded some peculiar qualifications, to constitute the surgeon of real merit & abilities.

Besides a competent acquaintance with the learn'd languages, which are to lay the foundation of every other acquisition, he must possess an accurate knowledge of the structure of the human body acquir'd not only by attending anatomical lectures, but by frequently dissecting dead bodies with his own hands. This practice can not be too warmly recommended to the students in surgery: 'tis from this source,

---

1. Kings College (later Columbia) Medical School was organized in 1767. It was the Colonies' second medical school, antedated by that of the College of Philadelphia (later the University of Pennsylvania), founded two years earlier.

& a knowledge of Hydraulics, they must derive any adequate notions of the laws of the animal oeconomy, or Physiology. Chymistry and the materia medica are very necessary to a right understanding of Pharmacy, or composition. To these shou'd be added some progress in the mathematics, & mechanics; which I will venture to assert, may be applied with much more safety & utility to the science of surgery than Physic. But there must be a happiness, as well as art, to compleat the character of the great surgeon.

He ought to have firm steady hands, & be able to use both alike, a strong clear sight, & above all a mind calm & intrepid, yet humane, & compassionate, avoiding every appearance of terror & cruelty to his patients amidst the most severe operations.

Though surgery is one of those sciences which have been cultivated with the utmost industry, & attention, & its progress, particularly during the present century, has been very rapid, new lights having been thrown upon it by a variety of different discoveries; yet none but very superficial minds can imagine that the limits of our present knowledge are the limits of the art.

The variety & multiplicity of our diseases, & the absolute impossibility of our being able to discover with certainty their primary causes, leads us into a vast extensive field where wee are frequently oblig'd to strike out into new, & untrodden paths. From this view of the subject arises a very natural & interesting question.

What method ought surgeons to follow, in order to give the highest degree of perfection to their art?

Is it from that experience which is acquir'd from practice alone wee are to expect this perfection? If that had been the case, the art wou'd many ages ago have been at its height.

But there is another source of improvement, equally essential to the perfecting our art, & perhaps with more difficulty acquir'd, than that wee obtain from practice alone.

I mean experimental Philosophy. It is very easy to demonstrate the necessity of that valuable information which wee derive from a well regulated course of Philosophical experiments. Nature shews herself but very imperfectly to the naked eye. Wee ought then to observe her with every assistance which wee can draw from the refinements of art, & the experience of ages. A mind of the most exalted powers is only capable of comprehending the superficial appearance of objects: & without calling in the assistance of Physical experiments can never penetrate into their original properties.

Observation, & Physical experiments which form the only basis of surgery have, then, two different objects.

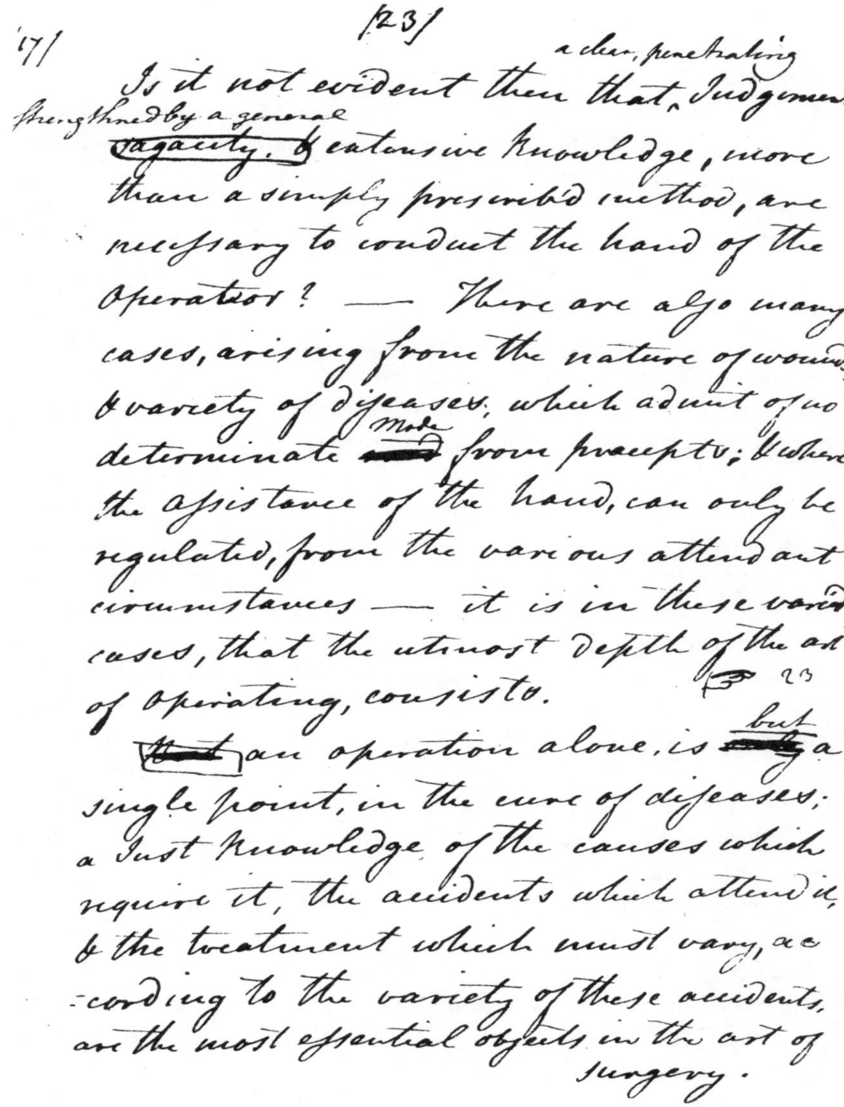

a clear, penetrating

Is it not evident then that, Judgment,
strengthened by a general
~~sagacity.~~ & extensive Knowledge, more
than a simply prescribed method, are
necessary to conduct the hand of the
Operator? — There are also many
cases, arising from the nature of wounds,
& variety of diseases; which admit of no
determinate *mode* ~~and~~ from precept; & where
the assistance of the hand, can only be
regulated, from the various attendant
circumstances — it is in these various
cases, that the utmost depth of the art
of operating, consists.   ☞ 23

~~That~~ an operation alone, is ~~only~~ *but* a
single point, in the cure of diseases;
a Just Knowledge of the causes which
require it, the accidents which attend it,
& the treatment which must vary, ac
-cording to the variety of these accidents,
are the most essential objects in the art of
surgery.

Figure 7. A page from John Jones's manuscript for a lecture to his class.
(Courtesy Philadelphia College of Physicians.)

Observation regards the sensible qualities of bodies, the course of diseases, their Phenomena, with the effects which result from the process of art. Physical experiments unravel the structure & uses of the parts; the composition of mix'd bodies, the properties of those fluids which circulate in the vessels, the nature of ailments, & the action of medicines; yet, these so necessary helps do not conduct us seperately to hidden truths which may serve to enrich our art.

Observation improves our experiments, & experiments influence our observations; they mutually assist each other, & are like lights united for the dissipation of obscurity.

Observation alone may be very imperfect, & fallacious; & has frequently been the source of error as well as truth. Opinions entirely opposite often produce an equal number of facts in support of their equivocal Judgements. The ancients were perswaded that taking blood from different veins in the same arm, produced very different effects, & two thousand years had elaps'd before mankind were disabused from so ridiculous an opinion; founded upon the observation of the greatest masters of the art.

But wee are very apt to fly, from one extreme to another.

When Harvey had discover'd the circulation of the blood, those Physicians who had been most blindly attach'd to the opinion of the ancients, on a sudden regarded them with the utmost contempt. They no longer acknowledg'd any elective remedies: the current of blood which flow'd to all parts must carry the remedies, equally to act upon all. But more exact observations have oblig'd the most obstinate minds to return to the ancient opinions, respecting the effects of certain medicines.

Thus physical experiments, which discover'd to us the circulation of the blood, led us into erroneous opinions which observation alone cou'd correct. Observation not only rectifies Physical experiments, but suggests new ones; for example, it taught surgeons that a ligature on the arm stops the course of the blood in the veins, that wee must afterwards loosen it to facilitate the passage of the blood, thro the orifice made in bleeding. But the cause of this Phenomenon remain'd a secret 'til the discovery of the circulation (this discovery threw a light upon the observation which was the origin of it). Thus surgeons who aim at perfection in their art must sometimes depart from observation, & return to it again, to confirm the conclusions which they draw from Physical experiments.

This course wou'd not be very difficult if wee had only a few observations & experiments to make, but at our first setting out difficulties present themselves from all parts. To obtain a knowledge of the most simple truths requires a long train of observations & experiments which only serve to extend our views, & shew us the necessity of continually repeating our experiments & observations, in order to make any true progress in knowledge.

The truth of this reasoning will be more clearly illustrated by example.

Blows on the head have frequently occasion'd death. The first step which the observation of such accidents requir'd was to seek out the cause from anatomical inspection, Opening dead bodies discovered it to be oweing to an extravasation of blood within the cranium, & evidently pointed out the necessity of perforating the skull to discharge the extravasated fluid. But further observations & inquiries have inform'd us that cases, & those very fatal ones, have occur'd where there is no extravasation; & where the application of the trepan, is entirely useless.

Such are the difficulties which arise in the progress of an art which requires the work of ages to perfect.

For this reason it becomes necessary to collect the observations of our predecessors & contemporaries; without whose assistance the greatest genius wou'd be nothing more than an ignorant & presumptuous practitioneer.

Continual study, therefore, is equally necessary to the surgeon as it is to the Anatomist & Physician who, in neglecting to inform themselves of the new discoveries made in different parts of the world, will become only servile imitators, & perhaps after twenty years labour be little wiser than their first masters. If the science of surgery requires so much pains & labour, how unjust & inadequate must the Ideas of those people be who wou'd reduce it to the art of operating alone. This art is without doubt very essential to it, & it is operation which principally characterises surgery, but the art of operating, consider'd in itself, depends chiefly upon anatomical knowledge, & address of the hands. Practice, indeed, gives this address in a great measure, but it does not bestow genius, nor the lights which are necessary to conduct it.

Those therefore who estimate surgery by operation alone, & believe that nothing but long habit & practice is necessary to form the great surgeon, are grossly ignorant of the art; & those surgeons who found their only merit upon this experience degrade themselves & their profession; the greatest operators having always been remarkable for the extent of their knowledge, & a contempt for the servile routine of those mean practitioners whose experience is of little more than heaping one blunder upon another.

This will more evidently appear from some examples: before the discovery of making a ligature upon the blood vessels after amputation, the only method of stopping the Haemorrhage was the cruel one of the actual cautery, or red hot iron, a method as terrifying as it was painful to the unhappy patient. Yet near a century elapsed before the surgeons, habitually bigotted to their old forms, wou'd adopt a more mild & gentle method, the offspring of a happy inventive genius.

The ancient surgeons, & particularly Celsus, boldly & successfully perform'd the operation for the Fistula in ano, yet to the shame & reproach of modern operators there was no one found to undertake it in the latter end of the last century. 'Till the danger to which the life of Lewis the fourteenth was expos'd by that disease excited the industry & genius of Falix,[2] his first surgeon, who after several experiments upon patients in Hospitals perform'd the operation with success upon the King, & was rewarded for his services with a munificence becoming a great Prince.

Thus men of more enlighten'd genius & more intrepid spirit must compose themselves to the risque of public censure, & the contempt of their jealous contemporaries, in order to lead ignorant & prejudic'd minds into more happy & successful methods.

How much have wee to apprehend from that servile road of imitation which is the sole guide to some men. Since it is very certain that a great many of those operations which appear to be so plainly describ'd in books require something more than a simple routine to execute.

How many varieties does the application of the trepan require? The accidents which render it necessary, the parts to which it is to be applied, & the number of applications are so various & different that wee are frequently oblig'd to quit the plain beaten road & boldly strike into a track entirely new, the propriety & necessity of which can only be discovered by those Rules of Analogy, which are to be found in the structure of the parts & nature of diseases.

Is it not evident, then, that a clear, penetrating judgement, strengthened by a general sagacity & extensive knowledge, more than a simply prescrib'd method are necessary to conduct the hand of the operator? There are also many cases arising from the nature of wounds & variety of diseases which admit of no determinate mode from pre-

---

2. "Falix" was Charles-Francois Felix (fl. 1686), surgeon to Louis XIV. The operation alluded to here was a most important one in the history of surgery, for the status of the lowly surgeons was greatly improved as a result of the regard that the monarch developed for his surgeon following the successful operation for an anal fistula.

cepts; & where the assistance of the hand can only be regulated from the various attendant circumstances. It is in these vari'd cases that the utmost depth of the art of operating consists.

An operation alone is but a single point in the cure of diseases; a just knowledge of the causes which require it, the accidents which attend it, & the treatment which must vary, according to the variety of these accidents, are the most essential objects in the art of surgery. And hence it will evidently appear how necessary a deep knowledge of anatomy, & the animal oeconomy, is to the just exercise of this science. 'Tis this knowledge which lays the foundation & constitutes a considerable part of the merit & difficulty of the art; & shews us from what hands wee are principally to expect its progress.

The mind therefore must be prepar'd, before its entrance into the study of surgery, by a previous acquisition of those branches of knowledge, which form the rules, by which wee ought to conduct ourselves in the cure of diseases. 'Tis to such cultivated geniusses, that surgery owes its greatest progress—such were a Serverinus, a Fallopius, a Hildanus, a Vesalius, a Scultetus, a Heister, a Le dran, a Wiseman, a Cheselden, a Monro, a Sharp. These illustrious surgeons, whose minds were prepar'd by the study of the learn'd languages, cultivated by the belles lettres, & enrich'd with the knowledge of Philosophy, have hung up the best lights to conduct us through the dark & intricate windings of our art.

To conclude Gentlemen: if the science of surgery, then, requires genius, knowledge, & indefatigable application to render its Professors truly respectable, what must wee think of the insolence & malevolence of those who represent it as a low mechanic art, which may be taught a butchers boy in a fortnight. Yet such false & absurd representations have been made of it by some who have enjoy'd no small share of medical reputation in this country, & what is equally reproachful, there have been men, who stil'd themselves gentlemen, ignorant & weak enough to credit such absurdities.

But we have some reason already to flatter ourselves that, under the protection of the liberal patrons of this medical institution, Ignorance and imposture will no longer be able to combat truth & error, and that the latest posterity may view with gratitude the benificent founders of an institution calculated to promote the health & happiness of Mankind.

Remarks on
the Management of
the Scalped-Head

JAMES ROBERTSON (1742–1814) communicated by
FELIX RANDOLPH ROBERTSON, M.D. (1781–1865)

The following article is presented as it appeared in The Philadelphia Medical and Physical Journal *(2, Pt. 2: 27–30, 1805–1806). It gives an unusual glimpse of rough-and-ready surgery as it was practiced on what was then our western-most frontier.*

Scalping was quintessentially an American injury, and one occasionally encounters references to individuals who survived being scalped (such a case is mentioned in Thacher's Military Journal, *see page 42 in this anthology). The following article, however, on the treatment of the scalped head, is unique for several reasons. First, there is no mention in the surgical literature of that era on the use of bone drilling to promote the formation of granulation tissue; the technique apparently was little known. The "proud flesh," which forms after drilling, becomes covered in time with epithelium ("skinning" in Robertson's article. These descriptive Anglo-Saxon words were then in general use in English medical writing; Latinization came later). This technique of drilling bone is occasionally useful today when sizable areas of the skull (or other bone) have been denuded. Second, the author of this paper was not a physician, but rather a pioneer frontiersman who founded the city of Nashville and has been referred to as the father of Tennessee.*

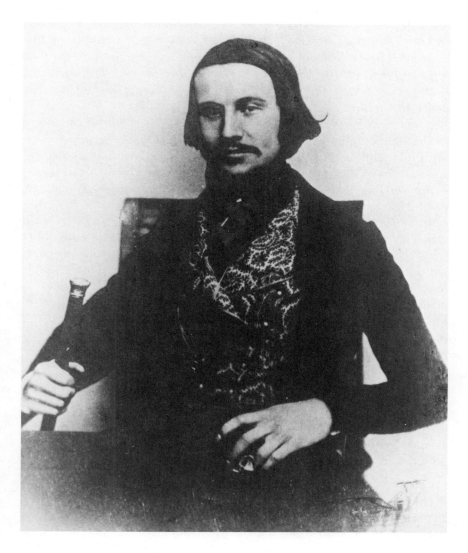

Figure 8. James Robertson (1742-1814). (Courtesy Tennessee State Library and Archives.)

James Robertson was born in Daniel Boone country—Brunswick County, Virginia—in 1742. In 1769 he led a party of settlers onto Cherokee lands to settle on the Holston River—one of the first permanent settlements in Tennessee—near present-day Knoxville. The "Cheerake-Indians" attacked in 1777; Frederick Calvit was a casualty of that warfare. The early settlers on the Holston River fought hard for their land and held off the Indians. The Treaty of Holston, signed in 1791, finally established the Cherokee Nation's boundaries and brought peace to the area.

Felix Robertson, M.D. (1781–1865), who submitted this paper to the Philadelphia Medical and Physical Journal *(it also appeared in the* Philadelphia Medical Museum, *vol. 3, 1807), was James Robertson's sixth child and the first white child to be born in the newly settled community of Nashville. (The settlers had arrived during the winter of 1779–1780 and named their new community after a North Carolinian, Francis Nash[ca. 1742-1777] who had fallen two years earlier in the Battle of Germantown.) The younger Robertson received his M.D. from the University of Pennsylvania in 1805, the year before this paper was published. After his graduation he returned to Nashville where he lived and practiced for the remainder of his life. Felix Robertson achieved considerable local prominence both as a practitioner (he limited his practice to the care of children—unusual in that era) and as a public figure, serving two terms as mayor of Nashville.*

Remarks on the Management of the Scalped–Head

In the year 1777, there was a Doctor Vance[1], about the Long-Islands of Holsten, who was then attending on the different garrisons, which were embodied on the then frontiers of Holsten, to guard the

---

1. Dr. Patrick (shortened from Kilpatrick) Vance (dates unknown) was a Scotsman who studied at (but apparently did not graduate from) the University of Edinburgh before coming to this country. As mentioned in the Robertson's article, Vance served as a military surgeon, stationed on the Long Island in the Tennessee River near present day Knoxville, Tennessee. The practice of boring the outer table of the skull, which he taught to James Robertson, has been traced down through surgical history by L. M. Strayer in an historical essay which appeared in the *New England Journal of Medicine* (220:901, 1939) and by Mary H. McGrath, M.D.—who brought this bit of history to my attention—in her dissertation (as yet unpublished) on the history of scalping and the treatment of scalping wounds.

inhabitants against the depredations of the Cheerake-Indians. This Doctor Vance came from Augusta–County, in Virginia. In March of the same year, Frederick Calvit was badly wounded, and nearly the whole of his head skinned. Doctor Vance was sent for, and staid several days with him. The skull-bone was quite naked, and began to turn black in places, and, as Doctor Vance was about to leave Calvit, he directed me, as I was stationed in the same fort with him, to bore his skull as it got black, and he bored a few holes himself, to show the manner of doing it. I have found, that a flat pointed straight awl is the best instrument to bore with, as the skull is thick, and somwhat diffi-cult to penetrate. When the awl is nearly through, the instrument should be borne more lightly upon. The time to quit boring is when a reddish fluid appears on the point of the awl. I bore, at first, about one inch apart, and, as the flesh appears to rise in those holes, I bore a number more between the first. The flesh will rise considerably above the skull, and sometimes raise a black scale from it, about the thickness of common writing paper. It is well to assist in getting off the scales of bone with the awl. These scales are often as large as a dollar, and some-times even twice as large.

It will take, at least, two weeks from the time of boring for it to scale. When the scale is taken off at a proper time, all beneath it will appear flesh, like what we call proud-flesh, and as if there was no bone under it.

The awl may, at this time, and indeed, for a considerable length of time, be forced through the flesh to the bone without the patient's feeling it; but after any part has united to that portion of the scalp, which has remaining original skin, it becomes immediately sensible to the touch.

The scalped-head cures very slowly, and if this kind of flesh rise, in places, higher than common, touch it with blue-stone water,[2] dress it once or twice a day, putting a coat of lint over every time you dress it, with a narrow plaister of ointment.

It skins remarkably slow, generally taking two years to cure up.

In the year 1781, David Hood was shot, at this place, with several balls and two [sic] scalps were taken off his head, and these took off nearly all the skin which had hair on it. I attended him, bored his skull and removed from almost the whole of his head, such black scales as I have described above.

---

2. Blue-stone water refers to a copper sulfate solution.

It was three or four years before his head skinned over entirely; but he is now living, and is well.

In 1789, Richard Lancaster and Joel Staines were both wounded, scalped, and left for dead. These persons were under my directions, and their heads were bored as above described. They both got well, in the course of two years

M. Baldwin, and some others, were scalped either in the year 1790, or 1791. Their sculls I also bored, or directed it to be done. They all recovered.

I never knew one that was scalped, and bored as above directed, that did not perfectly recover. There is always part of the scalped head over which but little or no hair afterwards grows.

In 1769, I saw a young man in South–Carolina, who had been scalped eight years before that time, and about twice the size of a dollar of the bone of his head was then perfectly bare, dry, and black. I am persuaded, that had his skull, even then, been bored, he might have recovered of the wound, which put an end to his life about a year after I saw him; the naked portion of bone having rotted, or mortified, and exposed the substance of his brain, a very considerable quantity of which issued out at the opening, at his death.

Nashville, April 10th, 1806

Excerpts from
a Military Journal During
the Revolutionary War

JAMES THACHER, M.D. (1754–1844)

James Thacher was born on February 14, 1754. He grew up to become a patriotic young man who had just finished his medical apprenticeship at the beginning of the Revolution. He joined the Continental Army and served as a surgeon through the entire war. Thacher's Military Journal *contains a great many personal observations of value and interest to students of Revolutionary history; but, unfortunately, there is little enough in it concerning wartime surgery. The excerpts that follow are a collection of items of surgical interest—virtually all that are to be found in the journal. These follow the young man from his enlistment in 1775 to his mustering-out in 1783.*

With the coming of peace, Thacher settled down to community practice in Plymouth, Massachusetts. He led a long and useful life as a physician and made several noteworthy contributions to American medical literature. The most important of these is his American Medical Biography *(Boston: Richardson & Lord and Cotton & Barnard, 1828), an important source book for the medical historian. Thacher lived to be 90. He died in Plymouth on May 24, 1844.*

The excerpts included here were taken from the second edition of A Military Journal During the American Revolutionary War from 1775–1783 *by James Thacher, M.D. (Boston: Cottons & Barnard, 1827).*

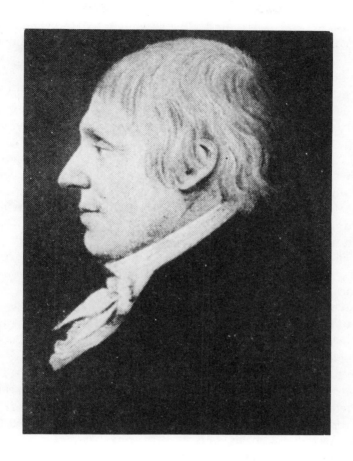

Figure 9. James Thacher (1754–1844) at about the age of 30, several years after the Revolution had ended. (Courtesy *Virginia Medical Monthly.*)

A Military Journal During the American Revolutionary War from 1775 to 1783

January 1775—At the precise period when my medical studies and education are completed, under the patronage of Dr. Abner Hersey,[1] of Barnstable, my native town, and I am contemplating the commencement of a new career in life, I find our country about to be involved in all the horrors of a civil war...

I shall venture, I hope not rashly, to enlist, and trust my destiny in the hands of a kind and over-ruling Providence. My contemplated enterprise, it is true, requires the experience and resolution of riper years than twenty-one...

[Thacher applied for an appointment in the Continental Army as a physician. He was instructed to appear for examination before an examining committee.]

On the appointed day, the medical candidates, sixteen in number, were summoned before the board for examination. This business occupied about four hours; the subjects were anatomy, physiology, surgery and medicine. It was not long after, that I was happily relieved from suspense, by receiving the sanction and acceptance of the board, with some acceptable instructions relative to the faithful discharge of duty, and the humane treatment of those soldiers who may have the misfortune to require my assistance. Six of our number were privately rejected as being found unqualified. The examination was in a considerable degree close and severe, which occasioned not a little agitation in our ranks. But it was on another occasion, as I am told, that a candidate under examination was agitated into a state of perspiration, and being required to describe the mode of treatment in rheumatism, among other remedies, he would promote a sweat, and being asked how he would effect this with his patient, after some hesitation he replied, 'I would have him examined by a medical committee...'

I was so fortunate as to obtain the office of surgeon's mate in the provincial hospital at Cambridge, Dr. John Warren[2] being the senior

---

1. Dr. Abner Hersey (1722–1787) and his brother, Ezekiel (1709–1770), were physicians in southeastern Massachusetts. Both these men left generous bequests to Harvard College for the professorships of physic and of anatomy that still bear their names.

2. John Warren (1753–1815) was a surgeon in the Continental Army. Subsequently he became the professor of surgery in Harvard's newly formed medical school. He was the first of a long line of distinguished Boston surgeons to bear the Warren name.

surgeon. He was the brother and pupil of the gallant General Joseph Warren,[3] who was slain in the memorable battle on Breeds (Bunker) Hill.

[Thacher stayed in the vicinity of Boston, reporting faithfully all that occurred. He was busy during the winter of 1775–1776 caring for the sick who suffered from "fevers and dysenteric complaints, which have proved fatal in a considerable number of instances." He entered Boston after the British evacuated the city on March 17, 1776, and subsequently was busily involved in inoculating the troops with smallpox. This method usually gave a mild form of the disease (inoculation with cow-pox was not introduced by Jenner until 1798). In the autumn of 1776 Thacher was transferred to Ticonderoga, where he remained until that fort was evacuated in July 1777. He was stationed near Saratoga, N.Y. and cared for the wounded of the battle fought there on October 7, 1777. Following the battle, he wrote]

October 12th, 1777—The wounded officers and soldiers of our army, and those of the enemy who have fallen into our hands, are crowding into our hospital, and require our constant attention. The last night I watched with the celebrated General Arnold,[4] whose leg was badly fractured by a musket ball while in the engagement with the enemy on the 7th instant. He is very peevish and impatient under his misfortunes, and required all my attention during the night. . . .

[Later, in Albany, he wrote]

October 24th, 1777—This hospital is now crowded with officers and soldiers from the field of battle; those belonging to the British and Hessian troops are accomodated in the same hospital with our own men, and receive equal care and attention. The foreigners are under the care and management of their own surgeons. I have been present at some of their capital operations, and remarked that the English surgeons perform with skill and dexterity, but the Germans, with a few exceptions do no credit to their profession; and some of them are the most uncouth and clumsy operators I ever witnessed, and appear to be destitute of all sympathy and tenderness toward the suffering patient. Not less than one thousand wounded and sick are now in this city; the

---

3. Joseph Warren (1741–1775), physician and patriot of Boston, played an active part in the political maneuvering that eventually led to the outbreak of the Revolution and to his death at Bunker Hill.

4. Benedict Arnold (1741–1801) had previously been wounded in the left leg at Quebec on New Year's Day, 1776. He was cared for by Continental Army surgeon Isaac Senter (1755–1799), who removed the musket ball. Thacher does not indicate whether the same leg was involved.

Dutch church and several private houses are occupied as hospitals. We have about thirty surgeons and mates; and all are constantly employed. I am obliged to devote the whole of my time, from eight o'clock in the morning to a late hour in the evening to the care of our patients. Some of our soldiers' wounds, which had been neglected while on their way here from the field of battle, being covered with putrified blood for several days, were found on the first dressing to be filled with maggots. It was not difficult however, to destroy those vermin by the application of tincture of myrrh. Here is a fine field for professional improvement. Amputating limbs, trepanning fractured skulls, and dressing the most formidable wounds have familiarized my mind to scenes of woe. A military hospital is peculiarly calculated to afford examples for profitable contemplation, and to interest our sympathy and commiseration. If I turn from beholding mutilated bodies, mangled limbs, and bleeding, incurable wounds, a spectacle no less revolting is presented, of miserable objects, languishing under afflicting diseases of every description— here, are those in a mournful state of despair, exhibiting those harbingers of approaching dissolution—there, are those with emaciated bodies and ghastly visage, who begin to triumph over grim disease and just lift their feeble heads from the pillow of sorrow. . .

It is my lot to have twenty wounded men committed to my care, by Dr. Potts,[5] our Surgeon General; one of whom, a young man, received a musket ball through his cheeks, cutting its way through the teeth on each side, and the substance of his tongue; his sufferings have been great, but he now begins to articulate tolerably well. Another had the whole side of his face torn off by a cannon ball, laying his mouth and throat open to view. A brave soldier received a musket ball in his forehead, between his eyebrows; observing that it did not penetrate the bone, it was imagined that the force of the ball being partly spent, it rebounded and fell out, but on close examination by the probe, the ball was detected, spread entirely flat on the bone under the skin, which I extracted with the forceps. No one can doubt but that he received his wound while facing the enemy, and it is fortunate for the brave fellow, that his skull proved too thick for the ball to penetrate. But in another instance, a soldier's wound was not so honorable; he received a ball in

---

5. Jonathan Potts (1745–1781) graduated in 1768 with the first class of the medical school of the College of Philadelphia (subsequently the University of Pennsylvania), the Colonies' first medical school. He had a distinguised career as a surgeon during the Revolution and became a director-general of the middle hospital department of the Continental Army.

the bottom of his foot, which could not have happened unless when in the act of running from the enemy. This poor fellow is held in derision by his comrades, and is made a subject of their wit for having the mark of a *coward*.

Among the most remarkable occurances which come under my observation, the following is deserving of particular notice. Captain Greg, of one of the New York regiments, while stationed at Fort Stanwix, on the Mohawk river, went with two of his soldiers into the woods a short distance to shoot pigeons; a party of Indians started suddenly from concealment in the bushes, shot them all down, tomahawked and scalped them, and left them for dead. The captain, after some time revived, and perceiving his men were killed; himself robbed of his scalp, and suffering extreme agony from his numerous wounds, made an effort to move and lay his bleeding head on one of the dead bodies, expecting soon to expire. A faithful dog who accompanied him, manifested great agitation, and in the tenderest manner licked his wounds. which afforded him great relief from exquisite distress. He then directed the dog, as if a human being, to go in search of some person to come to his relief. The animal, with every appearance of anxiety, ran about a mile, when he met two men fishing in the river, and endeavored in the most moving manner, by whining and piteous cries, to prevail on them to follow him into the woods; struck with the singular conduct of the dog, they were induced to follow him part of the way, but fearing some decoy or danger, they were about to return, when the dog, fixing his eyes on them, renewed his entreaties by his cries, and taking hold of their clothes with his teeth, prevailed on them to follow him to the fatal spot. Such was the remarkable fidelity and sagacity of this animal. Captain Greg was immediately carried to the fort, where his wounds were dressed; he was afterward removed to our hospital and put under my care. He was a most frightful spectacle; the whole of his scalp was removed; in two places on the fore part of his head, the tomahawk had penetrated through the skull; there was a wound on his back with the same instrument, besides a wound in his side and another through his arm by a musket ball. This unfortunate man, after suffering extremely for a long time, finally recovered, and appeared to be well satisfied in having his scalp restored to him, though uncovered with hair. The Indian mode of scalping their victims is this—with a knife they make a circular cut from the forehead quite round, just above the ears, then taking hold of the skin with their teeth, they tear off the whole hairy scalp in an instant, with wonderful dexterity. This they carefully dry and preserve as a trophy; showing the number of their victims, and they have a method of painting on the dried scalp, different figures, and colors, to designate the sex and age of the victim, and also the manner and circumstance of the murder.

December 20, 1777—The wounded soldiers committed to my care in October last have all recovered, and as a compliment for my assiduity, and attention to my patients, I have received from Dr. Potts, our Surgeon General, a generous and handsome present. The duties of our hospital being now greatly diminished, I have obtained a furlough for forty days, and shall commence my journey to visit my friends in New England.

[Thacher's hospital moved, in June of 1778, to Highlands on the Hudson, opposite West Point. He remained there and met many of the great men of the Revolution during this time: Kosciuzko, Washington, Lafayette, Steuben, and others. This was a period of relative inactivity for the young surgeon. In June of 1779 Thacher was transferred to New England for a time, but he returned to West Point in the fall of 1780. There was some skirmishing in this area and he was busy with the wounded. There is surprisingly little in his journal on the medical aspects of his life, but his note on one of the wounded throws some light on surgical practices of his day:]

March, 1781—One of our volunteers, named Hunt, received a dangerous wound through his shoulder and lungs, the air escaped from the wound at every breath. Dr. Eustis[6] came to the lines, and dilated the wound in the breast, and as the patient is athletic and had not sustained a very copious loss of blood, he recommended repeated and liberal blood letting, observing that in order to cure a wound through the the lungs, you must bleed your patient to *death*.[7] He eventually re-

---

6. William Eustis (1753–1825) graduated from Harvard College in 1772 and then learned his medicine as a pupil of Joseph Warren. Eustis served as a surgeon throughout the Revolution and remained with the army for several years afterward. Subsequently he served successively as a congressman, ambassador to Holland, and secretary of war during the War of 1812. He died in 1825 while serving as the governor of Massachusetts.

7. Bleeding was standard treatment for chest and belly wounds during the eighteenth century, and even later. John Jones wrote in his text, for the benefit of the military surgeons of the Continental Army, "The bleedings must be proportionate to the degree of hemorrhage, which if violent can only be restrained by large and repeated venesections.... " The therapeutic reasoning for this method of handling chest wounds is enlightening and apparently proceeded as follows: (1) active hemorrhage could be stopped by additional bloodletting (as exsanguination and shock appeared, both the volume and the pressure of the flow approached zero); (2) the treatment of inflammation in that day included bleeding, and chest wounds always became inflamed; and

covered, which is to be ascribed principally to the free use of the lancet and such abstemious living, as to reduce him to the greatest extremity. A considerable number of wounded prisoners receive my daily attention.

[In the autumn of 1781, Thacher marched to Yorktown. He wrote an excellent eyewitness account of the battle and the subsequent surrender of Cornwallis and his men. Following the battle, Thacher again returned to West Point. The war was essentially over. Other than a detailed description of the method used for inoculating for smallpox, there is little else in the journal of medical interest except for his meeting with Dr. John Jones, the author of America's first medical text, in Philadelphia.]

September, 1782—I returned last evening from Philadelphia. . . where I had the pleasure of being introduced to two celebrated characters, Dr. John Jones[8] of Philadelphia, and the honorable Robert Morris[9], the great American financier. Dr. Jones formerly resided in the city of New York where he was distinguished for his professional merit, urbanity of manners, and moral excellence. As a surgeon, Dr. Jones is considered at the head of his profession in the United States, and his reputation has been considerably extended by a valuable work entitled, "*Plain Remarks on Wounds and Fractures*" which he published in the year 1775 for the particular benefit of the surgeons of our army, and which has been received with universal approbation.

[On New Year's day, 1783, Jame Thacher left his country's service. He wrote:]

January 1st, 1783—This day I close my military career, and quit forever the toils and vicissitudes incident to the storm of war. . . .

---

(3) difficulty in breathing was sometimes relieved by phlebotomy, and persons wounded in the chest had difficulty in breathing.

Benjamin Rush (1745–1813), the best known American physician of his era, during his service as an army surgeon in the Revolution, bled one victim of a chest wound to a total of 140 ounces (almost 9 pints!) over a period of several weeks. His patient, like Eustis's, recovered.

8. John Jones (1729–1791); see page 22.

9. Robert Morris (1734–1806) was a patriot and financier who raised the funds with which the war was fought.

An Essay on
Wounds of the Intestines

THOMAS SMITH (1785?–1831)

The following essay, published in 1805, described the first experimental surgery ever to be performed in America. Its author, Thomas Smith, was a medical student at the University of Pennsylvania at the time that it was written. This selection, reprinted here in its entirety, was his inaugural thesis, required in those days for graduation from medical school. In it, Smith reviewed briefly what was known at that time about surgery of the intestine and went on to describe 12 experiments that he had carried out on dogs in an attempt to determine the best method of intestinal repair. A number of prosaic questions—unanswerable today—come to mind on reading his thesis: Where did he get his animals? Did he pay for them and for their care himself? Where was the surgery performed? Who helped him? Did he use any type of anesthesia or sedation?

The value of Thomas Smith's work did not go unrecognized. Samuel D. Gross, the greatest surgical educator of nineteenth century America had little use for inaugural theses, stating that most were without merit, but he did single out Smith's as one that had true value (Gross was especially interested in intestinal surgery and wrote extensively on the subject). In spite of this recognition we know little about Smith himself.

A few deductions can be made from his thesis, which was dedicated to his father, "William Smith, Esquire, of the island of St. Croix" and to Dr. John Ruan of Pennsylvania for the "polite attention conferred on me by the members of your family, during my residency in this country." (John Ruan [1771–1845] was a physician of Philadelphia, born in St. Croix, educated at Princeton and then at Edinburgh and presumably a family friend of the Smiths.) That Thomas may have been reasonably well-to-do is suggested by his nicely published and bound thesis and by the experiments that he probably paid for himself. We also know that he did return to his native St. Croix and was in practice in Fredericksted in 1809. He died in 1831 during a visit to the United States.

While bowel surgery was of less importance in 1805 than it is today, it did represent a frustrating problem for surgeons, particularly when dealing with strangulated hernia, a relatively common problem. Patients with wounded or strangulated intestine were expected to die even though intestinal suture was recommended—without much enthusiasm—in most texts. Occasionally it was possible to exteriorize the injured portion as an "artificial anus" with survival of the patient; rare cases of successful intestinal repair had also been recorded. The first meaningful experiments on intestinal repair were those reported by Astley Cooper (1768–1841) in his Anatomy and Surgical Treatment of Inquinal and Congenital Hernia (*London: Longman, 1804*) and in *Thomas Smith's elegant little thesis. Thus it was demonstrated, first, that intestinal suture could be carried out successfully, at least in animals; and, second, methods by which it could be done. Further progress would come; these were the foundations.*

An Essay on Wounds of the Intestines

INTRODUCTION

It is proposed in the following pages to take a brief view of the different methods which have been recommended for treating wounds of the intestines, to describe certain experiments, on brute animals which were made to ascertain the method most likely to prove successful, and to offer some doubts relative to the common opinions on this subject. I do not intend to enter minutely into the general mode of treating wounds of the intestines, but to confine myself entirely to the best manner of stitching them. Perhaps there are few accidents, to which surgeons are called, where they find themselves more at a loss on how to proceed, than in wounds of the intestines. These circumstances, as well as the frequent fatality of such injuries, evince the great importance of the subject. It is well known to surgeons, that the most trifling puncture, made into the cavity of the abdomen, is apt to induce very serious consequences, from the tendency which the peritonaeum has to inflame, when slightly injured; how much must the danger be increased when an intestine is wounded, and an opening produced, through which the contents may pass into the cavity of the abdomen. We are, however, told by a celebrated author (Mr. John Bell)[1], that there is very little to be apprehended from this circumstance, on account of the equable pressure which is always kept up in the abdomen by the viscera. But I hope to prove from experiment, that his ideas were not altogether correct on that subject. The invaluable work on hernia, of Mr. Astley Cooper, gave rise to this essay, and the ingenious observations of Messrs. Cooper and Thompson[2], respecting the difference between the consequences of longitudinal and transverse wounds of the intestines, induce me to attend particularly to that part of the subject.

AN INAUGURAL ESSAY

Wounds of the intestines may be known by a passage of blood from the mouth and anus, as well as by the discharge of faeces and foetid air from the external wound, and they ought to be suspected, when nausea, vomiting, violent gripping, pains through the abdomen, cold sweats or faintings occur after penetrating wounds of that cavity. The intestines are sometimes wounded without protruding through the external wound: in such cases it would be of very little advantage to know, whether the wound was transverse or oblique; for the methods to be pursued must be similar to that in simple penetrating wounds of the abdomen, viz. blood-letting and a low diet. Some authors recommend dilating the external wound, and searching for the injured bowel;

---

1. John Bell (1765–1820) of Edinburgh was the leading surgeon of that city during his professional life. A prolific writer, his *Principles of Surgery* in 3 volumes (London, 1808) was a popular text. He showed (independently of John Hunter) that arterial collaterals protected limbs when major vessels were ligated.

2. Astley Paston Cooper (1768–1841) was the greatest of John Hunter's many illustrious pupils. He was a dedicated anatomist and an excellent surgeon. Cooper's superb treatise on hernia incorporated detailed anatomy ("Cooper's ligament"), the results of animal experiments, and patient case reports. Cooper wrote comprehensive monographs on many other subjects (breast, testis, thymus, fractures, and dislocations).

John Thomson (1749–1806), surgeon and faculty member of the University of Edinburgh, also performed animal experiments on intestinal repair.

but to the danger arising from penetrating wounds in the abdomen, of all sizes, is so great, that in no instance ought it to be attempted, as there are cases on record of persons recovering from a wounded bowel, without having been under surgical treatment. It is, therefore, only in cases where the wounded intestine is protruded that the suture can be properly applied. The different kinds of sutures which have been recommended, have all had their advocates; the most ancient, and that which appears to have been most generally used is termed the glovers suture, which I shall now take the liberty of describing. In making this suture, a fine small round needle should be used armed with a silk thread, which has been previously waxed. The surgeon bringing the lips of the wound in contact, perforates both edges at the same time, and carrying the needle to the same side at which it entered, he must make a second stitch, at a small distance from the first, perhaps the eighth of an inch, and in the same manner by a proper number of stitches, must close the wound throughout its whole extent. This being done, a sufficient length of thread is left out at the external wound for the purpose of drawing it away, when we suppose the wound of the intestine to be united, which is generally completed in six or seven days: in withdrawing the ligature care should be taken to do it very gently, least we should destroy the adhesions which have taken place. This mode of stitching a wounded intestine, is certainly a very complicated process, and should be dispensed with in every instance for a more simple one.

A more modern method has been spoken of by Mr. Ledran[3], which is termed the looped suture. To make this suture, an assistant takes hold of one end of the wound whilst the surgeon does the same with the other, and the needles, which should be round, straight, and small, carrying each of them a thread a foot long, and not waxed, must be equal in number to the stitches intended to be made: as the threads are now to be passed through both lips of the wound as are thought necessary, taking care that they are a quarter of an inch distant from each other. All the threads being passed, the needles are to be withdrawn, and the ends of the threads on each side are tied, after which, joining them together they are twisted into a sort of cord: by this means,

---

His results were incorporated into Cooper's book. The dog was the animal used by all of these experimenters and has been used for this purpose up to the present time.

3. Henry Francois Ledran (leDran, LeDran, 1685–1770) was a surgeon, popular teacher, and author (military surgery, cancer, lithotomy) of Paris.

the divided portions of intestine are drawn into pleats, so that the stitches which were distant about a quarter of an inch are now brought together, and thus the lips of the wound are prevented from separating. The ligatures are to be fastened to the external dressing, afterwards they remain until the wound in the intestine is healed; they are then to be untwisted, and all the ends cut off on one side; after which they must be withdrawn slowly and separately. The same objection may be applied here as in the glovers suture, this is certainly a more complicated process, and it increases the danger of the operation, by lessening the diameter of the intestine, thereby occasioning dangerous obstructions.

Mr. John Bell has recommended in wounds of the intestines we should only use one single stitch which should be passed through the wounded bowel, and then drawn through the integuments of the abdomen at the external wound. But notwithstanding what Mr. Bell has said, of the equable pressure which is kept up among the viscera, preventing foeces from being shed into the cavity of the abdomen; I must, however, beg leave to differ from him, for in the experiments which I performed, I found that treating the intestine in this manner was not sufficiently secure for preventing the foeces from escaping into the abdominal cavity.

The following suture has also been proposed in a complete division of the intestine (Mr. Benjamin Bell speaks highly of it in his *System of Surgery*[4]). It was first recommended by Mr. Ramdohr,[5] in cases of hernia, where a portion of the intestine had been destroyed by mortification. In these cases, he has advised *to extirpate the diseased part*, and to introduce the upper portion of the sound intestine within the lower, for about an inch, and to confine it there by sewing it once or twice round with a fine needle and thread; but besides the difficulty of knowing which is the upper or lower portion in wounds of the intestines I find that it never can be performed on the living subject, as will appear by the ninth experiment, for immediately upon making the section of the intestine, the divided parts became so much inverted, as to render the introduction of one within the other utterly impossible. The method

---

4. Benjamin Bell (1749–1806) was the brother of Sir Charles Bell, unrelated to John Bell (fn. 1 above). He was a surgeon of Edinburgh and the author of an excellent, popular,and concise *System of Surgery*. The American edition (Philadelphia, 1791) is considered to be the first true surgical text to be published in this country.

5. Ramdohr, a German surgeon, apparently operated on a strangulated hernia in 1727 and successfully resected two feet of gangrenous intestine. He invaginated the proximal end into the distal and sutured these in place. This seems to have been his only claim to fame; I cannot identify him further.

which appears to promise most success, is that recommended by Mr. Astley Cooper, in his work on hernia, in that part wherein he treats particularly of mortification of the intestine. He directs that the injured part should be removed, and the divided portions brought into contact, and secured by four stitches, one being at or near the mesentery, and the others at equal distances from each other.

This method is certainly the most safe and simple of any that yet been spoken of, and will no doubt in time be generally adopted. Perhaps four or five stitches will be found sufficient in most instances of a complete division of the intestine. But we should be careful not to use more than are really necessary, for it has been observed, that puncturing the intestine frequently increases the danger of the operation very much.

In order to decide between these different methods, I determined to institute a series of experiments upon dogs by wounding them with the various sutures above stated. I am aware, that it is not easy to determine with precision the treatment proper for the human species, by inferences derived from the dog; but the analogy in the present instance appears to me very strong. I shall in the next place commence, by relating my experiments.

EXPERIMENT I

April 7.

ASSISTED by my friend Mr. Klapp[6], an incision was made into the abdomen of a dog, and one of the small intestines; having been brought into view, a transverse section was made into it, and the wound secured by four stitches, one at the mesentery, and the other three at equal distances from each other, the threads were then cut off at the knots, and the external wound closed by the interrupted suture. The animal did not appear to have suffered materially from the operation, for in twenty four hours he took food, and after the first day exhibited no symptoms of indisposition. On the 30th, he was killed, the wound of the intestine was found completely healed; the place at which the intestine had been divided, appeared somewhat thickened, considerable adhesions were observed among the small intestines. Three of the ligatures had disappeared, the other was still remaining loosely attached to the internal coat, and probably would have been discharged in the same manner as the others, had the dog been permitted to live a few days longer.

---

6. Klapp was a common medical name in nineteenth-century Philadelphia. I cannot identify this man, however. He presumably was a student at the University of Pennsylvania in 1805.

EXPERIMENT II

April 7.

On another dog, I repeated the same operation, with this difference that the ligatures which had been cut off in the preceding experiment at the intestine, were now left out at the external wound, in case it should be necessary to withdraw them. In consequence of the restlessness of the animal during the operation, considerable violence was done to the parts, before they could be reduced. On the second day after the operation, he appeared so ill as to make his recovery doubtful: on the 4th day, it was thought proper to remove the ligatures; after this he appeared better and took nourishment. On the 19th, he was killed: upon laying open the abdomen, the effects of inflammation were still obvious. The omentum was found adhering to the parietes of the abdomen, and very much indurated. Preternatural adhesions had taken place among all the viscera, but more particularly in the small intestines, which were knotted and twisted together in an astonishing manner. The intestine at the place where the wound had been made was not quite united.

EXPERIMENT III

April 9.

SEVERAL of my friends honoured me with their attendance, whilst the following experiments were performed; the abdomen of a dog having been opened, and the small intestines brought into view, a longitudinal incision of about an inch and a half was made parallel with the mesentery, which was secured by four stitches, and the intermediate spaces sewn with a fine thread to prevent the faeces from escaping into the cavity of the abdomen: the threads were cut off at the intestine. The animal died in about thirty six hours. On dissection the marks of inflammation were found much less than might have been expected. The wound in the intestine was completely torn open, excepting at one stitch.

EXPERIMENT IV

April 9.

A FULL grown dog was submitted to the same experiment as the former with this difference, that the intermediate spaces between each stitch were left unsewn. Six hours after the operation, the animal vomited stercoraceous matter, appeared dull and drowsy. On the 10th, in consequence of food being offered, of which he took a small quantity, vomiting was again excited. On the 12th, he took food, and from that time seemed to be doing well. Seven days after he was killed; on opening the abdomen the omentum was found adhering to the site of the external wound, being considerably indurated. The mesenteric glands were enlarged. The wound in the intestine was not completely united, two of the ligatures had disappeared. The other two still remained; the wounded gut had adhered to the mesentery and adjoining portion of intestine.

EXPERIMENT V

April 10.

ON a full grown tarrier, I repeated the former experiment wishing to see, whether a longitudinal incision could not by great care and attention, be so managed, as to do away the opinion of its being universally fatal. To effect which, a very small opening was made through the parietes of the abdomen, and a portion of intestine, being brought into view, it was divided longitudinally for about two inches, and afterwards secured by six stitches which were cut off at the knots. The parts having been returned, the lips of the external wound were brought together and secured by adhaesive plaister (for it was observed, that the ligature used for securing the external wound increased the inflammation very much). The animal did not appear to have suffered in the least from the operation, for in less than twenty four hours he took food and has continued doing well ever since.

EXPERIMENT VI

April 16.

PLEASED with my success in the preceding experiment, I obtained another dog and opened his abdomen, in one of the small intestines, I made a longitudinal wound for about three inches, and treated it in every respect similar to that related above. This animal appeared to have suffered very little more than the other considering the extent of the wound, for in about twenty eight hours he eat [sic] and continued doing so untill the tenth day after the operation, when he refused nourishment. Two days after he died, on examination it was found that the wound had healed completely, but directly above the wound a bone half an inch long, and nearly as broad, was discovered to have perforated the intestine. (This must have been owing to a diminution of the intestinal canal which is always produced by longitudinal wounds of the intestines.)

EXPERIMENT VII

April 16.

WISHING to know how much of the intestine might be removed, without endangering the life of the animal, I performed the following experiment: having obtained a full grown dog, an incision was made into the cavity of the abdomen, two inches of one of the small intestines were removed; the divided portions were then brought together, and the wound was treated as the transverse incisions had been. In dissecting off the divided portion of intestine; some of the branches of the mesenteric arteries were wounded, but did not bleed during the operation. On visiting him in the afternoon, I found there had been a considerable hemorrhage which still continued. I did not open the wound, but applied a piece of wetted linen to the parts, which had the desired effect. On the 18th, the belly being somewhat tense, two of the external ligatures were cut away, that the blood, should any have collected, might be discharged; but the wound did not open, and the dog soon resumed the appearance of perfect health, which continued without interruption until May 6, when he was killed. The divided portions of intestine were found united, and the ligatures had been all discharged. (The viscera in this experiment appeared much more natural than in any other, probably from the hemorrhage that took place, which shews the propriety of bleeding largely in such cases.)

EXPERIMENT IX

April 18.

HAVING divided the intestine of a dog transversly, I attempted to treat it in the manner spoken of by Mr. Ramdohr, viz. by introducing the upper extremity of the divided intestine within the lower; after having procured a piece of candle, as directed by him, it was inserted into that portion of intestine, which was supposed to be the uppermost. I then endeavoured to introduce the superior within the inferior, but the extremities of each became so inverted, that it was found utterly impossible to succeed, it was therefore given up and treated in the way recommended by Mr. John Bell, using only one stitch, and fastening it to the parietes of the abdomen. The dog took food the day after. On the 20th, it was observed that the faeces were discharging at the external wound, when the animal appeared very weak, but still continued to take food. On the 21st, he was much worse, and the abdomen being tense, the ligatures at the external wound were removed to facilitate the discharge of faeces which gave a temporary relief. On the 22nd, he died. On examination there was found a considerable quantity of faeces and water in the abdominal cavity. One portion of the intestine had united to the external wound through which part of the faeces were discharged.

EXPERIMENT X & XI

April 28.

WISHING to give Mr. John Bell's method of stitching an intestine a fair trial, I made the following experiments: having obtained two full grown dogs, a transverse incision was made into the intestines of each of them, which was secured by one stitch and fastened to the wound. No. 10, died in about twenty-four hours. The marks of inflammation were very great, and the faeces had been discharged into the abdomen. No. 11, died on the 2nd of May. The intestines appeared very much inflamed, faeces as in the other instances were found in the abdomen, also water which the animal had drank. The large intestines appeared gangrenous and tore very easily.

EXPERIMENT XII

A POINTER pup of about two months was submitted to the following experiment: a triangular piece was cut out of one of the small intestines, and the wounded intestine sewn to the parietes of the abdomen. The animal very soon showed symptoms of indisposition and died in thirty hours. On examination the peritonaeum and all the viscera of the abdomen were found considerably inflamed, a quantity of water was also in the cavity.

It appears then from the result of my experiments on dogs, that not only the intestine may be returned into the cavity of the abdomen, but that the ligatures may be cut off and returned with the intestine, and that we need not be under any apprehension to their being discharged into the cavity, for by some process of the animal oeconomy of which we are ignorant, the ligatures have in every instance either been discharged with the faeces or been found loosely attached to the internal coat of the intestine. It has been said by Messrs. Cooper and Thompson, that there is a curious difference in the facility with which a longitudinal and transverse wound of the intestine unites. But in all the experiments which I have made, it was found that with care the longitudinal united as kindly as the transverse, only requiring a little more attention to the diet of the animal, which should be very sparing and liquid until the wound has had time to heal. It certainly requires more pains to close a longitudinal wound of the intestine completely, than one which is transverse. The longitudinal incision always occasions a diminution in the diameter of the intestinal canal, thereby producing dangerous obstructions. If it should be of any considerable extent, probably the surgeon would be justified in cutting out the wounded portion and treating it as a transverse division. This may be done without much endangering the life of the animal, as appears by two experiments where three inches of the intestine were removed.

Remarkable Case of the Swallowing of a Silver Spoon

SAMUEL WHITE, M.D. (1777–1845)

The following case report appeared in the New York Medical Repository, *the first medical journal published in the United States. The
author, Samuel White of Hudson, N.Y., described a surgical operation
that he had performed to remove a spoon from the small intestine. This
apparently represents the first description of a successful case of open
intestinal surgery in America. White's operation was daring; that his
patient survived was miraculous.*

*Samuel White and his operation have been lost to sight over the
years, and his name is to be found in none of the standard medical biographical sources. He was born in Coventry, Connecticut, and learned
his medicine and surgery as an apprentice in nearby Norwich. He practiced in Hudson, N.Y., for the remainder of his life. Although White
became known as an alienist in later life and organized one of this
country's first institutions for the insane (1830), he never lost his love
of surgery and continued to operate up until his death. Many of his
operations were of considerable magnitude and included the successful
removal of a parotid gland in 1808—one of the earliest recorded cases.*

*The following report has been abstracted from Samuel White's
article as it appeared in the* Medical Repository *(4:367, 1807). White's
case report also appeared in a fascinating book devoted to surgical
curiosities entitled* Remarkable Cases in Surgery *(1857) by Paul Fitz-
simmons Eve (1806–1877), the professor of surgery at Nashville.*

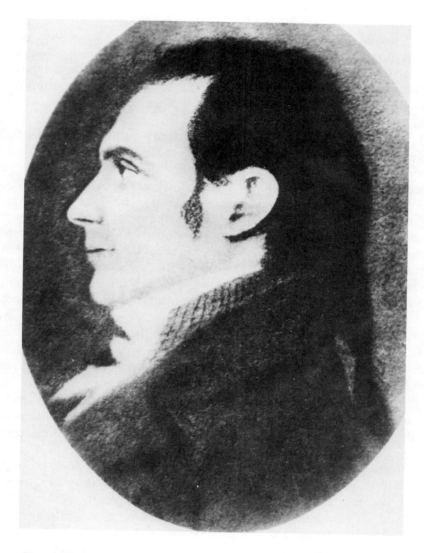

Figure 10. Samuel White (1777–1845). (Courtesy New York Academy of Medicine.)

Remarkable Case of the Swallowing of a Silver Spoon, and of the Excision of It from the Intestinal Canal with the Recovery of the Patient

Having noticed in some of your introductory observations, your decided approbation of practical remarks in preference to those of a speculative nature, and noticing that *chirurgical* cases were comparatively small in number, with those of a medical kind; I communicate for your Repository, if judged worthy a place, a surgical case, which fell under my care last year.

May 22d, 1806, George Macy, aged twenty-six became a patient of mine, with a *rheumatic white swelling*[1] of the left knee; an *exostosis* of the left tibia, about two inches above the inner ancle; with extensive ulcers, situated on the anterior and middle part of each leg.

Mr. M. informed me that the complaint of his knee took its rise from a violent sprain, on a passage from London to New York, in July, 1804. His knee continued swollen and painful for several months subsequent to the injury; after this it was at times more comfortable; but every exciting cause roused to action a strong predisposition to rheumatic affections, and his knee was the part which generally suffered. In December, 1805, after a severe attack of intermitting fever, his knee became more sensibly affected, and he gained only temporary alleviation from external applications. He visited the Balltown springs in March, 1806, but derived no benefit from the waters; and returned to his father's, in this place, the May following, and became my patient as above.

The knee was now nearly twice its natural size, owing principally to a morbid thickening of the tendinous and ligamentous expansion, with a puffy elastic state of the *bursæ mucosæ* and surrounding teguments. The rest of the limb was much emaciated, with considerable contractions of the flexor tendons, and immobility of the diseased joint. The ulcers on the legs were to be considered as a secondary complaint, receiving their primary cause from the rheumatic diathesis. They discharged an albuminous matter, which operated as a drain for the morbid accumulation, and was probably one great cause why abscesses did not form around the joint.

July 1st. The inflammatory complaint progressing with extreme pertinacity, the nervous system became sensibly agitated.... The violence of his disease, and his inability to receive medicine, seemed to

---

1. "Rheumatic white swelling" implied tuberculous arthritis.

thwart every exertion to give relief, and palliatives only were admissible. He seemed to be rapidly sinking, and but small hopes were entertained of his exhausted powers withstanding any longer this extreme torture; an imperfect crisis, however, was unexpectedly formed, followed by a watchful delirium, and an artful disposition to procure some instrument of death. Being unable to turn himself in bed, there was no suspicion of danger.

July 7th. The night following this extraordinary change, he procured a full tea-spoon with some fruit jelly, and impractical as it may appear, forced it down his throat, while his attendant was gone, by his request, to the opposite side of the room for water. His struggles were violent, and he was apparently suffocating, when, by the force of his fingers against the handle of the spoon, he crowded it so far as to suffer it to pass into the stomach before his friends could be gained to give his attendant assistance.

In this deplorable situation I was immediately requested to visit him. He was greatly agitated—talked much—believed he had gained his point, and declared that no attempt of ours could rescue him; which, at the time, I considered too true. The morning following he had some irregular sleep, continued through the 8th under a slight delirium, and complained of no uneasiness of the stomach. 9th. Continued the same until evening, when a spasmodic affection of the stomach alternated every fifteen minutes with a stupor; throwing himself, as often as the spasm returned, with great violence from one side to the other, for about two hours (while the spoon probably passed the pylorus), when he suddenly fell asleep, and rested well through the night, extending the diseased leg, the flexor tendons of which had been greatly contracted, especially through the last complaint. He now became rational, his fever formed a perfect crisis; he recounted the past transaction with extreme sensibility, and expressed great anxiety for relief.

I waited the efforts of nature, assisting her with oily and mucilaginous substances, which served to remove the constipated state of the bowels, and to guard against any corroding effect of the metal. His ulcers soon healed, and he continued to gain in health and strength until the 25th, when a cutting sensation, confirmed by pressure of the hand, when in a stooping position, led to discovery of the situation of the spoon in one of the last circumvolutions of the intestinum ilium, near the line dividing the right iliac and hypogastric regions. It remained in this fixed position with increased heat and irritation in the adjacent parts, till August 7th.

Fearing that any further delay might endanger success, and he being resolutely determined to suffer everything for relief, accompanied by the consulting physician, I had recourse to an operation as the dernier resort. I made an incision of about three inches, parallel with the epigastric artery, extending upwards to near a transverse line with the top of the os ilium—penetrating the inner edges of the obliquus externus descendens, internus ascendens, and transversalis abdominis –opened the peritonaeum with a lancet, protruded the lower part of the intestines containing the handle of the spoon, with my fore finger; pierced the intestine with the lancet over the end of the handle, and extracted it in the same direction with the forceps. I then laid the divided edges of the intestine directly opposite, and secured them with the glover's switch[2]—dressing the external wound with slips of adhesive plaster and lint.

After this I made use of simple dressings to the wound; applied a liniment composed of camphorated oil, volatile spirits of ammonia, and laudanum, equal parts, to the diseased joint and limb, which became more painful and contracted while labouring under the irritation of the spoon. Under this treatment, his wound healed by the first intention; his knee became almost free from pain, and with the use of mild preparations of bark, he was soon able to move on his crutches, and ride abroad.

In September I applied a large stimulating plaster to the knee, and he soon after left this place for Nantucket, to gain the benefit of a sea-breeze; since which I learn he continues to recover, though much doubt remains in my mind as to the security of the limb.

---

2. It seems unlikely that White would have been familiar with the previous selection (Thomas Smith's "An Essay On Wounds of the Intestine," 1805). Intestinal suture was mentioned briefly, however, in every work on surgery that had been published in America up to 1807, when White's paper appeared. Benjamin Bell (*System of Surgery*, Philadelphia, 1807) recommended the glover's stitch as had John Jones (1775). Jones also recommended that the sutures be left long to attach the repaired intestine to the wound in the abdominal wall. This might have been of value in localizing infection if a leak had occurred.

Extracting Poisonous
Substances from the Stomach

and

The Use of Animal Sutures

PHILIP SYNG PHYSICK, M.D. (1768–1837)

Philip Syng Physick, "the father of American surgery," was a favored pupil of London's great John Hunter (1728–1793). Physick brought the principles of Hunter's conservative surgery with him when he returned to his native Philadelphia. His pupils, in turn, carried these same precepts to all corners of the growing United States.

Physick was born in Philadelphia on July 7, 1768. He attended the University of Pennsylvania (A.B., 1785) and afterward studied medicine there under Dr. Adam Kuhn (1741–1817), the professor of materia medica. Physick subsequently went to London where he was John Hunter's pupil and associate for two years. The young American next went on to Edinburgh where he received his M.D. in 1792. After his return to the United States, Physick earned the reputation of being this country's leading surgeon. He became the professor of surgery at the University of Pennsylvania and inspired a number of very capable pupils. These men, in turn, went on to become the surgical leaders of this country. Physick continued to practice in Philadelphia and died there on December 15, 1837.

Physick made several significant contributions to surgical practice. These were described in brief papers published from time to time during his professional years. The first of the two selections that follow is of interest in view of the present widespread use of gastric intubation

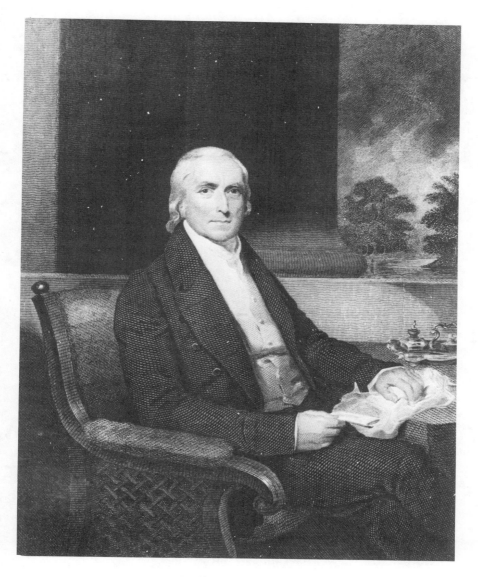

Figure 11. Philip Syng Physick (1768–1837). Engraved from a painting by Henry Inman.

in surgery. This paper introduced and popularized the stomach tube for removing substances from the stomach. The second describes the use of "animal ligatures," which could be cut short to remain in the depths of the wound, in contrast to the usual practice of leaving uncut ends dangling to be withdrawn at a later time. The catgut sutures used today are the immediate descendants of Lister's "carbolized gut" and more remotely are descended from Physick's animal ligatures.

The first of the two papers that follow appeared in the Eclectic Repertory *(3:111) in 1812. The second appeared in the same periodical (6:389) in 1816.*

Account of a New Mode of Extracting Poisonous Substances from the Stomach

On Thursday 6th June, 1812, I was sent for in much haste at nine o'clock in the evening, to visit two children of Mr. S. B. each three months old. They were twins, and had been affected with hooping cough for several weeks. The mother informed me that in consequence of her children having been very restless the night before, she had this evening given them some laudanum. To William she had given one drop at seven o'clock, and the same dose to Edmund forty minutes afterwards.

I found William in a state of stupor or very profound sleep, from which he could not be roused, and was informed, that just before my arrival, his whole body had been strongly convulsed; his breathing was laborious and his pulse feeble and slow. On inquiry, I found that the vial out of which the drop of laudanum had been given, had contained, several weeks before, nearly one ounce of that medicine, but having been left without a cork, it had dried away so much that one drop only could be obtained for William; in order to procure another drop, two drops of water had been put into the vial and stirred about, by which another drop had been obtained and given to Edmund, forty minutes having intervened between the two doses.

About a quarter of an hour before my visit, the mother had given to William fifteen drops of antimonial wine, but as it had produced no effect I prescribed an emetic of ipecacuanha, and directed it to be given immediately; this however was found impracticable, as the child was incapable of swallowing.

At half past nine o'clock, Edmund, who had appeared to be in a very easy sleep, became convulsed, and his pulse and breathing were affected in the same way that his brother's had been. We attempted to give him ipecacuanha, but could not make him swallow it. The countenances of the children became livid,—their breathing very laborious; with long intervals between the times of each inspiration, and the pulse in each very feeble.

Under these circumstances it clearly appeared no time was to be lost, and therefore, as they could not swallow any thing, I determined to inject an emetic into their stomachs. For this purpose a large flexible catheter[1] was passed through the mouth down the oesophagus into the stomach, and through this, one drachm of ipecacuanha mixed with water was quickly injected by means of a common pewter syringe. In hopes that the emetic would operate, I waited some time without any effect being produced. William exhibited now every symptom of speedy dissolution,—his face became very livid;—the pulse and respiration had almost ceased; and indeed the pulse could not be perceived, except for a faint stroke or two, after that kind of imperfect and convulsive inspiration which is commonly observed in children just before actual death, accompanied with a convulsed action of the muscles of the mouth and neck. In this situation I passed the catheter again, and by applying the syringe to its projecting end, drew up the fluid contents of the stomach, and immediately injected warm water which was again withdrawn. These operations were alternated two or three times, but when completed no sign of life remained. Hopeless as the case now appeared, I injected some spirit and water mixed with a little vinegar through the catheter;—in less than one minute the child again inspired, the pulse became perceptible at the wrist, and in four minutes, with the aid of external stimuli, both went on so perfectly that there was every reason to believe the child would recover.

By the time that these operations were performed on William, Edmund was observed to have passed into the same condition of apparent death, from which his brother had just recovered. The same measures were adopted in his case, and with the same happy effect. I now flattered myself that the children would do well, but in this expec-

---

1. The concept of introducing a tube into the stomach is an old one and reaches back into antiquity. The first recorded use of a stomach tube, however, was by John Hunter, who passed an eel skin into the stomach of a woman who was unable to swallow. This "tube" was used to feed the patient. Physick was a pupil of John Hunter in 1790, at the time that Hunter carried this out.

Charles Bell's *System of Operative Surgery*, 1st American edition (Hartford, 1812, 2:13) mentions Hunter's case and states that, "for the same purpose we now use the flexible gum tube", but makes no note of actually using such a tube for the removal of substances from the stomach.

tation I was disappointed. In about half an hour, Edmund's breathing became very slow and laborious, and his pulse which had before been very much excited became so feeble, that he appeared to be sinking very fast. Supposing that the effects observed, might be produced by the spirit which had been given, occasioning intoxication, I determined to extract it from the stomach and to inject warm water, removing it again. This operation was very quickly performed, but at the conclusion of it I was much distressed by seeing the little patient to all appearance lifeless. Observing in this case, that the actions of life ceased so immediately after the extraction of the spirit, I determined to try it again, and injected a little weak brandy and water. In less than a minute this occasioned a repetition of breathing and of the action of the heart, and in about five minutes both were regularly performed. The symptoms of ebriety took place also in William, but observing that his brother had been nearly lost by extracting the spirit from his stomach, I did not attempt the removal of it in William's case.

Doctor Austin,[2] who kindly assisted me on this occasion, remained all night with my little patients. He informed me, that after some time they became better, though they both had slight convulsive motions occasionally through the night. Their bowels were moved several times by castor oil. After five o'clock in the morning Edmund had no convulsions, but they continued with William until twenty-five minutes after nine, when he struggled a little, sighed, and expired. Edmund was troubled for two or three days with a diarrhoea, but soon recovered completely.

The Use of Animal Sutures

Having repeatedly experienced considerable delay in the healing of wounds from ligatures applied on divided arteries remaining a long time in the sore before they could be removed, I have for many years been very desirous of avoiding such an inconvenience in the use of ligatures. With this view, the first idea that occurred was that of drawing the ligature tight on the vessel by the assistance of a double canula; unfortunately, the first patient on whom it was employed for securing the femoral artery, died of tetanus; and though I by no means believe the disease to have been occasioned by the instrument, yet the event discouraged from further trials of it.

---

2. "Dr. Austin" cannot be identified with certainty, but he was probably one of Physick's pupils. A John Austin is listed as a graduate of the University Pennsylvania Medical School in 1811, but no further information is available.

Several years ago, recollecting how completely leather straps, spread with adhesive plaster, and applied over wounds for the purpose of keeping their sides in contact, were dissolved by the fluids discharged from the wound, it appeared to me that ligatures might be made of leather, or of some other animal substance, with which the sides of a blood-vessel could be compressed for a sufficient time to prevent hemorrhage; that such ligatures would be dissolved after a few days, and would be evacuated with the discharge from the cavity of the wound.

Under this impression, I requested Dr. Dorsey[3] to try an experiment on a horse, by using a ligature of buckskin. This was found to answer every purpose, and came away in a few days.

This fact was mentioned at the time to several of my medical acquaintances; and I understand that Dr. Hartshorne[4] has lately tied up some of the arteries after amputating the thigh, with ligatures of parchment. They were found dissolved at the first dressing. Dr. Dorsey, in several operations, in which I have assisted, has used ligatures of French kid, which he finds stronger than any other leather. He has it cut into narrow strips, stretches them and peels off the coloured polished surface. No hemorrhage has taken place in any instance, and the ligatures are found dissolved at the end of two or three days.

With the view of ascertaining what animal substance would withstand the solvent power of pus for the longest time, I suggested the plan of trying different articles, by applying them over the surfaces of ulcers. Buckskin, kid, parchment, and catgut, have been tried in this way. The buckskin and kid dissolved first; then the parchment; when at the same time the catgut was but little changed. From an apprehension that in tying large blood-vessels the leather might dissolve too soon, I have requested Dr. Dorsey, to try leather impregnated with the varnish used by Mr. Bishop of this city, in making elastic catheters; in the hope that when so prepared it will be somewhat more durable. Perhaps tendon would be found to answer the purpose. Future experiments will probably place at the command of the surgeons a variety of ligatures,

---

3. John Syng Dorsey (1783-1818); see p. 74.

4. Joseph Hartshorne (1779–1850) was an apprentice under George Washington's physician, Dr. James Craik (1731–1814), and then graduated from the University of Pennsylvania Medical School in 1805. In 1815 Hartshorne became a surgeon to the Pennsylvania Hospital and an associate of Physick and Dorsey. He became a very successful surgeon in Philadelphia and accumulated a large fortune in the practice of his profession.

which may be so selected as to remain the exact length of time he may require.

This hasty notice on the subject is given, because it is thought important that these facts should be made public without delay.

Philadelphia, July 9, 1816.

Of Femoral and Inguinal Aneurisms

and

Of Stone in the Bladder

JOHN SYNG DORSEY, M.D. (1783–1818)

In 1813 John Syng Dorsey, a young surgeon of Philadelphia, published the first text by an American author that attempted to encompass the entire field of surgery as it was then practiced. Dorsey was the nephew and protege of Philip Syng Physick; his book, Elements of Surgery, *was based on what he had seen of his uncle's practice but included as well much from the teachings of the great European masters. Dorsey's text therefore was truly eclectic.* Elements of Surgery *was popular both with the students of this country, for whom it had primarily been written, and with practicing physicians and surgeons. It went through three editions in a decade.*

Dorsey was born in Philadelphia on December 23, 1783. He trained in his uncle's office and then received his doctor's degree in medicine from the University of Pennsylvania in 1802. Dorsey traveled and studied in Europe before returning to Philadelphia to go into practice with Physick. He embarked on a distinguished, although brief, life devoted to the practice and teaching of surgery. His premature death on November 12, 1818, ended a promising career.

The first of the following selections describes a case in which Dorsey successfully tied the external iliac artery for aneurysm—the first time the operation had been performed in America. It is taken from the first edition of Dorsey's Elements of Surgery *(Philadelphia: W. Brown,*

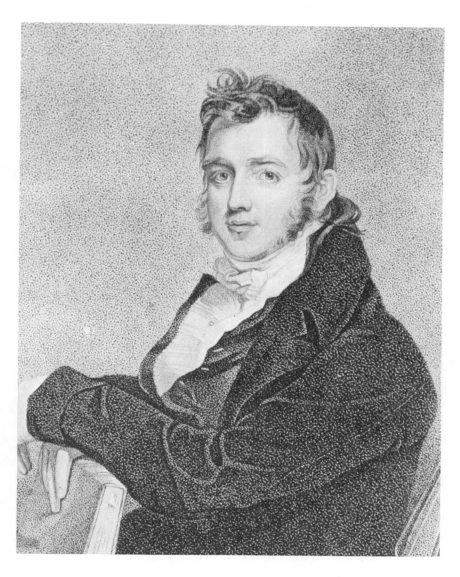

Figure 12. John Syng Dorsey (1783–1818). This portrait was engraved from a painting by Thomas Sully.

printer, 2:180, 1813). This case had previously been published in the Eclectic Repertory *(2:111) in 1811. The second selection describes the operation of lithotomy as it was performed by Physick, the most capable lithotomist in America at that time; this selection is taken from the same volume (page 148).*

Of Femoral and Inguinal Aneurisms

On the 15th of August 1811, I was consulted by Alexander Patton on account of a tumour in his right groin. The patient was a native of Aberdeenshire in Scotland, aged about thirty years, the last ten of which he had passed in America. He followed the trade of a cooper; was accustomed to hard labour and to athletic exercises, jumping, running and the like. He was six feet in height, of a robust but not corpulent habit.

Two years ago he perceived, for the first time, a small tumour in the right groin. Having never had the venereal, nor indeed any other disease, and not having met with any accident, he was at a loss to account for this appearance. From its commencement it throbbed with considerable violence. For a year and four months it increased very slowly; during the last eight months much more rapidly. In January it was no bigger than a walnut; in August its shortest diameter was four inches, its longest, nearly five. It occasionally gave him severe pain, and at length incapacitated him from all labour. In June last (1811) he applied to Dr. Irwin[1] of Easton, the place of his residence, who instantly apprised him of the nature and importance of the complaint, and advised him to come to Philadelphia. He arrived here the 14th of August, and was admitted next day into the Pennsylvania hospital.

On examination, an aneurism was found, situated immediately below Poupart's ligament, forming a regular tumour in the groin, nearly hemispherical with a kind of apex, where the skin appeared extremely thin, and discoloured as if by ecchymosis. The patient had used a good deal of exercise previously to his admission into the hospital, and had taken a drink of rum, in consequence of which his arterial system was greatly excited, and the tumour pulsated so violently that the bed clothes were bounced up with great force. He was confined to bed, was purged, and kept to a low diet. A consultation was called; and the

---

1. "Dr. Irwin" of Easton may have been Dr. Handy Irwin, who graduated from the University of Pennsylvania in 1810.

surgeons of the house concurred in recommending the operation of tying the artery as high as practicable above the tumour.[2] It was determined to perform the operation promptly; as the disease was progressing, and no benefit was to be expected from delay.

On Monday 19th of August, at noon, in presence of Dr. Physick[3] and Dr. Hartshorne,[4] surgeons to the hospital, and a number of medical gentlemen, I proceeded to the operation. The patient, having previously taken fifty drops of laudanum, was placed on the table. An incision, three inches and a half long, was made, beginning an inch and a half higher than the superior anterior spinous process of the ilium, and one inch distant from that process internally; being also four inches and a half distant from the umbilicus, extending obliquely downward and terminating about one inch above the basis of the tumour. This incision, which was nearly in the direction of the fibres of the tendon of the external oblique muscle, divided the skin and adipose membrane, and exposed that tendon, which was next cut through, the whole length of the external incision. The internal oblique muscle now protruded at the wound and was carefully cut through; the inferior edge of the transversalis abdominis was next divided, but not so far upward as the top of the external wound. My finger was then introduced, and the cellular texture readily yielded it a passage to the external iliac artery, the trunk of which I distinctly felt pulsating very strongly. With my finger I separated it gently from the neighbouring parts; but took care to denude only a very small portion of the vessel. The peritoneum I was equally careful to detach as little as possible; and not more than a square inch of it was disturbed. The only remaining difficulty in the operation was to pass the ligature round the vessel; and this having been anticipated, was readily surmounted. Before commencing the operation, I had secured an aneurismal needle (a blunt bodkin of silver properly bent) in a pair of curved forceps, by tying the handles of the forceps firmly together. The needle

---

2. John Hunter was the first to treat aneurysms by tying off a normal femoral artery above a popliteal aneurysm. Other surgeons borrowed his principle and ligated for aneurysm occurring almost anywhere among the various branches of the aorta.

Aneurysms of the extremities occur relatively infrequently today and when encountered are usually the result of arteriosclerosis or of trauma. In former years, however, most aneurysms were the sequelae of infection— usually syphilis, but probably also from typhoid, tuberculosis, and other pathogens. With the control of these diseases the number of aneurysms, especially those involving extremities, has declined.

3. "Dr. Physick"; see p. 66.

4. "Dr. Hartshorne"; see p. 71.

was armed with strong bobbin; and thus connected with the forceps, resembled a tenaculum, which could easily be managed outside of the wound. With one finger in the wound I found it very easy to direct the extremity of the needle, and with the forceps in my other hand, to push it through the fascia surrounding the vessel. The string connecting the handles of the forceps was now cut, and the needle was left under the vessel. The forceps being removed, the needle was drawn out, leaving the ligature round the artery. Convinced, by careful examination, that nothing but the artery was included in the ligature, and that it was, to the best of my judgment, natural in size and texture, I tied it very firmly, as high up as possible. The pulsation of the tumour instantly ceased. Three knots were made, and the ends of the ligature were left out at the external wound. No blood-vessel of magnitude was divided, and not half an ounce of blood was lost. No stitches were employed to close the wound; a strip of adhesive plaster effectually answered this purpose. A pledget of lint was applied, and the patient was put to bed, his thigh being moderately flexed upon the pelvis. He complained of extreme pain during the latter part of the operation, the whole of which occupied eleven minutes.

The patient's pulse, for several days before the operation, was 80; after the operation it was 88, and rose in the afternoon to 100. At four o'clock he was bled ten ounces. At seven he complained of extreme pain in the back and belly, and also of some pain in the limb. He was not permitted to take any sustenance except toast and water. The superficial veins of the leg and foot were filled; and the whole of the limb was covered all the evening with perspiration. Its temperature was examined repeatedly by a thermometer, and was five degrees colder than the other. It was covered with flannel and carded wool.

Tuesday 20th. Passed a restless night, in great pain. To use his own language, in expressing his sensations, "he felt as if his loins were tearing apart." He was also troubled with pain of the bowels. Three grains of calomel and ten of rhubarb were given, but without procuring a stool. In the afternoon he was bled ten ounces, and a purgative injection was ordered; after which his bowels were freely opened, and his pain subsided. An enema, consisting of a hundred drops of laudanum and two ounces of water, was administered, and he soon after fell asleep. The weather, on the day of the operation and several days after, was very hot. The mercury of the thermometer in the patient's room stood at 86° Fahrenheit. Placed between the toes of the aneurismal limb, it rose to 88°; between those of the sound limb 90°; at both knees it stood at 92°. His pulse was 100 and tense.

Wednesday 21st, *third day* after the operation. The sleep procured by the anodyne injection continued all night. In the fore part of the day he was easy; but in the evening his pain returned with considerable fever. He was bled ten ounces and took ten grains of magnesia and as much rhubarb; this with the assistance of a clyster, brought away a large quantity of faeces and flatus, and procured relief of all his pain. The anodyne injection was again administered, and he soon slept. His pulse 100 and somewhat tense.

Thursday, *fourth day.* He slept all night, and was much better; being quite free from pain and fever. His pulse 90. He ate some boiled rice with great relish. The wound was examined, and it was found that nearly all of it had united: a little healthy pus surrounded the ligature. The limb was four degrees colder than the sound one.

From this time no change of importance occurred until Sunday, 1st Sept. when the ligature came away; viz. on the fourteenth day after the operation. In a few days more the wound cicatrized, without the occurrence of a single unpleasant symptom. On the twentieth day after the operation, his nurse being absent, he arose from bed and walked across the room, and has taken exercise every day since without inconvenience. The tumour in the groin diminishes slowly, and at this time is much reduced in size.

REMARKS

The operation of tying up the external iliac artery above Poupart's ligament was first performed by Mr. Abernethy,[5] under circumstances in which immediate death was the only alternative. He repeated it afterwards in cases of aneurism seated so high in the femoral artery as to preclude all prospect of a cure by any other means. He performed the operation four times. In the first two instances his patients died; in the succeeding cases they recovered. Mr. Freer,[6] in the Birmingham hospital, performed the operation in a case of inguinal aneurism with complete success; and soon after another case was treated successfully by Mr. Tomlinson, of the same hospital. These six cases are all that I have

---

5. John Abernethy (1764–1831) was a pupil of John Hunter and his immediate clinical successor. Hunter had observed the formation of collateral circulation in animals after the interruption of major arteries and deduced that man would survive arterial ligation as well. He first ligated the femoral artery for popliteal aneurysm in 1786, thus saving his patient's leg. Abernethy was the first to tie the external iliac for a high femoral aneurysm in 1796.

6. George Freer, surgeon of Birmingham, England, was the author of a text, *Observations on Aneurysm* (1807). Mr. Tomlinson has not been further identified.

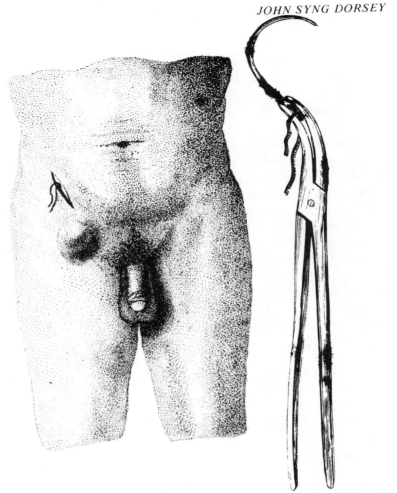

Figure 13. An inguinal aneurysm and Physick's needle holder. This figure was drawn and engraved by John Syng Dorsey for his *Elements of Surgery*. It illustrates the case report included here. Physick's needle holder is also depicted.

seen related, in which the operation has been tried. The case I have now detailed is the seventh; and it has failed in only two of these. In every instance the limb has been supplied with blood, which does not uniformly happen after the operation for popliteal aneurism.

I wish, before closing this paper, to call the attention of those surgeons, who may have occasion to perform the operation, to the forceps, of which an engraving is annexed. This instrument was contrived several years ago by Dr. Physick for the purpose of passing a needle under the pudic artery, when wounded in lithotomy, and has since been used by him for securing bleeding arteries in deep narrow wounds. Mr.

Abernethy complains of "the great difficulty of turning a common needle in a deep narrow wound:" and Mr. Freer was unable to pass his aneurismal needle round the iliac artery, until he punctured the fascia surrounding it with his knife, which he confesses was the most "difficult and dangerous part of the operation." These dangers and difficulties are entirely obviated by means of the curved forceps; and I think the operation greatly simplified by the use of this contrivance.

Should this meet the eyes of Mr. Abernethy, I hope he will be gratified with the additional testimony of the importance of an operation for which the world is indebted to the intrepid efforts of true genius; and he will no doubt learn with pleasure, that one individual on this side of the Atlantic owes to it, his life.

To this account I have only to add that the operation has been since performed in Dublin and London with success; it certainly affords a strong proof of the courage derived from our increased knowledge of the resources of the animal oeconomy. The extent to which anastomosing vessels are capable of enlarging when a main artery is obliterated, is perhaps not yet fully developed. Mr. Astley Cooper[7] has made some experiments upon dogs, by which it appears that the aorta, both carotids, and the subclavian arteries may be tied without destroying the life of the animal.

Of Stone in the Bladder

Without entering into a history of the operation of lithotomy which would occupy a volume, I shall proceed to describe the manner of performing the operation which I consider most advantageous.[1]

The instruments necessary for performing the operation, are, strong garters or bands for securing the patients hands and feet,—a grooved staff or director, adapted to the urethra,—a scalpel,—a sharp-

---

7. Astley Cooper (1768–1841) ligated most of the major arteries including even the aorta in the abdomen (1817); his patient did not survive. See also fn. p. 52.

1. The operation of lithotomy plays such a prominent part in the history of surgery that this selection—one of the best available descriptions of the procedure—is included here. This operation as described by Dorsey is, in all essentials, identical to that described by William Cheselden (1688–1752) in 1727.

Lithotomy was one of the earliest of surgical operations and is mentioned in the Hippocratic Oath (c. 400 B.C.): "I will not cut persons laboring under stone, but will leave this to be done by men who are practitioners of this work."

pointed straight bistoury,[2]—a gorget or knife for dividing the neck of the bladder,—forceps of various sizes for seizing and extracting the stone,—scoops or levers of different degrees of curvature,—a sharp-pointed curved bistoury, for enlarging the wound in the bladder, if necessary,—strong forceps with a screw in the handle to break the stone if it be too large for extraction,—a glystering syringe and pipe, together with warm barley water, to wash out any fragments of stone,—sponges, warm water, needles, ligatures, tenaculum,—a needle and curved forceps, for tying the pudic artery if it be cut, and warm olive oil for the purpose of lubricating the instruments.

All the instruments which the surgeon can possibly need should be at hand, and carefully put in order before the operation. The beak of the gorget should be adapted to the groove of the staff, and should move readily in it. The gorget should have a perfectly keen edge, especially at that part which commences the incision, which is the part immediately connected with the beak of the instrument. There is no method of having this part of the gorget perfectly keen, but by having the beak and blade separable, and Dr. Physick has accordingly for many years had his gorgets constructed in this manner.

The patient about to submit to lithotomy should if practicable choose the spring or autumn in preference to the cold or hot months. The operation should never be performed during a paroxysm of stone. A temperate diet should be directed for some time previously, and if plethoric the patient should be bled. It is well to administer, on the day preceding the operation, a dose of castor oil, and to empty the rectum two hours before the appointed time by an injection. The perineum should be shaved, after which an enoema of laudanum and water may be administered, an hour or more before the operation, and the patient

---

The earliest and simplest method of performing lithotomy was "cutting on the gripe." This consisted of holding the stone forcibly on the perineum by two fingers in the rectum ("gripe" is an obsolete word meaning to seize and hold) and then cutting on the perineal bulge. This procedure was far simpler to perform in children than in adults. The grooved staff was introduced about the year 1500 and the "high [suprapubic] operation" was first performed around the same time. Cheselden and several others used the high operation during the first part of the eighteenth century. Cheselden soon gave this up in favor of the lateral (perineal) operation, which he perfected. See also the introduction to *Joseph Baker's Bladder Stone*, p.8.

Bladder stone was a relatively common affliction up to the present century. It undoubtedly was related to poor diet and associated vitamin deficiency.

2. A bistoury is a long slender scalpel, curved or straight, sharp—or blunt—pointed. It was often made as a pocket instrument in the form of a penknife.

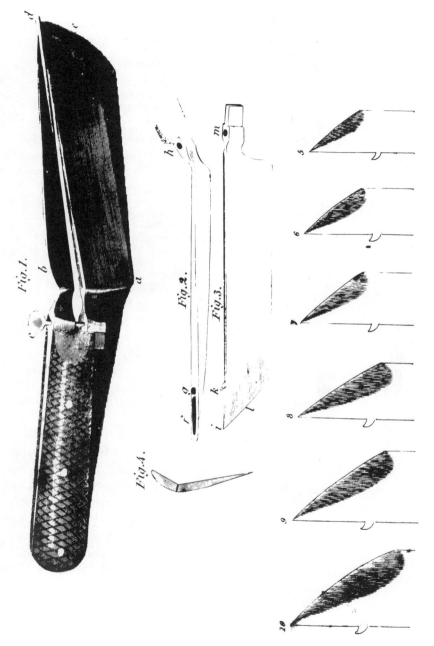

Figure 14. Physick's gorget. This instrument was forced along the grooved staff (sound) in the urethra during lithotomy. In so doing, the prostatic urethra, the prostate gland, and the bladder neck were divided, affording rapid entry into the bladder for extraction of stones.

should void no urine for several hours before the time affixed for operating.

OPERATION

The patient is to be placed on the end of a common dining table, with the leaves down, covered with blankets. The staff is to be well oiled and introduced; the different surgeons present take hold of it and satisfy themselves that they feel the stone. A strong fillet or garter is fastened by means of a noose, round each wrist, the patient is directed to grasp his feet with his hands, and by means of the fillets they are securely bound together.

The patient is now placed close upon the edge of the table, his head and back being supported by pillows in such a manner as to present the perineum in a convenient manner to the operator. In this posture he is to be held by two assistants who stand along side of the table (which of course should be narrow) and place the knees of the patient in their armpits, separating his limbs and firmly holding his feet.

Another assistant takes hold of the staff with one hand and with the other raises the scrotum so as to expose the perineum. He is to hold the staff in such a manner that it may project a little towards the left side of the perineum. The usual attempts to make its convexity very prominent, are however, attended with risk of forcing the staff out of the bladder, and there is no advantage in it, because the first incision should be made without any reference to the staff.

The surgeon being seated conveniently, commences the first incision with a scalpel, the point of which he inserts through the skin, at that part of the perineum which is immediately opposite the lower end of the arch of the pubis, of course the incision begins at the raphe of the perineum just behind the scrotum; the knife is to be carried steadily in a right line terminating midway between the lower margin of the anus and the tuberosity of the ischium of the left side. The first incision should be deeper than it is commonly made, as there is no danger to be dreaded at this stage of the operation, except a wound of the rectum which is easily avoided. This incision in an adult should be between three and four inches in length. By two or three successive strokes of the knife the incision is to be deepened, and the transversales perinei muscles completely divided—when this is done the groove of the staff is readily felt, and the prostate gland at the bottom of the wound. The surgeon now exchanges his scalpel for a sharp straight bistoury the point of which he inserts with the back towards the rectum into the membranous part of the urethra; with this instrument he slits up the membranous part of the urethra by cutting in the groove of the staff from the prostate gland to the bulb and effects in this manner by one stroke of the knife what I have known [to take] surgeons half an hour in accomplishing by repeated attempts to dissect down to the staff with a scalpel. It is of no consequence whether the bulb be cut or not by this incision, it is unnecessary to do it, unless the surgeon should have difficulty in seeing or feeling the groove of the staff, and in that case, no danger attends his slitting the urethra freely forwards, always, however, cutting from the staff, the point of the bistoury being in its groove. The division of the urethra is greatly facilitated by the use of the bistoury, and one simple incision is made instead of twenty. The staff is now laid bare to a considerable extent, and is generally visible, but is always readily felt by the surgeon's finger; it only remains now to divide the prostate gland and neck of the bladder, which may be readily effected by a bistoury, scalpel, or gorget, but far most conveniently by the last named instrument. The surgeon therefore after laying bare the staff places the nail of the left index finger in the groove of the staff and introduces the beak of his gorget previously dipped in warm oil, into the situation where his nail had been, and now rising from his chair, he takes the handle of the staff in his left hand and moves the beak in its groove, ascertaining that no membrane or other substance intervenes between the staff and beak of the gorget. He should be certain also at this moment that the staff has not slipped out of the bladder. With a gentle steady motion he passes the gorget along the groove of the staff into the bladder, depressing the handle of the gorget in such a manner that the beak may move along the convex part of the staff nearly at a right angle, and the beak of the gorget will consequently take a direction nearly in a line from the anus to the umbilicus. In introducing the gorget Dr. Physick recommends to push the staff and gorget as far towards the right side of the perineum as possible, in order to avoid wounding the pudic artery. The urine gushing from the bladder and flowing along the gorget announces the division of the neck of the bladder. The gorget is instantly removed (and there is no risk of making a wound in withdrawing it unless by great carelessness) and the forefinger of the left hand introduced and brought in contact with the stone. The staff may now be taken out, and the forceps introduced, or if the surgeon have any fears from the smallness of his opening into the bladder, that he will not readily find the passage, he may leave the staff in as a guide for the forceps, but this *ought never to be necessary*. When the forceps dipped in warm oil are introduced, the surgeon should touch the stone before he opens them, and then with one handle in each hand he separates the blades and grasps the stone. It is best to use small forceps at first as they enter more easily, and in general, answer as well as the large ones.

This part of the operation is sometimes very embarrassing.[3] Surgeons have been baffled in their attempts to find a stone with the forceps which with the staff they could readily touch, and sometimes an hour has been consumed in fruitless searches for the calculus. In general the most depending part of the bladder contains the stone, and this is commonly immediately on the rectum, or a little to one or the other side of it, the elevation of the handles of the forceps, therefore commonly brings them in contact with the stone. The introduction of a finger into the rectum frequently facilitates very much this part of the operation. In some cases the stone is situated near the fundus of the bladder; in these cases a scoop may be used to draw it towards the wound in the bladder. In all cases of difficulty in finding the stone, it is better to search with a finger or a female catheter, than with the forceps. The bladder is often filled with clotted blood, this should be rinsed out with warm barley water if it prevent the extraction of the stone.

The surgeon having grasped the stone with his forceps, should be careful that he has taken hold of it in the shortest diameter so that it may occasion as little laceration as possible whilst it is extracted. The use of a simple lever which is contained in all lithotomy cases, assists greatly in placing the stone in a position convenient for extraction. When this is done a regular but forcible effort is to be made and the stone extracted. The extraction may often be facilitated greatly by moving the forceps from side to side, using in this maner each blade as a lever. It sometimes breaks in the grasp of the forceps, and then the larger fragments are to be successively taken out by the forceps, the smaller ones by means of a scoop, and the detached sandy matter is to be washed out by injecting forcibly a stream of warm barley water into the bladder, which will be evacuated through the wound, pleno rivo, and with it all the smaller particles of calculus.

Sometimes the stone is too large to be extracted, and then it is to be broken, by means of a strong pair of forceps with a screw in the

---

3. Embarrassment might have been difficult for the surgeon but was, of course, excruciating for the patient. The severity of the pain experienced by a patient undergoing lithotomy without anesthesia can hardly be imagined. Speed was merciful: the faster the operator, the less the agony. A skillful lithotomist could often complete the operation in three minutes or less, and sometimes in under a minute. Skill and speed were of such importance that relatively few surgeons performed this operation during the pre-anesthetic era, and their successes (or failures) did much to influence their reputation.

handles, and the pieces extracted as we have just directed, but if a small enlargement of the wound in the neck of the bladder will enable the surgeon to effect the extraction without recourse to this expedient, it will be better to introduce the index finger of the left hand into the bladder, and then a curved bistoury with a sharp point may be used in such a manner as to enlarge the wound, the surgeon cutting down upon his finger, runs no risk of wounding any important part, the prostate gland may be thus divided with great facility to any necessary extent, and the extraction of a very large stone may in this manner, in general, be conveniently effected. The surgeon should always remember, that it is better to *cut* than to *tear*, and the maxim of Celsus should never be forgotten "plaga, paulo major quam calculus sit."[4]

The surgeon should next examine if any other stone remains. If the stone have a rough surface it is generally considered a proof that no other remains, the finger however or a female catheter should be introduced for the purpose of ascertaining this fact.

One of the chief subjects now demanding attention is the hemorrhage. It always happens that some considerable blood vessels are divided and bleed freely in this operation. The arteria transversalis perinei is always cut, as it runs directly across the perineum in the course of the incision. This artery is easily secured with a ligature if it bleed freely, but commonly it stops after the operation is completed.

The artery of the bulb of the urethra is occasionally divided, and sometimes it is necessary to tie it up, but the chief danger arises from the pudica interna, a very large artery running along the ramus of the ischium which is sometimes wounded by the edge of the gorget. When this happens the hemorrhage is profuse, and in many cases has proved fatal. I am happy in being able to describe a method of securing this vessel which obviates in great measure this danger from lithotomy.

In the year 1794 I assisted Dr. Physick in his first operation for stone, and it happened that in passing the gorget he divided the pudic artery. He immediately placed a finger upon the spot, the bleeding ceased, and he felt distinctly the trunk of the vessel pulsating between his finger and the ramus of the ischium. It was evident that if the flesh between his finger and the bone could be compressed, the hemorrhage

---

4. "Plaga paulo major quam calculus sit"—"the wound should be a little larger than the stone."

Although lithotomy was mentioned early in antiquity, it was first described in detail by Celsus (A.D. 30). His works, written during the reign of Tiberius, were lost for 14 centuries. They were then rediscovered and published under the auspices of Pope Nicholas V in 1478.

would be commanded. He accordingly passed a tenaculum under the trunk of the artery, the point of which came out near the bottom of the wound. A strong ligature was then passed under the projecting point and handle of the tenaculum, and was firmly tied, it included consequently a portion of flesh, in which the wounded artery was contained, and effectually stopped the bleeding. This measure, which was contrived and executed in as short a time as I have consumed in describing it, can no doubt be applied in similar cases with equal advantage: the plate [Fig. 15] conveys an idea of the manner in which this was effected. Another mode however which promises to be more easily executed, consists in passing an armed needle contained in curved forceps under the artery, bringing it out near the bottom of the wound and then tying the ligature. This operation I have never seen performed, but have no doubt that it could easily be done.

After the operation is completed, the patient is to be placed on his side in bed, without any dressing to the wound, a folded sheet being laid under him in such a manner, that as fast as it becomes wet by the urine, a dry part may be substituted. A low diet and rest are the only remedies necessary.

In some cases the patient has no unpleasant symptom in consequence of the operation, and in other instances death results without any evident cause. Mr. Charles Bell[5] says he has known "the violence of the operation, without hemorrhagy or inflammation, to kill the patient in about ten hours." I have seen patients die in three or four days without inflammation. Sometimes gangrene results from the escape of urine into the surrounding cellular texture, and sometimes the bladder inflames violently and death results from this cause. Peritoneal inflammation in some instances comes on, terminating very speedily in death. In cases where inflammation runs high, bleeding, and evacuating remedies are to be used and large blisters are to be applied over the abdomen.

In general the urine flows for the first few days after the operation through the wound, but in two instances in which I performed lithotomy it was my good fortune to witness the healing of the neck of the bladder by the first intention. In the first case (which occurred in private practice) not one drop of urine ever flowed through the wound after the operation was completed, a circumstance which I ascribed to

---

5. Charles Bell (1774–1842), surgeon and anatomist of Edinburgh and London. His *System of Operative Surgery* had been published in this country in 1812 and Dorsey quotes here from this text. See also fn. page 69.

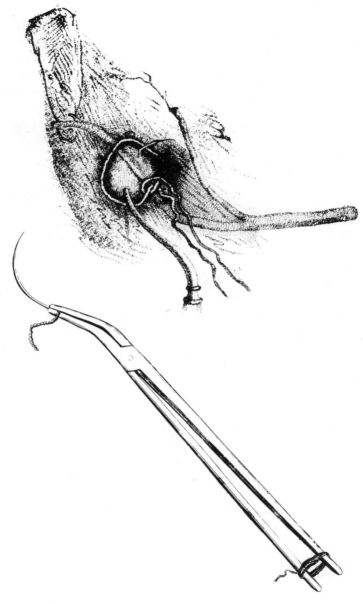

Figure 15. Methods of hemostasis: tenaculum and Physick's needle holder. The upper figure depicts the method used for seizing and tying vessels during any major procedure—in this case the vessel is the internal pudendal during lithotomy. The vessel was seized and elevated by the tenaculum and a ligature then was passed around it and tied. The lower figure illustrates Physick's needle holder. The instrument is similar in principle to that used today. Physick's method of securing vessels gradually supplanted the tenaculum.

smallness of the stone, and the consequent absence of contusion. This patient walked about in two weeks, and his wound was healed before three weeks had elapsed. The other case occurred in the Pennsylvania hospital, the stone was much larger, and it required great force to extract it. The urine in the patient flowed during the afternoon and evening of the day on which I operated, through the wound, but never again, and the wound healed as if in one of the limbs. I have no hesitation in ascribing the successful termination of these cases to the use of a gorget which is so perfectly keen, as to pass without any resistance through the prostate gland and neck of the bladder.

I have purposely avoided noticing the various modes of operating, now in use in Europe. The knife has many advocates, and the lithotome cache[6] some. I have seen a very celebrated surgeon in Paris, cut off an arm; cut out an eye, and perform lithotomy with the same bistoury, but I confess this simplification of apparatus is carried farther than I approve, and since I am persuaded that most of the objections to the gorget have originated from the use of bad gorgets, I have no hesitation in recommending a sharp gorget as the most convenient knife with which the bladder can be opened in lithotomy.

6. The lithotome cache was a long guard containing a thin blade, which could be made to spring open. It was used for dividing the prostate and bladder neck.

Extirpation of Diseased Ovaria

and

Observations on Diseased Ovaria

EPHRAIM McDOWELL (1771-1830)

The following two articles by Ephraim McDowell of Danville, Kentucky, record the birth of abdominal surgery. True, the peritoneal cavity had been successfully entered on a number of isolated occasions by various operators during the history of surgery; but McDowell's contribution was exceptional for two reasons. First, he presented a series of cases associated with a respectable success rate (only one death among his first five operations); and second, his reports encouraged other surgeons to follow his example. Ovariotomy became an established procedure even before the arrival of aseptic surgery in the latter part of the nineteenth century.

Ephraim McDowell was born in Rockbridge County, Virginia, on November 11, 1771, and then traveled to Kentucky with his family while he was still a youngster. Later he returned to Virginia to learn medicine as an apprentice under Dr. Alexander Humphreys of Staunton, a graduate of Edinburgh. McDowell went abroad in 1793 to study at Edinburgh, where he remained for two years, although he did not take his degree—probably because of insufficient funds. He returned to Danville, Kentucky, where he remained for the rest of his life, practicing both medicine and surgery. He died there on June 20, 1830.

The following two papers on ovariotomy were McDowell's only significant contributions to medical literature. Both are included here in their entirety. The first appeared in the Eclectic Repertory *(7:242) in 1817. The second was published in the same journal in 1819 (9:546).*

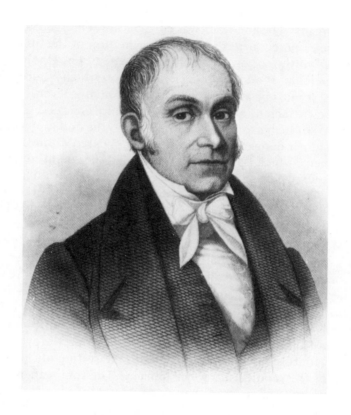

Figure 16. Ephraim McDowell (1771–1830). (Courtesy New York Academy of Medicine.)

Three Cases of Extirpation of Diseased Ovaria

In December 1809, I was called to see a Mrs. Crawford,[1] who had for several months thought herself pregnant. She was affected with pains similar to labour pains, from which she could find no relief. So strong was the presumption of her being in the last stage of pregnancy, that two physicians, who were consulted on her case, requested my aid in delivering her. The abdomen was considerably enlarged, and had the appearance of pregnancy, though the inclination of the tumor was to one side, admitting of an easy removal to the other. Upon examination, per vaginam, I found nothing in the uterus; which induced the conclusion that it must be an enlarged ovarium. Having never seen so large a substance extracted, nor heard of an attempt, or success attending any operation, such as this required, I gave to the unhappy woman information of her dangerous situation. She appeared willing to undergo an experiment, which I promised to perform if she would come to Danville (the town where I live), a distance of sixty miles from her place of residence. This appeared almost impracticable by any, even the most favourable conveyance, though she performed the journey in a few days on horseback. With the assistance of my nephew and colleague, James McDowell, M.D.,[2] I commenced the operation, which was concluded as follows: Having placed her on a table of the ordinary height, on her back, and removed all her dressing which might in any way impede the operation, I made an incision about three inches from the musculus rectus abdominis, on the left side, continuing the same nine inches in length, parallel with the fibres of the above named muscle, extending into the cavity of the abdomen, the parietes of which were a good deal contused, which we ascribed to the resting of the tumor on the horn of the saddle during her journey. The tumor then appeared full in view, but was so large that we could not take it away entire. We put a strong ligature around the fallopian tube near to the uterus; we then cut open the tumor, which was the ovarium and fimbrious part of the fallopian tube very much enlarged. We took out fifteen pounds of a dirty, gelatinous looking substance. After which we cut through the

---

1. Mrs. Jane Todd Crawford was seen by McDowell at her home near Greensburg, Kentucky. At that time she was about 46 years old and the mother of five children. She lived to be 79 and apparently remained in good health until her death in 1842. She outlived her surgeon by 12 years.

2. Very little information is available concerning most of the doctors (including this nephew) mentioned by McDowell in his two papers. Whenever possible, further identification is included in the footnotes.

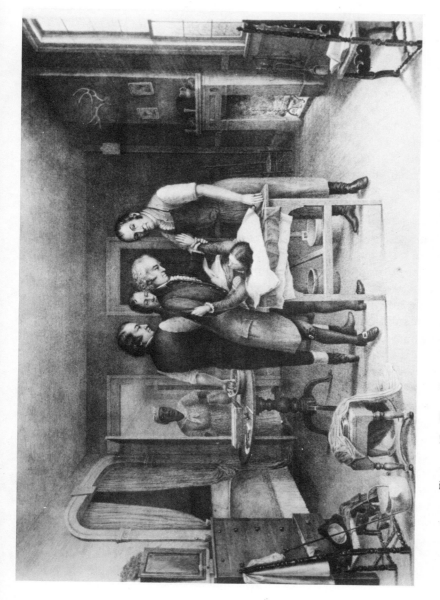

Figure 17. The first ovariotomy. (Courtesy National Library of Medicine.)

fallopian tube, and extracted the sack, which weighed seven pounds and one half. As soon as the external opening was made, the intestines rushed out upon the table; and so completely was the abdomen filled by the tumor, that they could not be replaced during the operation which was terminated in about twenty-five minutes. We then turned her upon her left side, so as to permit the blood to escape; after which, we closed the external opening with the interrupted suture, leaving out, at the lower end of the incision, the ligature which surrounded the fallopian tube. Between every two stitches we put a strip of adhesive plaster, which, by keeping the parts in contact, hastened the healing of the incision. We then applied the usual dressings, put her to bed, and prescribed a strict observance of the antiphlogistic regimen. In five days I visited her, and much to my astonishment found her engaged in making up her bed. I gave her particular caution for the future; and in twenty-five days, she returned home as she came, in good health, which she continues to enjoy.

Since the above case, I was called to a Negro woman,[3] who had a hard and very painful tumor in the abdomen. I gave her mercury for three or four months with some abatement of pain; but she was still unable to perform her usual duties. As the tumor was fixed and immovable, I did not advise an operation; though from the earnest solicitation of her master, and her own distressful condition, I agreed to the experiment. I had her placed upon a table, laid her side open as in the above case; put my hand in, found the ovarium very much enlarged, painful to the touch, and firmly adhering to the vesica urinaria and fundus uteri. To extract I thought would be instantly fatal; but by way of experiment I plunged my scalpel into the diseased part. Such gelatinous substance as in the above case, with a profusion of blood, rushed to the external opening, and I conveyed it off by placing my hand under the tumor, and suffering the discharge to take place over it. Notwithstanding my great care, a quart or more of blood escaped into the abdomen. After the hemorrhage ceased, I took out as nearly as possible the blood, in which the bowels were completely enveloped. Though I considered the case as nearly hopeless, I advised the same dressings, and the same regimen as in the above case. She has entirely recovered from all pain, and pursues her ordinary occupations.

---

3. S. D. Gross, one of McDowell's biographers, was able to document eight certain cases of ovariotomy performed by McDowell, although there may have been as many as five more. Of the eight, four operations were performed on Negroes.

In May 1816, a Negro woman was brought to me from a distance. I found the ovarium much enlarged, and as it could be easily moved from side to side, I advised the extraction of it. As it adhered to the left side, I changed my place of opening to the linea alba. I began the incision, in company with my partner and colleague Dr. William Coffer, an inch below the umbilicus, and extended it to within an inch of the os pubis. I then put a ligature around the fallopian tube and endeavored to turn out the tumor, but could not. I then cut to the right of the umbilicus, and above it two inches, turned out a scirrhous ovarium (weighing six pounds), and cut it off close to the ligature, put round the fallopian tube. I then closed the external opening, as in the former cases; and she complaining of cold and chilliness, I put her to bed prior to dressing her—then gave her a wine glass full of cherry bounce,[4] and thirty drops of laudanum, which soon restoring her warmth, she was dressed as usual. She was well in two weeks, though the ligature could not be released for five weeks; at the end of which time the cord was taken away; and she now, without complaint, officiates in the laborious occupation of cook to a large family.

Observations on Diseased Ovaria

Sept. 1819

DEAR SIR, I am induced to make this statement, principally, in consequence of the observations of Dr. Henderson,[1] which appeared in a number of the Repertory, published twelve or fifteen months since; on ovarian disease, and abdominal steatoma.

Since my former communication, I have twice performed the operation of excision; which cases are subjoined.

I shall in the first place take some notice of the remarks of Dr. Michener,[2] which Dr. Henderson in his dissertation has thought

---

4. Cherry bounce, a favorite drink of McDowell's, was made by steeping crushed cherries in whiskey and then adding sugar and spices.

1. Dr. Thomas Henderson of Georgetown, D.C. (1789–1854), wrote a paper describing a case of abdominal steatoma (vol. 8 of the *Eclectic Repertory*, 1818). He supported McDowell and wrote that the Kentucky surgeon's cases proved ". . . that an operation may be successful in cases which have, I fear, too frequently been allowed to proceed undisturbed to a fatal termination. . . ."

2. Ezra Michener (1794–1887) graduated from the medical school of the University of Pennsylvania in 1817, the year that McDowell's first paper was published. Michener, rather brashly, wrote in the *Eclectic Repertory* (1818) to

worthy of notice. The number of the Repertory, containing the above mentioned remarks, I have unfortunately lost; but believe that I remember most of his principal strictures. In the first case related by me, in Vol. VII. the Doctor appears to take exception to the length of the incision, by pointing out the sentence which stands thus; "I made an incision about three inches from the musculus rectus abdominis on the left side, continuing the same about nine inches in length." As I did not actually measure the incision, it would, perhaps, have been better to have said, an incision was made, about three inches to the left of the musculus rectus, extending from the margin of the ribs to the os pubis, on a woman whose abdomen was distended by a tumour, to an enormous size. He likewise objects to the parieties of the abdomen being contused, in consequence of the tumour resting on the horn of the saddle, during the patient's journey to Danville. Observing that the "horn of the saddle is on the right side, and the tumour was on the left." Now, with all due deference to the Doctor's knowledge in surgery, and the structure of *side saddles,* I think it would not be difficult to conceive, that a tumour weighing upwards of twenty pounds, would fill the whole abdomen, and although attached to the left ovarium, the weight and bulk must have been almost, if not quite as great, on the right side as on the left. I would observe, that my patient was a woman of small stature; her abdomen had become so pendulous, as to reach almost to her knees; the size of the tumor was ascertained from actual weight. Had the left side of the abdomen been contused, I would either have delayed the operation until the contusion was removed, or operated on some other part. I never have been of opinion, that bruised flesh would heal so readily as sound; which matter I esteem of essential importance to success in this operation. The Doctor also objects to another assertion in this case, viz: "When I visited her on the fifth day, I found her engaged in making up her bed." The Doctor's scepticism, alone, appears to have carried him through the statement, and I am surprised that he will even admit the fact of her returning home, in five and twenty days after the operation, on horseback; a distance of seventy miles, and in the depth of winter.

---

criticize McDowell for not presenting his cases in more detail. He doubted the possibility of making accurate enough diagnoses in abdominal disease to warrant surgical interference and stated that this alone would "prove an insurmountable barrier to the use of the knife." Michener went on to predict that "few persons will be likely to venture their reputation on such uncertain data."

Dr. Michener became a practitioner in Chester, Pennsylvania. He was better known as a botanist than as a physician.

Dr. Henderson thinks I was entirely too inconsiderate in my detail of the cases of diseased ovaria; I thought my statement sufficiently explicit to warrant any surgeon's performing the operation when necessary, without hazarding the odium of making an experiment; and I think my description of the mode of operating, and of the anatomy of the parts concerned, clear enough, to enable any good anatomist, possessing the judgment requisite for a surgeon, to operate with safety. I hope no operator, of any other description, may ever attempt it. It is my most ardent wish, that this operation may remain, to the mechanical surgeon, for ever incomprehensible. Such have been the *bane* of the science; intruding themselves into the ranks of the profession, with no other qualification but boldness in undertaking, ignorance of their responsibility, and indifference to the lives of their patients; proceeding according to the special dictates of some author, as mechanical as themselves, they cut and tear with fearless indifference, utterly incapable of exercising any judgment of their own cases of emergency; and sometimes, without possessing even the slightest knowledge of the anatomy of the parts concerned.

The preposterous and impious attempts of such pretenders, can seldom fail to prove destructive to the patient, and disgraceful to the science. It is by such this noble science has been degraded in the minds of many, to the rank of an art.

No case of diseased ovaria has come under my observation, similar to the one described by Dr. Henderson. The tumours extracted by myself, I have kept by me, in a state of preservation; they have been submitted to the inspection of most, if not all the physicians who have visited me. Their opinions, as to the nature of the disease, have all accorded with my own. In our most scrupulous examinations, we were never able to discover any portion of the tumours to be of a natural or healthy structure; the whole exhibition was that of a morbid undistinguishable mass, which myself and others of the faculty, who were present at the operations, were of opinion, had once been the natural ovaria; in as much as no ovarium remained on the side from whence the tumour was extracted. This was as clearly evident as it could have been on dissection after death; my incisions were made so free and extensive, that I have always performed every part of this operation by sight.

Such ovaria as I have described as dropsical, contained a gelatinous fluid in a sac about half an inch in thickness, and of a spongy texture; such as I have denominated scirrhus, were of a spongy texture throughout, and some what elastic. Those affected with scirrhus, complained of lancinating pains in the parts affected; which, from their description, were similar to the pains in other scirrhous glands. The drop-

sical ovaria, are attended with a dull pain, and produce a most oppres-
ive sense of weight in the abdomen. By these symptoms, and by a nice
sense of touch, the species may generally be distinguished from one
another. How to distinguish them from steatoma and other affections
which those organs are liable to. I shall not pretend to define, nor, in
the present state of knowledge, do I think it at all necessary; nor even
the distinction from one another.

Excision I esteem less perilous than any other mode of treatment;
and the only certain cure for either of them. For scirrhus and steatoma,
no other relief, within our knowledge, is practicable.

The dropsical ovaria may be relieved by tapping with a large trocar. But the relief is only temporary, and would be attended with no inconsiderable danger. Some further reasons for my aversion to the trocar, I will relate hereafter.

The second case in which I operated for diseased ovaria, was the
case of a Negro woman in this neighborhood. On exposing the tumour
(as related in the Repertory, Vol. VII.) it adhered so firmly to the neighboring parts, that I did not attempt its extraction, but made a free incision into it with the scalpel, and discharged its contents; she recovered
of the operation, and I thought her well of the disease; but, she informed me some short time since, that it had been growing for the last
twelve or eighteen months, and says it is now, about the size it was
when I opened her six years ago.

None of my patients have been able to give me any satisfactory account as to the origin of the disease; with some it commenced some
months afer delivery. The first supposed herself pregnant, and went on
to make the necessary preparation for her lying-in; the time for her delivery being protracted to a great length, and her anxiety and doubts increasing, I was called in, and immediately, on examination, per vaginam, found she was not with child.

CASE I

In April, 1817, I operated on a Negro woman from Garard county;
extracting a scirrhous ovarium, weighing five pounds. The incision was
made near the linea alba; as in cases formerly related, I tied a cord firmly round the ligament attaching it to the uterus, and cut away the ovarium; but owing to the shortness and sponginess of the part, the cord
slipped off, before I laid the ovarium out of my hands, and a profuse
discharge of blood took place, I immediately drew the uterus to the external incision, and commenced tying up the bleeding mouths separately. This also, in consequence of the diseased state of the parts,

proved only of partial efficacy, as several of the ligatures cut through, on tying them. I now thought it all over with my poor patient, but arming a needle with a strong ligature, I passed it round the ligaments; securing it in its place by taking several stitches over its surface as I passed it round, and firmly tied it. By turning her nearly on her stomach, I was able to get most of the blood out of the abdomen, using my hand to extract the coagulated portion. The incision was then closed by the interrupted suture, and strips of adhesive plaster. She recovered happily; but, I am told her health is not good; the account I had of her was awkwardly given; from what I could learn, her complaint is hysterical. This, though the smallest ovarium I have ever extracted, was much more troublesome to the patient than in any previous case. Besides experiencing severe lancinating pains in the parts, she was seldom able to discharge her urine, without getting almost on her head, in consequence of the tumour falling down into the pelvis, and compressing the urethra.

CASE II

A Negro woman from Lincoln county, was brought to me in April, 1818, supposed, by the different physicians who had attended her, to be affected with ascites; she had been under their care about eighteen months. On examining her, I could very plainly discover the fluctuation of fluid in the abdomen, and for some months administered medicines for ascites, without effect; despairing of the power of medicines, I at length tapped her, and discharged thirteen quarts of gelatinous fluid, such as I had before met with in dropsical ovaria, of so thick a consistence, that I found it extremely difficult and tedious to discharge it. In two months after, I found it necessary to tap again; during the process of discharging it a second time, the opening was frequently stopped by viscid portions of the jelly, which were broken by introducing a probe; when the abdomen was pretty well evacuated, I discovered, with the probe, a firm substance, which, on minute examination, I found to be of considerable size. I at once supposed the existence of a dropsical ovarium, in which I was confirmed, on finding the uterus empty by examination per vaginam. Some months after she was again tapped; at which time, I made the opening large enough to admit my finger; by which means, I was able to ascertain the nature of the disease beyond a doubt. I informed her master what was certainly her situation, and that nothing but excision could affect a cure. My advice was not immediately followed, nor until after she was tapped a fourth time; a week or two after which, she was brought to Danville, to undergo the operation, which was performed May 11, 1819. The diseased ovarium being on the left side, and evidently dropsical; the incision was of course made on the left side. On exposing the tumour, it was found to adhere to the parietes of the abdomen; and to the intestines, by slender cords which were easily separated with the hand, and which caused a slight effusion of blood. To the uterus, two strong ligaments adhered; one, the natural ligament, attaching the ovarium to the uterus, the other, an artificial one, attached to the fundus uteri: which appeared to be composed of the above mentioned slender cords, compacted together. I then tied fine cords of silk firmly round each of these ligaments, discharged the contents of the tumour, and cut it away.

There was sixteen quarts of gelatinous fluid discharged from the tumour and abdomen. The dressings and precautions were the same as in other cases. The second day after the operations, she was affected with violent pain in the abdomen; together with an obstinate vomiting. She was blooded as copiously as her strength would allow, but without producing any abatement of the pain or vomiting. On the third day she died. On examination after death, the uterus, contrary to expectation, appeared natural and uninflamed, the right ovarium healthy, the silken cords were securely, and properly fixed, and not in a situation likely to injure the adjoing parts. Her death had proceeded from peritoneal inflammation. This membrane, throughout its whole extent, appeared greatly inflamed, and the intestines largely inflated.

I was assisted in this operation by my nephew, Dr. William A. McDowell. Doctors Weizegar, Tomlinson, and Horr were present.[3]

On examining the substances we had removed, the contents of the sac presented a variety; different portions of the fluid were of different colours: semitransparent, white, brown, and yellow. There was also contained in the sac, a considerable quantity of hair; which grew from the inner surface. Enveloped in the inner substances of the sac, we found a bone, resembling, very much, in shape, the front tooth of a cow.

From the circumstances of the hair and bone, one or two of the physicians present, were inclined to believe the disease originated from an extra uterine conception; and that all of the foetus had been absorbed, save the hair, and single bone, which was found. As for myself, I think it as reasonable to suppose, the hair and bone in this unnatural

---

3. The only one of this group who has been identified is McDowell's nephew, William Adair McDowell (1795–1853), who received his M.D. from the University of Pennsylvania in 1818. He practiced for a while with his uncle. In later life he became interested in tuberculosis and wrote several papers on this disease.

situation, was the result of a morbid action. She had been delivered of a child two years before the operation, her health during that time was never good, but she had no reason to believe herself pregnant; and if it were the case, I doubt whether a whole foetus could be so nearly absorbed in two years. There was likewise a round hole in the sac, which, from the levelled appearance of its edges, appeared of long standing; the hole was about the size of a musket ball. And there is no doubt, that the gelatinous fluid escaped through this aperture into the abdomen. This ovarium, when brought into view, was of a large size; which is the more remarkable, when we consider the enormous quantity of fluid which had been drawn off at different times, by the operation of paracentesis abdominis. During the evacuation, a bandage was kept bound tightly round the abdomen; and considerable pressure was made with the hands, in order to evacuate its whole contents. In an attempt to draw off the contents of such a tumour with the trocar, it would be impossible to perforate all the vesicles; and such only, as were pierced, would discharge their contents. While one portion of the vesicles of the ovaria would discharge themselves into the abdomen, another portion would remain diseased in the original way. Thus componding in the system, two of the most deplorable diseases to which it is liable.

EPHRAIM McDOWELL.

A New Instrument for the Extraction of Coins and Other Foreign Substances from the Oesophagus

and

A Case of Ovarian Dropsy Successfully Removed by Surgical Operation

NATHAN SMITH, M.D. (1762–1829)

Nathan Smith of New England was one of this country's great medical figures. He was not only an excellent physician, a popular teacher, a capable administrator, and the founder or cofounder of four medical schools, but he was also a fine and able surgeon whose contributions to surgery are often overlooked.

Nathan Smith was born in Rehoboth, Massachusetts, on September 30, 1762, and then moved with his family to Vermont while still a boy. He learned his medicine first as an apprentice under Dr. Josiah Goodhue (1759–1829) of Putney, Vermont, and then took his degree in medicine at Harvard in 1790. After practicing in New Hampshire for several years, Smith went to London for further training. The remainder of his life was spent as a teacher, and he founded or aided in the founding of medical schools at Dartmouth (1797), Yale (1812), Bowdoin (1821), and the University of Vermont (1821). In spite of his teaching duties, Nathan Smith actively practiced medicine and surgery until his death on January 26, 1829.

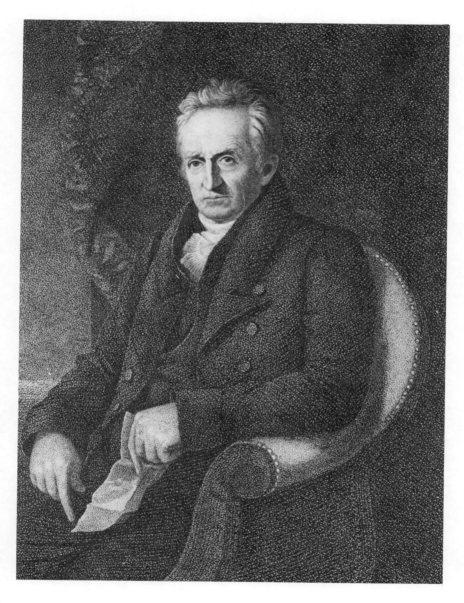

Figure 18. Nathan Smith (1762–1829). An engraving made from a portrait by Samuel F. B. Morse.

The two following selections were published in Nathan Smith's posthumous volume of Medical and Surgical Memoirs *(Baltimore: William A. Francis, 1831). The first briefly describes a device that he used to remove foreign bodies from the esophagus—an unusual and ingenious accomplishment in that era. The second report describes an ovariotomy that he performed in 1821. Smith's operation differed from McDowell's in that he used a buried "animal ligature" of leather to tie the ovarian pedicle. This case had previously been published in the* American Medical Recorder *(5:124, 1822).*

Description of a New Instrument for the Extraction of Coins & Other Foreign Substances from the Oesophagus

I have twice been called upon to remove coins from the throats of children. In both instances, they had descended to near the inferior extremity of the oesophagus; where the passage is a little narrowed, just before entering the stomach. Of course, they were entirely beyond the reach of forceps, or any instrument which might be employed to grasp and thus withdraw them.[1]

The instrument which the exigencies of the case suggested, and with which I succeeded, was unlike any thing which I have known to be employed for a similar purpose. A very few words, with the acompanying plate, will be sufficient to give an idea of it.

The shaft of the instrument is a rod of whalebone, twenty inches in length, and of the size of a small quill. Half an inch from one extremity there are attached, at acute angles, like the barbs of an arrow, two wings of silver, an inch and a quarter in length, a quarter of an inch wide, and so thin as to be very elastic and flexible. The extremity, which stands off from the instrument, is convoluted so as to render it blunt, and is a little curved inward toward the shaft of the instrument. The two wings are pinned to the shaft of the instrument, and may be continued over its extremity, which should terminate with a bead, or obtuse point.

From the position of the oesophagus between the trachea and

---

1. The usual methods used in Smith's day for removal of foreign bodies in the esophagus were (1) "fingers and forceps" for high obstructions; (2) relaxation of the spasm by swallowing tartar emetic (antimony and potassium tartrate); (3) a sponge tied to a string and swallowed to entangle the object; (4) a probang, whalebone, or bougie to force the foreign body into the stomach (J. S. Dorsey, *Elements of Surgery* [Philadelphia, 1813] 1:366).

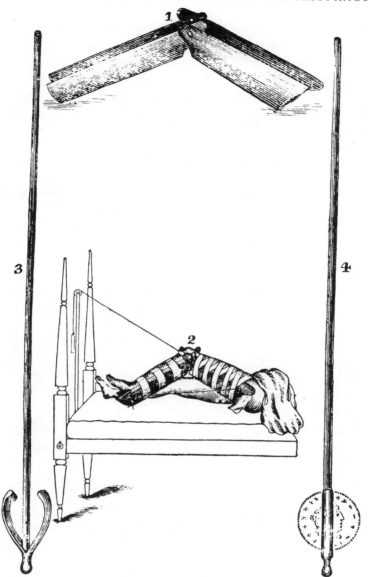

Figure 19. Nathan Smith's splint and his instrument for removal of foreign bodies from the esophagus. The apparatus for removing coins from the esophagus is illustrated on either side. This figure also depicts Smith's method of treating thigh fractures. The weighted traction device was far ahead of its day and is functionally quite similar to present-day methods.

spine, the faces of the coin present forward and back. When the instrument is thrust down the oesophagus, avoiding the glottis, as may be done without difficulty, and presenting the barbs one forward and the other back, it will pass either behind or before the coin, and the barb will spring beyond it, and catch it between itself and the shaft, when it may be very easily withdrawn. The manner in which the shaft is embraced by the esophagus above, prevents its slipping off laterally. In both the cases alluded to, I accomplished the extraction of the coin without any difficulty, and at the first trial. In the second case, after I had once raised the coin into the mouth, the child instantly swallowed it again, though I had almost seized it with my fingers. It returned to the same place, and I again withdrew it at the first trial.

The barbs are made so thin that should they catch in any of the follicles of the oesophagus, they would be everted sooner than rupture the membrane.

A Case of Ovarian Dropsy Successfully Removed by Surgical Operation

The subject of this operation was a Mrs. Strobridge, of Norwich, Vermont, aged 33 years.

The following account of the case, previous to the operation, was taken from the patient:—Seven years before, she had perceived a small tumour in her right side, situated in the right iliac region; when about the size of a goose's egg, she could move it with her hand to the opposite side of the linea alba, and to some distance above the umbilicus. The patient had borne five children, two previous and three subsequent to her discovering the tumour. The youngest child was 10 months old, and was nursed at the breast when she submitted to the operation. Soon after her first pregnancy, from the commencement of the tumour, and when, as she thinks, it was about four or five inches in diameter, it suddenly disappeared, probably burst into the abdomen. In four or five weeks it was as large as before. Before and after the bursting of the tumour she had turns of faintness, which lasted from two hours to half a day. During parturition of her second child, after the commencement of the tumour, it having acquired a considerable size, it burst again, and nothing was perceived of it till eight months had elapsed. In four days from its reappearance it was as large as it had ever been. It was again burst by fall; great soreness of the abdomen, and confinement of the patient for several weeks were the consequence. The tumour filled again in a fortnight and from this time continued to increase; it did not burst in the delivery of her last child, which was ten months previous to the operation. The patient's health was not much affected by the tumour. She was costive; and the size of the tumour incommoded her in the ordinary duties of her family, especially in stooping. On examination I found a large tumour in the right side of the abdomen; it was considerably moveable, and I could produce a distinct fluctuation through it.

Having decided on the operation, and determined the mode of operating, on the 5th of July, 1821, in the presence, and with the assistance of Doctors Lewis, Mussey, Dana, and Hatch,[1] I commenced the operation as follows:—

The patient being placed on a bed with her head and shoulders somewhat raised, an assistant rolled up the tumour to the middle of the abdomen, and held it there. I then commenced an incision about an inch below the umbilicus, directly in the linea alba, and extended it downwards three inches. I carried it down to the peritoneum, and then stopped till the blood ceased to flow, which it soon did. I then divided the peritoneum the whole extent of the external incision.—The tumour, now exposed to view, was punctured; a canula introduced, and seven pints of a dark coloured ropy fluid was discharged into a vessel. About one pint was spilt, so that the whole fluid was about eight pounds. Previous to tapping the tumour, by inserting my finger by the side of it, I ascertained that it adhered to some extent to the parietes of the abdomen, on the right side, between the spine of the ileum and false ribs. After evacuating the fluid I drew out the sack, which brought out with it, and adhering to it, a considerable portion of the omentum. This was separated from the sack with the knife; and two arteries which we feared might bleed, were tied with leather ligatures, and the omentum was returned. By continuing to pull out the sack, the ovarian ligament was brought out, this was cut off, two small arteries secured with leather ligatures,[2] and the ligament was then returned. I then endeavoured to separate the sack from its adhesions to the parietes of the abdomen, which occupied a space about two inches square; this was ef-

---

1. Reuben Dimond Mussey (1780–1866) was one of Smith's early pupils and had graduated from the Dartmouth Medical School in 1805. He had a distinguished surgical career, during which he performed a number of truly formidable operations (closure of a vesico-vaginal fistula, antedating Sims; bilateral carotid ligation for a vascular tumor of the scalp; a fore-quarter amputation, etc.). He held professorships in at least five medical schools. He was professor of surgery at Dartmouth at the time that he witnessed Smith's ovariotomy.

I am unable to identify Doctors Lewis, Dana, or Hatch with certainty. They may have been medical students at Dartmouth who had accompanied Dr. Mussey to watch the operation.

2. Cf. p. 66, "The Use of Animal Ligatures," by P. S. Physick.

fected by a slight stroke of the knife at the anterior part of the adhesion, and by use of the fingers. The sack then came out whole, excepting where the puncture was made, and I should think it might weigh between 2 and 4 ounces. The incision was then closed with adhesive plaster, and a bandage was applied over the abdomen. No unfavourable symptoms occurred after the operation; in three weeks the patient was able to sit up and walk, and has since perfectly recovered.

I was induced to undertake this operation from the following considerations:—The patient, though her health was not greatly impaired, was sensibly affected by the disease. She was quite certain that the increase of the tumour, in a given time, was augment'd; probably, at no very distant period, it would have destroyed her. I had, also, had an opportunity to dissect the body of a patient, who had died of ovarian dropsy, after being tapped seven times. In this case the sack was found to be in the right ovarium, which filled the whole abdomen; but it adhered to no part except the proper ligament, which was not larger than the finger of a man. I have seen two other ovarian sacks which were taken from patients after death. They had been tapped several times; the sacks were equally unattached, except to their own proper ligaments. Hence, I inferred, that in a case of ovarian dropsy, while the tumour remained movable, it might be removed with a prospect of success. The mode of operating, practised in the above case, is the same that I have described to my pupils in several of my last courses of lectures on surgery. The event has justified my previous opinions.[3]

---

3. It is universally stated that Smith was unaware of McDowell's ovariotomies at the time that this operation was performed. I find this most unlikely. The *Eclectic Repertory,* in which McDowell's reports were published, was not an obscure journal. McDowell's cases were well known and discussed, and many doctors had visited him to watch him operate or examine his specimens. Smith would have been well aware of progress made in a field in which he was vitally interested.

Excerpts from William Beaumont's Journal

WILLIAM BEAUMONT (1785–1853)

William Beaumont was an army surgeon and a pioneer physiologist who kept a detailed journal during much of his life. The first of the following selections was written while Beaumont served during the War of 1812 and describes vividly both the military action and the wartime surgery practiced during the landing at York (Toronto) on Lake Ontario in 1813. The second selection describes the famed gunshot wound of the young voyageur Alexis St. Martin. Beaumont's journal not only gives a good description of wound surgery as practiced in America in his day but also reveals him to be a capable surgeon who deserved the fame that came to him in later years as the result of his dedication to his patient.

Beaumont was born in Lebanon, Connecticut, on November 21, 1785, and migrated as a young man to Champlain, New York. He later studied medicine as a pupil of Dr. Benjamin Chandler (1772–1818) in St. Albans, Vermont. Beaumont joined the army during the War of 1812 and then, during peacetime, served in a succession of frontier posts. Although he is known primarily as a physiologist, Beaumont practiced medicine and surgery, both in the army and later in St. Louis, Missouri. after resigning from the service. He died on April 25, 1853, in St. Louis.

The following excerpts were taken from the Life and Letters of Dr.

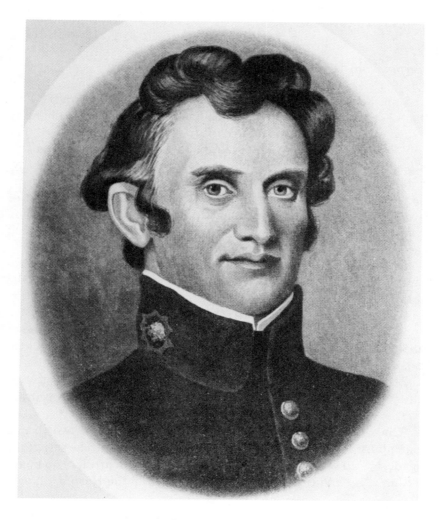

Figure 20. William Beaumont (1785–1853). From Myer's *Life and Letters of Dr. William Beaumont* (St. Louis: C.V. Mosby, 1912).

William Beaumont, *by Jesse E. Myer (St. Louis: C. V. Mosby, 1912). A shorter and more polished account of St. Martin's wound may be found in the introduction to the recently reprinted edition (New York: Dover, 1959) of Beaumont's* Experiments and Observations on the Gastric Juice and the Physiology of Digestion *(Plattsburgh: F. P. Allen, 1833).*

Excerpts from William Beaumont's Wartime Diary

Sept. 8th, 1812. Quit my Preceptor, Dr. Benjamin Chandler,[1] St. Albans, Vt., under whose friendly inspiration and instruction I happily pursued my medical studies for 2 years to my own satisfaction and that of my Preceptor. Came to Plattsburgh. Joined the Army as Surgeon's mate of the 6th Infty. on the 13th inst. Continued duty as such till Jany. 1st, 1813, at which period I suspended duty on account of the unfavorable prospects of the army at that time, and proposed to the people of Plattsburgh to commence private practice in that and the neighboring vicinities. Met with good encouragement during six weeks, in which time visited my respected friends at St. Albans.

On the fifteenth Feby. recommenced service in the 6th Infty. on account of the prospect there was then of an engagement with the Enemy. . . . .

Sacketts Harbor, 20th April, 1813. The first Brigade, with several detachments from other corps, in readiness and waiting in suspense to embark on board the navy for an expected attack on the enemy. Genl. Dearborn arrived in Town tonight.

21st. Weather rainy, wind southeast. Sick mending. Troops waiting for orders to embark. 11 o'clock, nothing remarkable has occurred today. Wind south, weather rainy.

22nd. Embarked with Capt. Humphreys, Capt. Walworth and Muhlenburg and Compy. on board the Schooner Julia. The rest of the Brigade, the 2d with Fourth rifle Regts. and the light artillery on board the Ship, Brig and other Schooners, remained in the Harbor till next morning.

23rd, 11 Ock. A. M. Weighed Anchor and put out under impression of going to Kingston. Got out 15 or 20 miles. Came on a storm. Wind ahead and the fleet returned in to harbor. No one permitted to go on shore.

---

1. Benjamin Chandler (1722–1818) of St. Albans, Vermont, was a practitioner "skilful in his medical practice and notably in surgery." Beaumont had been his pupil from 1810 to 1812.

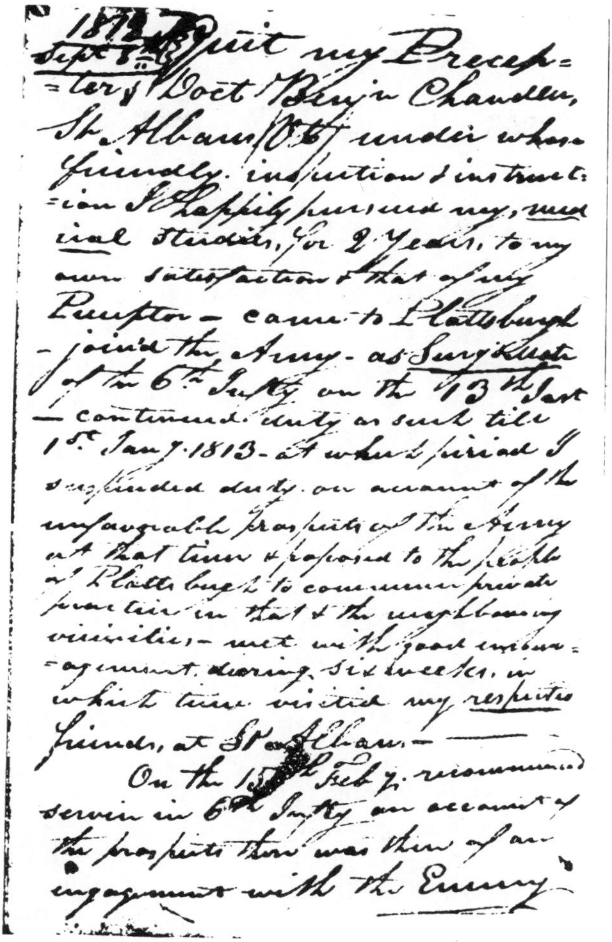

Figure 21. The first page of William Beaumont's wartime diary. From Myer's *Life and Letters of Dr. William Beaumont* (St. Louis: C. V. Mosby, 1912).

24th, 6 Ock. A.M. Put out of harbor with a fair wind, tho mild and pleasant, the fleet sailing in fine order, affording a very pleasant scene Thro the day.

25th, 6 Ock. A. M. Morning most delightful. Wind fresh and increasing, not fair, obliging us to beat. Getting along slowly.

27th. Wind pretty strong in the morning, increasing to a strong blow so that the swells run high, tossing our vessels smartly about. Everyone seasick—was myself. At half-past four o'clock passed by the mouth of Niagara River. This circumstance baffled our imagination where we were going. We were first impressed with the idea of Kingston then to Niagara, but now our destination must be Little York. At sunset came in view of York Town & the Fort, where we lay off all night within 3 or 4 leagues.

27th. Sailed into harbor and came to anchor a little below the British Garrison. We now filled the boats and affected a landing though not without some difficulty and the loss of some men. The British marched their troops from the Garrison down the hill to cut us off in landing, and then they had every advantage. They could not effect their plan. A hot engagement ensued, in which the enemy lost nearly a third of their men and were soon compelled to quit the field, leaving their dead and wounded strewed in every direction. We lost but very few in the engagement. The enemy returned into garrison, but from the loss sustained in the 1st engagement, the undaunted courage of our men, and the brisk firing from our fleet into the Garrison with 12 and 32-pounders, they were soon obliged to evacuate it and retreat with all possible speed. Driven to this alternative, they devised the inhuman project of blowing up their Magazine (containing 300 Bbls. powder), the explosion of which, shocking to mention, had almost totally destroyed our Army. Above 300 were wounded, and about 60 killed dead on the spot by stones of all dimensions falling like a shower of hail in the midst of our ranks. The enemy had about 20 killed and wounded by the explosion, tho the main body had retreated far out of the Garrison. After this sad disaster our Army marched into the Garrison, hawled down the British coat of arms (which they were too haughty to do), and raised the American Standard on its place. Our Army was about 1,500 strong—Theirs about the same. Encampt in Garrison this night, mounting a guard 500 strong to secure our safety through the night. A most distressing scene ensues in the Hospital—nothing but the Groans of the wounded and agonies of the Dying are to be heard. The Surgeons wading in blood, cutting off arms, legs, and trepanning heads to rescue their fellow creatures from untimely deaths. To hear the poor creatures crying, "Oh, Dear! Oh, Dear! Oh, Dear! Oh, my God, my God! Do, Doctor, Doctor! Do cut off my leg, my arm, my head, to relieve me from misery! I can't live, I can't live!" would have rent the heart of steel, and shocked the insensibility of the most hardened assassin and the cruelest savage. It awoke my liveliest sympathy, and I cut and slashed for 48 hours without food or sleep. My God! Who can think of the shocking scene when his fellow-creatures lie mashed and mangled in every part, with a leg, an arm, a head, or a body ground in pieces, without having his very heart pained with the acutest sensibility and his blood chill in his veins. Then, who can behold it without agonizing sympathy!

28th, 10 Ock. A. M. Just got time to suspend capital operation, whilst I can take a little refreshments to sustain life, for the first time since four o'clock yesterday. Return again to the bloody scene of distress, to continue dressing, Amputating, and Trepanning. Dressed rising of 50 patients, from simple contusions to the worst of compound fractures, more than half of the last description. Performed two cases of amputation and one of trepanning. 12 Ock. P. M., retired to rest my much fatigued body and mind.

29th. Dressed most of wounds over, Trepanned two. This day ordered to get the sick and wounded on board the fleet, to be transported to Sacketts Harbor. Sent them to the ships, and the most of them were sent back again, very much to the injury of the patients. One of those amputated yesterday does well; the other died in about 12 hours, the fracture being in the thigh and very much contused.

30th. Dressed the wounded, most of them doing well; the two cases of trepanning doing well. The Militia and people giving themselves up to be paroled, nearly 1,700 since the 27th.

May 1st. About my professional employment, dressing the wounded, the most of them doing well. Amputated an arm. On orders for getting all the sick and wounded on board prevents any more operations today. Several more will have to be performed. The wounded on board. All the troops ordered to embark. All on board at six o'clock. Brought off public property taken from his Majesty's stores, estimated to the amount of 2,000,000 and a half dollars. Burnt the ruins of the Government house, the Block-house, one or two public stores and an old sloop.

2nd. Wind unfavorable to sailing out—consequently we remain in the fleet where we were today. The sick and wounded lying distributed among the fleet. I can not note their several conditions—those on board this (The Julia) doing well.

Case History of Alexis St. Martin's Wound from William Beaumont's Journal

Alex Samata, St. Martin, San Maten,[1] a Canadian lad about 19 years old, hardy, robust and healthy, was accidentally shot by the unlucky discharge of a gun on the 6th of June, 1822. The whole charge, consisting of powder and duck shot, was received in the left side at not more than 2 or 3 feet distance from the muzzle of the piece, in a pos-

---

1. Alexis St. Martin became one of the most famous patients in the history of medicine. As is so often the case with famous patients, he outlived his

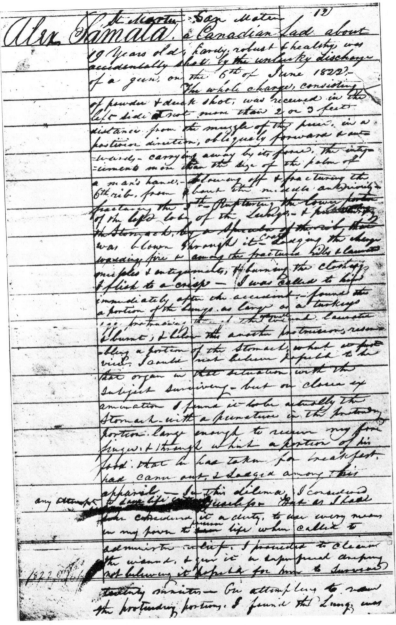

Figure 22. Beaumont's notebook describing St. Martin's wound. This is the first page of Beaumont's original case record on the wound of Alexis St. Martin. From Myer's *Life and Letters of Dr. William Beaumont* (St. Louis: C. V. Mosby, 1912).

terior direction, obliquely forward and outwards carrying away by its force the integuments more than the size of the palm of a man's hand; blowing off and fracturing the 6th rib from about the middle anteriorly, fracturing the 5th, Rupturing the lower portion of the left lobe of the Lungs, and lacerating the Stomach by a spicula of the rib that was blown through its coat, Lodging the charge, wadding, fire in among the fractured ribs and lacerated muscles and integuments, and burning the clothing and flesh to a crisp. I was called to him immediately after the accident. Found a portion of the Lungs as large as a turkey's egg protruding through the external wound, lacerated and burnt, and below this another protrusion resembling a portion of the Stomach, what at first view I could not believe possible to be that organ in that situation with the subject surviving, but on closer examination I found it to be actually the Stomach with a puncture in the protruding portion large enough to receive my forefinger, and through which a portion of his food that he had taken for breakfast had come out and lodged among his apparel. In this dilemma I considered any attempt to save his life entirely useless. But as I had ever considered it a duty to use every means in my power to preserve life when called to administer relief, I proceeded to cleanse the wound and give it a superficial dressing, not believing it possible for him to survive twenty minutes. On attempting to reduce the protruding portions, I found the Lung was prevented from returning by the sharp point of the fractured rib, over which its membrane had caught fast, but by raising up the Lung with the front of the forefinger of my left hand I clipped off with my penknife, in my right hand, the sharp point of the rib, which enabled me to return the Lung into the cavity of the Thorax, but could not retain it there on the least efforts of the patient to cough, which were frequent.

After giving the wound a superficial dressing, the patient was moved to a more convenient place, and in about an hour I attended to dressing the wound more thoroughly, nor supposing it probable for him to survive the operation of extracting the fractured spicula of bones and other extraneous substances, but to the utter astonishment of every one he bore it without a struggle or without sinking.

After taking away the fragments of the ribs, old flannel, wad and the principal charge of shot, all driven together under the skin and into the muscles, and replacing the lungs and stomach as much as practicable, I applied to the wound the carbonated fermenting poultice, com-

---

doctor, dying in 1880. Dr. William Osler attempted to obtain his stomach as a postmortem specimen, but the family made certain that the "stomach with the lid on it" went with its owner to his grave.

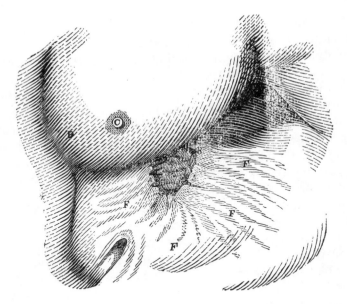

Figure 23. St Martin's wound. This illustration of St. Martin's wound is from Beaumont's *Experiments and Observations.* The letters A and B outline the aperture, C is the nipple, D is the anterior portion of the breast, and E and F show surrounding scar tissue.

posed of flour, hot water, charcoal, and yeast,[2] changing once every 8, 10, or 12 hours, according to the quicker or slower process of fermentation, keeping the parts around constantly bathed with a solution of muriate of ammonia in Spirits and vinegar. This was done with an intention to excite local reaction as soon as possible upon the surface and occasional sloughing of contused, lacerated and burnt muscles and integuments, which had the desired effect in less than 48 hours, with assistance of the Camphorated Aq. Amon. Acet.[3] given internally in liberal quantities. Under the above treatment a lively reaction commenced in about 24 hours, accompanied with strong arterial action and high inflammatory symptoms of the system generally, more specially of violent pneumonia and inflammation of the Lungs, with great dyspnoea and distressing cough. At the commencement of those symp-

---

2. Yeast poultice was a popular dressing in Beaumont's day. The United States *Dispensatory* praised it as "very useful in foul and sloughing ulcers, the fetor of which it corrects, while it affords a gentle stimulus to the debilitated tissue."

3. Camphorated solution of acetate of ammonia was used as a diaphoretic in febrile and inflammatory illnesses.

toms I opened a vein and took 12 or 14 oz. of blood from the arm. Gave a mild cathartic. The bleeding abated the action and gave relief. The cathc. had no effect having escaped from the stomach through the wound. I continued the Caphd. Aq. Acetat. every hour for the first 72 internally and the carbonated poultice and wash externally, omitting the muriate. The fever continued for 8 or ten days, running into the Typhoid type and the wound becoming very fetid. Nothing passed his bowels after the 2d day, and they became impervious and inactive, scarcely to be excited by stimulating injections. From the 2d day till the 10th nothing passed, no reaction from his bowels at all, everything he took into his stomach was either absorbed or made its exit at the wound externally.

About the 5th day a partial sloughing took place in the wound and the febrile symptoms abated. The protruded portion of the lungs and the small lacerated piece of the stomach also sloughed off, and left the puncture of the Stomach plain to be seen, and large enough to admit my forefinger its whole length directly into the cavity of the stomach, and a passage into the cavity of the Thorax half as a large as my fist, exposing to plain view the action of the left lobe of the Lungs, and admitting at every respiration full escape of air, bloody mucus, froth, etc.

About the 10th day a more extensive sloughing took place. The febrile symptoms all subsided, and the whole surface of the wound put on a healthy, granulating appearance. The fractures of the ribs commenced exfoliating, and nature kindly performing what human foresight viewed as hopeless and professional skill might calculate upon with dubious odds. All that entered his stomach came out again at the wound for 12 or 15 days, and the only means of sustaining him was by nutritious injection given per anus until all was sloughed, and compresses and adhesive strap could be applied to stop the orifice in the stomach and retain the food and drinks.

A lucky and perhaps the only circumstance to which his miraculous survival can be attributed was the protruded portion of the Stomach, instead of falling back into the cavity of the abdomen to its natural position, adhered by the first intention to the intercostal muscles, and by that means retained the orifice in the wounded stomach in contact with the external wound, and afforded a free passage out and a fair opportunity to apply the dressings. The carbon poultice was continued constantly until the sloughing was complete and the granulating process established. They were afterwards occasionally applied as a corrective when the wound was becoming ill conditioned or languid. The Aq. Am. Acetat. was continued for several weeks, in proportion to the febrile symptoms or fetid condition of the wound.

No sickness or peculiar irritability of the Stomach was ever experienced, not even nausea, during the whole time; and after 3 weeks the appetite regular and healthy, alvine evacuation became regular, and all the functions of the system seemed as regular and healthy as in perfect health, except the wounded parts.

Cicatrization and contraction of the external wound commenced about the 5th week, and continued gradually and almost uninterruptedly. The Stomach at the wounded part became more and more firmly attached to the intercostals by its external coats, but showed not the least disposition to close its puncture by granulations forming from its own lacerated coats any more than is in the anus or mouth. By applying the nitrate of silver to the edges of the wounded muscles of the stomach, I could extend the attachments by its external and cellular coats more firmly to the intercostals or external integuments, which seemed rather to enlarge than contract the orifice in the Stomach, bringing it more and more external as its adhesions to the external wound increased, resembling in its appearance (all but the Sphincter) a natural anus, with a slight prolapse every time I removed the dressings, and the contents of the Stomach would run out fairly in proportion to the quantity received. If the Stomach happened to be empty when I dressed it, a prolapse and partial invertion of the Stomach would follow the removal of the compresses of lints from the wound, unless prevented by the application of my thumb, finger, or something else to its orifice while the dressing was reapplying. Frequently upon removing the dressings, when they had become looser than usual by some derangement of the bandages, the stomach would be inverted and the inner coats protruded through the orifice large as a hen's egg. No difficulty occurred in reducing it; a gentle pressure with the thumb or finger upon the protruded portion would quickly return it to its place without giving the least pain and almost without sensation. Nitrate of silver, applied so as to produce sloughing, occasioned less sensation than when applied to the most common fungus or ulcer upon the surface of the body or limbs, a conclusive evidence in my opinion that the Stomach is not so exquisitely sensible an organ as is represented by anatomists and Physiologists in general.

About the 6th or 7th week exfoliation from the fractured ribs and the separation of the ribs from the cartilagenous ends began to take place; spiculae of bones and fragments of old cloth and shot also were working out from among the muscles and integuments. The 6th rib, that was worst injured and blown off entirely in the first place, was also abraded of its periostium for about three inches back of the fracture towards the Spine and became carious at its fractured extremity. So that I was obliged to amputate it about midway between sternum and spine, which I did by dissecting around, separating and retracting the intercostals to the sound portion of the rib, and then sawing it off by introducing between the ribs a very narrow, short saw, which I had made for the occasion. In this operation I succeeded admirably, beyond my most sanguine expectations, taking the rib off smoothly without injuring any parts whatever. The granulations shot immediately out and formed soundly over the amputated end. About half of the interior edge of the other rib exfoliated longitudinally from about the center to the Sternum, and then the healthy granulation formed soundly over the other part and continued so.

After removing all the exfoliations and extraneous substances that were to be found about the wound, my next object was to contract the external wound and close up the puncture in the stomach if practicable, which I attempted by drawing the edges of the wound as near together as I could by adhesive straps laid on in radiative form, the circumference of the external wound being at least 12 or 14 inches, the orifice in the Stomach about in the center. To retain the food and drink as much as possible, I kept to the orifice a firm compress of lint, fitted to the shape and size of the puncture, and confined by the straps. Under these dressings and management cictrization went on rapidly, his health improving, and all functions of the system regular. Digestion was as completely performed as in the most healthy person in the vicinity (and I could even see it go on every time I dressed the wound). I kept the granulating surface duly stimulated by applying sometimes Cincona pulv., sometimes Mirc. precip. Rub., and sometimes Nit. Silver,[4] as the state of the granulation indicated.

After trying every means within my power to close the puncture of the Stomach by exciting adhesions between the lips of the wound of its own proper coats, without the least appearance of success, I gave over trying, convinced that the Stomach of itself will not close a puncture in its coats by granulations, and the only alternative left seemed to be to draw the external wound together as fast as cicatrization would form and contracting as much as possible the orifice in the Stomach, and make the granulations from the intercostal muscles and integuments shoot across and form over and close it that way. But to this method there seemed an insuperable difficulty, for, unless there be kept constantly upon the orifice a firm plug of lint compound, all the contents

4. These substances, in order, were powdered Peruvian bark (quinine); red oxide of mercury (mercuric oxide), used as an escharotic and stimulant; and silver nitrate, used then as now to cut back exuberant granulations.

of the Stomach flow out and the patient must die for want of aliment, and this lint, intersepting, prevents the granulation from forming across.

The lacerated portion of the lungs sloughed off and digested away, leaving a surface suppurating in the lobe of the lungs large as the concave surface of a teacup, from which continued to issue much purulent matter for two or three months until it became completely filled up with healthy granulations and cicatrized over externally, with the lower portion of the left lobe firmly adhering to the Pleura costalis. Four months after the injury an abscess formed about two inches below the wound, anteriorly, over the cartilaginous ends of the 1st and 2d false ribs, very painful and extremely sore, producing a violent symptomatic fever, checking the process of cicatrization, rendering the granulation languid and pale, and the wound ill-conditioned and unfavorable to the prospects of recovery. After applying emolient poultices for several days, the swelling pointed externally, and I punctured and laid it open with the bistoury and director for about 2 or 3 inches. It discharged copiously very fetid, purulent matter for the first 2 days. On the 3d I could feel with the probe a small extraneous substance, which in the course of 3 or 4 days, by the use of the soap plaster and compresses, proved to be a shot and a small portion of the wad. After the exit of these I could introduce a common pocketcase silver probe nearly its whole length in the longitudinal direction of the ribs, and a great soreness and pain extended from the opening in the abscess upon the track of the cartilaginous ends of the false ribs to the spine, with a copious discharge from a long fistulous sinus. In the course of about 5 or 6 days appeared the cartilaginous end of a rib about an inch long; soon after this followed some small spicula of bone. The discharge, soreness and inflammation continued in the same direction. In about 6 or 7 days longer came away another similar cartilage about an inch and a half long, and in about the same length of time another 2 inches, and so continued to come away every 5 or 6 days, increasing in length in about the same proportion until five had made their exit through the same passage. The last was about three inches long, and seemed to be separated from the last false rib, as the soreness terminated at that point, and after which the sinus commenced closing, the discharge diminished, and the soreness subsided from that point forward with regular progression. The discharge, pain and irritation during the 4 or 5 weeks all those cartilages were working out reduced the strength of the patient very much, induced a general febrile habit, and stopped the healthy healing process of the original wound. Directly after exit of the last mentioned cartilage an inflammation appeared at the lower end of the sternum, about over the ensiform cartilage, from the anterior end of the original wound, extremely irritable and very painful. By the use of emolient poultice a few days it terminated in a large abscess, which I punctured and laid open an inch or two with the bistoury. About half a pint of very offensive matter discharged from this, and in a few days followed a cartilaginous substance about 3 inches long, after which the inflammation subsided. In a day or two after this came away another small cartilage and the discharge abated. To support the patient's strength under all these debilitating incidents, I gave him the diluted muriatic acid and wine, which very much improved his health and increased his strength.

It is now going on the 7th month since the injury was received, and the orifice in the stomach is still visible and but little contracted. The integuments are all cicatrized, smooth to within the circumference of a half eagle, immediately around the wound in the Stomach. His health daily improving, his spirits good, his appetite regular, his sleep refreshing, and all the functions of the system natural and healthy.

Dec. 2, 1822. Can the puncture of the Stomach be successfully closed by mechanical means until the granulations have time to form over and across it?

Dec. 3d. Omitted dressing wound myself, though dressed by the nurse.

Dec. 4th. On dressing today found a portion of the new cutis vera at the anterior extremity of the cicatrix raised up and separated from the pectoral muscle by the matter forced back from the sinus above in consequence of an obstruction in its usual outlet. On puncturing and laying it open about an inch and a half, found a small piece of cartilage loose and took it away and a large piece which seemed to be separating from the Sternum.

Dec. 5th. Dressed it today. Found it in better condition than yesterday. Inflammation and soreness subsiding, discharge less.

Dec. 6th. Dressed today. Still doing well.

Dec. 7th. Dressed. Still improving.

Dec. 8th. Dressed. Still improving.

Dec. 9th. Dressed. Original wound diminishing, sinuses discharge less, condition better.

Dec. 10th. Dressed. Condition of the wound, sinuses, etc., improving. Keep them dressed with cincona pulv., dry lint and adhesive straps, bathing the parts around with camphorated Spts. and water, and continue the muriatic acid.

Dec. 11th. Dressed. Improving, in healthy condition.

Dec. 12th. Dressed. Sores lessening in circumference and filling up with granulations. All healthy, except the one in front of the Sternum, which seems to have something extraneous behind yet—a piece of cartilage no doubt.

Dec. 13th. Dressed. To facilitate the closing of the puncture of the stomach, and remove the impediments to the granulations, which the constant pressure of compresses necessary to retain the food in the Stomach from day to day cause. I made fast a piece of lint to a ligature, just large enough to pass through the orifice into the Stomach, and then with the end of the probe pushed it on the inside, and, suspended by the ligature, drew it up against the inside of orifice, so as to stop the food, etc., from flowing out upon the inner side, and by this means suffering the granulations from the edges of the wound to contract nearer each other around the small ligature.

Dec. 14th. Dressed in the same manner as yesterday.

Dec. 15th. Dressed as yesterday, excepting the introduction of a small silver canula introduced instead of the ligature and lint.

Dec. 16th. Dressed as yesterday. Find the canula will not answer the purpose so well as the plug of lint suspended by the string.

Dec. 17th. Removed the canula and dressed as usual.

Dec. 22d. The above manner of dressing continued without any variation since the 17th. Continued the wash around the wound of Camphorated Spirits, water and vinegar, injecting frequently into the sinuses the same wash more diluted.

Dec. 23d. Added to the Muriatic acid, diluted, about one-third of the tincture of ———, to be taken three times a day in doses of a half teaspoonful. The discharge still purulent and healthy, and diminishing in quantity. The orifice in the Stomach remaining about the same as it has been for 3 months, tho the wounds of the muscles continue to contract and are fast cicatrizing upon the Stomach. The food still makes its exit whenever the dressings are removed.

Jany. 3d, 1823. Dressed every day since the 23d last mo., condition continuing nearly the same until, 3 or 4 days, an inflammatory redness appeared around the lower part of the Sternum, with considerable heat and some swelling, and today appeared another cartilage, which I took out–about one inch and a half long.

Jan. 6th. Swelling and inflammation subsiding. Took away at the opening of the sinus another cartilage 2 and half inch in length.

Jan. 10th. Since extracting the last cartilage the sinus has closed and the discharge ceased, excepting a very little from the sternal end, where some small pieces of diseased cartilage still remain undetached and keep up a small discharge.

Jan. 19th. Small piece of cartilage came from the ulcer on the sternum; other sinuses all closed; orifice in the Stomach about the same as ever.

Feb. 1st. Dressed every day since last date; all the ulcers and sinuses closed sound; the patient in perfect health; the orifice in the stomach in Statu quo.

March 10th. Dressed daily since last date; much in same condition; orifice in the stomach a little diminished.

March 25th. Dressed daily since last date; no alternative in condition; orifice in the stomach the same.

Apl. 1st. Dressed daily; continues in same condition; general health good.

May 30th. Continued daily dressing as usual since last date; no essential variation in the wound; health good until within a few days past. Having complained of pain in the head, nausea, a cathartic of Rhei and sulphur administered, it is presumed, as never medicine was before administered to man since the creation of the world–to wit, by pouring it in through the ribs at the puncture into the stomach. I administered it in the form of dry powder. It occasioned a slight nausea in less than 10 minutes and operated briskly as a cathc. in less than two hours.

May 31st. Feels relieved by the operation of the medicine given yesterday. Administered in the same manner today 11 oz. manna, 1 oz. magnesia.

The County refusing any further assistance to the patient (who has become a pauper from his misfortune), I took him into my own family from mere motives of charity and a disposition to save his life, or at least to make him comfortable, where he has continued improving in health and condition, and is now able to perform any kind of labor from the whitling of a stick to the chopping of Logs, and is as healthy, active and strong as he ever was in his life, or any man in Mackinac, with the aperture of the Stomach in much the same condition as it was at the last mentioned date. June 1, 1824.

Reflections on Securing in a Ligature the Arteria Innominata

VALENTINE MOTT, M.D. (1785–1865)

The following is the account of an audacious but well-conceived and well-executed operation that stunned the entire medical profession of the United States. This single procedure brought fame and acclamation to Valentine Mott, the 33-year-old surgeon of the New York Hospital who performed it, although his patient survived for less than a month. Mott went on to become one of the world's best-known surgeons, particularly in the field of vascular surgery. He lived long enough to hear of the first successful innominate artery ligation, performed by Andrew Woods Smyth (1833–1916) of New Orleans, in 1864.
Valentine Mott was born in Glen Cove, Long Island, on August 20, 1785. He served as an apprentice under his uncle, Valentine Seaman (1770–1817) and then took his M.D. degree from Columbia in 1806. Mott next traveled to England. There, he learned surgery as a dresser under London's most capable surgeon, Astley Cooper (1768–1841). A year studying in Edinburgh completed the young American's training. The fame gained by his feats of arterial surgery, performed after returning to New York, brought an endless stream of patients to him. Mott operated, taught, and traveled; he was the first American surgeon to be accepted on equal terms by the great surgeons of Europe. He brought a luster to American surgery as had no man before him. Valentine Mott died in New York City, April 26, 1865.

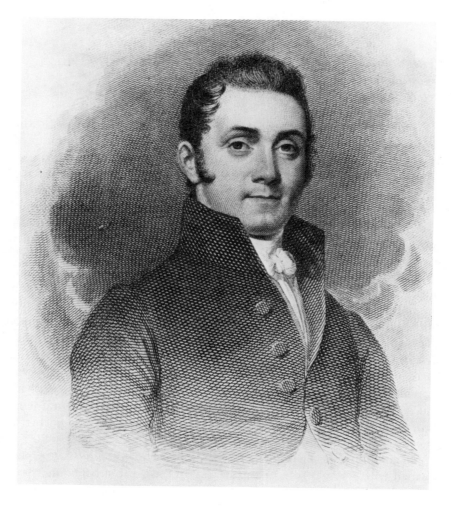

Figure 24. Valentine Mott (1785–1865). An engraving made from a drawing by Henry Inman.

*Mott's account of his most famous operation follows. It was pub-
lished in the* Medical and Surgical Register *(1:9) in 1818. This very
complete case report reveals a great deal about the practice of surgery
in the early nineteenth century. It is reproduced here in its entirety.*

Reflections on Securing in a Ligature the Arteria Innominata: to Which Is Added, a Case in Which This Artery Was Tied by a Surgical Operation

Since the publication of Allan Burns's[1] invaluable work on the
Surgical Anatomy of the Head and Neck, I have been in the habit of
showing in my surgical lectures the practicability of securing in a ligature the Arteria Innominata; and I have had no hesitation in remarking
that it was my opinion, that this artery might be taken up for some
condition of aneurisms; and that a Surgeon, with a steady hand and a
correct knowledge of the parts, would be justified in doing it. I felt myself warranted in this, from the singular success which this celebrated
anatomist informs us attended his injections, and from my own investigations of this subject. If the right arm, right side of the head and
neck, can be filled with injection, after interrupting its passage through
the innominata, as we believe they can, who can doubt the possibility
of the blood to find its way there also, as it will pass through thousands
of channels, which art could not penetrate even by the finest injections?
The well known anastomoses of arteries, and the great resources of the
system in cases of aneurism, encouraged me to believe, that this operation might be performed with reasonable prospects of success. With all
this sanction, and the analogy of the other great operations for aneurism, I could not for a moment hesitate in recommending and performing the operation.

The following operation, as the steps of it will show, was performed with the two-fold intention: 1st, of tying the subclavian artery
before it passes through the scaleni muscles, if it should be found in a fit

---

1. Allan Burns (1781–1813), of the eponymous suprasternal space, was a
surgeon and anatomist of Glasgow who made many pioneer observations in
anatomy and pathology, especially concerning diseases of the heart. His popular book, *Surgical Anatomy of the Head and Neck* (Edinburgh: T. Bryce) appeared in 1811. Burns discussed the possibility of ligating the innominate artery and decided that the operation was both feasible and proper in certain
cases of subclavian aneurysm and concluded wisely that "it is an operation
which ought not to be rashly undertaken."

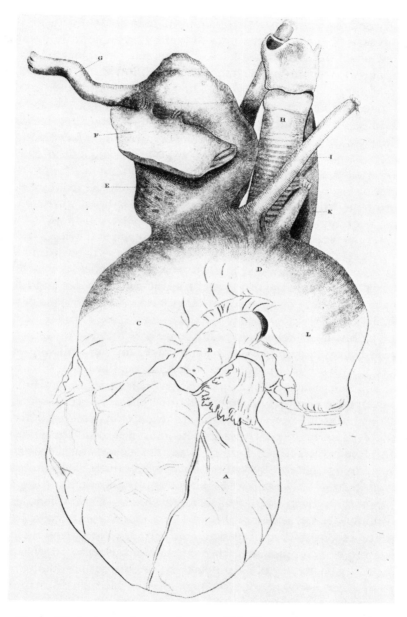

Figure 25. An innominate aneurysm. This illustration appeared in Allan Burns's *Surgical Anatomy of the Head and Neck* (Edinburgh: T. Bryce, 1811), the book that inspired Mott to attempt his operation for the ligation of this vessel. In Mott's case the aneurysm was higher, with a normal sized innominate artery. The letters, C, D, and L outline the arch of the aorta; E is the aneurysm; F is the first rib. A, of course, is the heart. (Courtesy National Library of Medicine.)

state; and 2dly, to tie the arteria innominata in case the former should be diseased or too much encroached upon by the aneurismal tumour.

Michael Bateman, aged 57 years, was born in Salem, Massachusetts, and by occupation a seaman. He was admitted into the New York hospital on the 1st of March, 1818, for a catarrhal affection, having at the same time his right arm and shoulder much swollen. At the time of his admission the catarrh being thought the most considerable disease of the two he was received as a medical patient and placed under the care of the physician then in attendance. During the three first weeks of his residence in the house, the catarrh had greatly yielded to the remedies prescribed. The inflammation, which had produced an enlargement of the whole superior extremity, extending itself to the muscles of the neck on the right side, was also gradually subsiding.

A tumefaction, however, situated above and posterior to the clavicle, at first involved in the general swelling, and not to be distinguished from it, began to show itself. This resisted the remedies which were effectual in relieving the other, and became more distinct and circumscribed as the latter subsided; at length assuming the form of an irregular tumour.

The history which he gave of the case is as follows: He said, about a week before he entered the hospital, while at work on ship-board, his feet accidentally slipped from under him, and he fell upon his right arm, shoulder, and the back part of his head; that he felt but little inconvenience from the fall, and after a short time returned to his duty. Two days subsequent to this, however, he felt pain in the shoulder, and the succeeding night was unable to lie upon it in bed. The whole arm and shoulder then began to swell, and became so painful that he was unable any longer to perform his duty as a seaman. The ship having arrived in New York, he was admitted into the hospital.

For some time after the general swelling had subsided, leaving the tumour distinct and circumscribed, no circumstance occurred which gave rise to a suspicion of its being aneurismal. The enlargement was thought to be a common indolent tumour, and was repeatedly blistered, with a view to discuss [i.e., to dispel] it. The tumor gradually diminished under this treatment; though a considerable time elapsed before any very striking change took place.

At length a faint and obscure pulsation was perceived; still it was a matter of doubt whether the tumour was aneurismal, or whether the pulsatory motion was communicated to it by the subclavian artery, immediately over which it was situated. From its firm unyielding nature upon pressure, the latter was considered as the most probable, and the blisters were continued as before. During the whole of this time the patient had worn his arm in a sling, the motions of it being very limited, and always attended with pain.

The patient remained in this state for several days, without any marked change either in his feelings or in the appearance of the tumour.

On the 3d of May, at 6 o'clock in the afternoon, the patient complained that he "felt something give way in the tumour," that his shoulder was very painful, and that he was able to raise it only a few inches from his side. The tumour at this time suddenly increased, about one third, and a pulsation was distinctly perceptible. Its most prominent part was below the clavicle; at which place the pulsation was also much enlarged; it still however had its usual firmness, except in one point near its centre.

May 4th.—The tumour is evidently increased, that portion of it more particularly which is below the clavicle; it is not as firm and resisting as it has been. Pulsation is not so distinct as yesterday, but appears to be more diffused.

He was this day transferred to the surgical side of the house, and became my patient. The cough having become comparatively slight, the tumour appeared to be the most urgent disease, and, in my opinion, to call for prompt attention. The arm is now perfectly useless, and any motion at the shoulder joint gives him severe pain. The patient is naturally of a spare habit, and from the nature of his disease, and the confinement to which he has been subjected, has become much reduced in strength.

May 5th and 6th.—The tumour is still progressing and the pain in the shoulder is also more severe. During the three last days his medicines have been discontinued, except that he is allowed to rub the parts about the clavicle with volatile liniment.

On the 7th I directed a consultation of my colleagues to be called, consisting of Drs. Post, Kissam and Stevens.[2] I now stated to them that I wished to perform an operation which would enable me to pass a ligature around the subclavian artery, before it passes through the scaleni muscles, or the arteria innominata, if the size of the tumour should prevent the accomplishment of the former. This I was permitted to do, provided the patient should assent, after a candid and fair representation was made to him of the probable termination of his disease; and that

---

2. Philip Wright Post (1766–1828) had studied with John Hunter in London after completing his medical apprenticeship in this country. He became one of America's best known surgeons, second only to Hunter's other American pupil, Philip Syng Physick of Philadelphia. Post was the first American

the operation, though uncertain, gave him some chance, and, as we thought, the only one of his life.

Dr. Post, at my request, communicated with him privately on this subject, and after a full explanation of the nature of the case, my patient requested to have any operation performed which promised him a chance for his life, saying that in his present state he was truly wretched.

May 8th, 9th, and 10th.—The tumour is acknowledged by all to be increasing, and it is thought proper not to defer the operation any longer. I therefore requested that preparation be made for performing it tomorrow.

It is difficult to give an idea of the size of a tumour so irregular in its form, and so peculiarly situated. A thread passed over it, from the lower part of that portion of it which is below the clavicle, extending upward obliquely across the clavicle toward the back of the neck, will measure five and a quarter inches.—Another crossing this at right angles one inch above the clavicle, will measure four inches; two and a half inches of the thread are on the sternal side of the former, and one and a half on the acromial. It rises fully an inch above the clavicle, which, added to the depression below the clavicle on the opposite shoulder, will make the size of the swelling above the natural surface about two inches.

May 11th.—One hour before the time assigned for the operation, the patient appeared perfectly composed, and apparently pleased with the idea that the operation afforded him a prospect of some relief. He was directed to take of Tinct. Opii. 70 drops.

No difference can be perceived in the pulsation of the arteries in the two extremities; his pulses are uniform and regular, each beating 69 in a minute.

He was placed upon a table of the ordinary height, in a recumbent posture, a little inclining to the left side, so that the light fell obliquely upon the upper part of the thorax and neck. Seating myself on a bench

---

surgeon to tie the femoral artery in the femoral canal (1796). He also was the first surgeon ever to tie the subclavian artery with success (1817).

Richard S. Kissam (1763–1822) was a graduate of Edinburgh. He practiced surgery in New York and was well known especially as a lithotomist.

Alexander Hodgdon Stevens (1789–1869) received his M.D. in New York in 1811 and then studied in Europe. He had just been made a member of the attending staff of the New York Hospital at the time that Mott's operation was performed. He later became professor of surgery at the College of Physicians and Surgeons of New York.

of a convenient height, I commenced my incision upon the tumour, just above the clavicle, and carried it close to this bone and the upper end of the sternum, and terminated it immediately over the trachea; making it in extent about three inches. Another incision about the same length, extended from the termination of the first along the inner edge of the sterno cleido mastoid muscle. The integuments were then dissected from the platisma myoides, beginning at the lower angle of the incisions, and turned over upon the tumour and side of the neck.

Cutting through the platisma myoides, I cautiously divided the sternal part of the mastoid muscle, in the direction of the first incision, and as much of the clavicular portion as the size of the swelling would permit, and reflected it over upon the tumour. The internal jugular vein was encroached upon by the swelling, which made this part of the operation of the utmost delicacy, from the morbid adhesion of that part of the clavicular portion of the muscle to it, which was detached. I separated this portion of the muscle to as great an extent, however, as the case would possibly allow, to make room for the subsequent steps of the operation; only a part of the vein was exposed. The sterno hyoid muscle was next divided, and then the sterno thyroid, and turned upon the opposite side of the wound, over the trachea. This exposed the sheath containing the carotid artery, and separated the par vagum from it; then drawing the nerve and vein to the outside, and the artery towards the trachea, I readily laid bare the subclavian about half an inch from its origin. In doing this, the handle of a scalpel was principally used, nothing more being required but to separate the cellular membrane, as it covers the artery. I judged it would be very imprudent to introduce a common scalpel into so narrow and deep a wound, especially as it would be placed between two such important vessels or parts, as the carotid and par vagum, and where the least motion of the patient might cause a wound of one or the other of them. The proper instrument, in my opinion, for this part of the operation, is a knife, the size of a small scalpel, with a rounded point, and cutting only at the extremity; this was used, and found to be very convenient for this stage of the operation. It can be introduced into a deep and narrow wound, among important parts, without the hazard of dividing any but such as are intended to be cut. This knife is contained in a set of instruments admirably calculated for this and other operations on arteries deeply seated, and which I shall mention more particularly hereafter.

On arriving at the subclavian artery, it appeared to be considerably larger than common, and of an unhealthy colour; and when I exposed it to the extent of about half an inch from its origin, which was all that the tumour would permit, to ascertain this circumstance more satisfactorily, my friends concurred with me in opinion that it would be highly injudicious to pass a ligature around it. The close contiguity of the tumour would of itself have been a sufficient objection to the application of the ligature in this situation, independent of the apparently altered state of the artery. Art in this case could not anticipate any thing like the institution of the healthy process of adhesive inflammation in an artery in the immediate vicinity of so much disease. The Pathology of arteries has long since taught us, that ulcerative inflammation, and all its train of consequences, would have been the inevitable result. This was the fate of the only case, in which a ligature has been applied to the artery in this situation. The operation was performed by that eminent Surgeon of Dublin, Dr. Colles.[3]

While separating the cellular substance from the lower surface of the artery, with the smooth handle of an ivory scalpel, a branch of artery was lacerated, which yielded for a few minutes a very smart hemorrhage, so as to fill the wound perhaps six or eight times. It was about half an inch distant from the innominata, and from the stream emitted, was about the size of a crow-quill. It stopped with a little pressure. I can scarcely believe this to have been the internal mammary, from the hemorrhage ceasing so quickly; though, from its situation, it would appear so; and if from some irregularity it were not the superior intercostal, it must have proceeded from an anomalous branch.

With this appearance of disease in the subclavian artery, it only remained for me either to pass the ligature around the arteria innominata, or abandon my patient. Although I very well knew, that this artery had never been taken up for any condition of aneurisms, or ever performed as a surgical operation, yet with the approbation of my friends, and reposing great confidence in the resources of the system, when aided by the noblest efforts of scientific surgery, I resolved upon the operation.

The bifurcation of the innominata being now in view, it only remained to prosecute the dissection a little lower behind the sternum. This was done mostly with the round edged knife, taking care to keep directly over and along the upper surface of the artery. After fairly denuding the artery upon its upper surface, I very cautiously, with the handle of a scalpel, separated the cellular substance from the sides of it, so as to avoid wounding the pleura. A round silken ligature was now readily passed around it, and the artery was tied about half an inch be-

---

3. Abraham Colles (1773–1843), of the eponymous Colles's fracture and Colles's fascia, was professor of surgery at Dublin.

low the bifurcation. The recurrent and phrenic nerves were not disturbed in this part of the operation.

As most surgeons who have performed operations upon large arteries, in deep and narrow wounds, complain of the embarrassment which has attended the application of the ligature, I am happy in the present opportunity to have it in my power to recommend an instrument, or contrivance, which, in my opinion, is calculated to surmount all difficulties. This set of instruments consists of several needles of different sizes and curvatures, with sharp and blunt points, and having in each two eyes. The needles screw into a strong handle or shank of steel: two strong instruments in handles, with a ring or eye in the extremity similar to a tonsil iron, and perhaps they may be called ligature irons: a small knife rounded at the extremity like a lancet for scarifying the eyes, and a small hook at the extremity of a steel shank, also fixed in a strong handle. These instruments are the invention of Drs. Parish, Hartshorne, and Hewson,[4] of Philadelphia. They are the result of investigations made upon the dead body, as to the best mode and place for tying the subclavian artery on the acromial side of the scaleni muscles.

With the ligature introduced into the eye of one of the smallest blunt needles, which was nearest the shank of the instrument, I pressed down the cellular substance and pleura with the convex part, and very carefully insinuated it from below upwards, under the artery. The point of the needle appearing on the opposite side of the artery, I introduced the hook into the other eye of it; then unscrewing the shank, the needle was drawn through with the utmost facility, leaving the ligature underneath the artery.

In the application of the ligature to this artery, I would invite the attention of those who perform it, to a circumstance which, in my opinion, is somewhat important: it is to pass the ligature from below upwards, in order to prevent the pleura from being wounded. From the use of these instruments repeatedly, I would also recommend that the

---

4. Surgeons of the Pennsylvania Hospital:

Joseph Parrish (1779–1840) received his M.D. degree from the University of Pennsylvania in 1805. He gave popular lectures on surgery and other subjects in Philadelphia and wrote several papers on hernia. Parrish succeeded Physick as surgeon to the Pennsylvania Hospital in 1816.

Joseph Hartshorne (1779–1850); see note 4, p. 71.

Thomas Tickell Hewson (1773–1848) attended Edinburgh (1796). He was best known as an anatomist and became professor of comparative anatomy at the University of Pennsylvania in 1818.

hook be fixed in the eye of the needle before the shank is unscrewed, otherwise very considerable difficulty will be experienced in finding it, and even when felt, not easily introduced, from the want of firmness which the handle part of the instrument would afford.

I now made a knot in the ligature, and with my forefingers carried it down to the artery, and drew it a little so as partly to close its diameter and arrest the column of blood gradually. This was continued for a few seconds to observe the effect produced upon the heart and lungs; when no change taking place, it was drawn so as to stop the circulation entirely, as was shown by the radial artery of the right arm, and the right temporal immediately ceasing to pulsate. The knot was drawn more firmly by the ligature irons, and a second knot applied in the same manner.

In no instance did I ever view the countenance of man with more fluctuations of hope and fear, than in drawing the ligature upon this artery. To intercept suddenly one fourth of the quantity of blood, so near to the heart, without producing some unpleasant effect, no surgeon, a priori, would have believed possible. I therefore drew the ligature gradually, and with my eyes fixed upon his face, I was determined to remove it instantly if any alarming symptoms had appeared. But, instead of this, when he showed no change of feature or agitation of body, my gratification was of the highest kind.

Dr. Post now asked him if he felt any unpleasant sensation about his head, breast, or arm, or felt any way different from common, to which he replied, that he did not.

Immediately after the ligature was drawn tight, the tumor was reduced in size about one third, and the course of the clavicle could be distinctly felt.

The parts were now brought into coaptation, and the integuments drawn together by three interrupted sutures and straps of adhesive plaster; a little lint and additional straps completed the dressing. Three small arteries were tied in the course of the operation: the first was under the sternum, and divided with the sternal part of the mastoid muscle, and from its course may have been a branch of the internal mammary reflected upwards; the second, in raising the inner edge of the mastoid muscle, about the upper angle of the longitudinal incision, and must have been the most descending branch of the superior thyroid; and the third, was a branch of the inferior thyroid, and cut while raising the sternothyroid muscle. The patient lost perhaps from two to four ounces of blood, most of which came from the ruptured branch of the subclavian. The operation occupied about one hour.

The curved spatulas recommended by Dr. Colles, I found of great use in the operation. I provided three for this purpose, two broad, and one narrow, bent at right angles, and sufficiently firm. After raising the muscles, they were of the greatest advantage in keeping separated the carotid artery and par vagum, as likewise the divided muscles; they served also another very useful purpose, that of preventing by their equable pressure the constant oozing from the smaller vessels; and the little room taken up in a small and deep wound, will give them a great superiority over the fingers introduced.

Ten minutes after the operation the pulse is regular, and not the least variation can be perceived; it beats 69 strokes in a minute; the patient says he is perfectly comfortable, and has no new or unatural sensation, except a little stiffness of the muscles of the neck, which he thinks is owing to the position in which his head was placed during the operation; the temperature of the right arm is a little cooler than the left; his breathing has not been the least affected by the operation, but is perfectly free and natural.

2 o'clock, P.M.—Patient expresses a desire to eat, and is directed a little thin soup and bread; the temperature of both arms is very nearly the same; breathing perfectly natural; pulse as before.

3 o'clock P.M.—There is still a trifling difference in the temperature of the two arms; ordered the right to be wrapped in cotton wadding; not the least unpleasant symptom has as yet made its appearance.

6 o'clock P.M.—Complains of a little pain in his head, not more on one side however than the other; describes it as a common head-ache: the pain of the shoulder and arm much less than before the operation: no difference can now be perceived in the temperature of the two arms; pulse a little accelerated, and perhaps a little full.

9 P.M.—Patient complains of head-ache; skin is rather hotter than natural; pulse strong and full, and beats 75 in a minute; the carotid on the left side of the neck is observed to be much dilated and in strong action; tongue moist and clean.

9½ P.M.—Symptoms continuing the same, directed him to be bled from the left arm to ℥xvj. After bleeding the pulse fell 7 beats, and was less full. Complains of some thirst; let him drink common tea.

12 P.M.—Patient has slept a little; is free from pain; pulse full and less frequent, beats 60; skin moist and of a natural temperature.

Second day, 2 o'clock A.M.–Patient enjoys a natural and undisturbed sleep; respiration free, and performed without the least difficulty.

5 A.M.—He has rested well the last three hours. Says he has a slight head-ache, and a little pain in the right elbow; the latter he attributes to the position in which his arm has lain during sleep; pulse full, but

not so tense as before the venesection; skin natural and moist; temperature of both arms the same. He states that he can now incline more upon the right shoulder than he has been able to do since the second day after he received the injury.

9 A.M.—Pain in the head no way troublesome; skin moist and of natural temperature; tongue clean; says his neck feels stiff, but is not painful; has no difficulty in swallowing. His cough has thus far been much less frequent than before the operation; expectoration is also attended with less difficulty; pulse 75, full, but not tense; has taken a dish of coffee, and some bread; complains of some thirst; directed a solution of supertartrite of potass, to be drank occasionally.

10 A.M.—Symptoms as before; the veins of the fore-arm and hand since the operation have been as much distended as previous to it, and upon compressing them so as to stop the circulation, and allow the vein to become empty for some distance above, the column of blood is seen to distend the vein immediately upon the removal of the pressure, plainly showing that the circulation is going on with considerable rapidity, although no pulsation has been felt in the brachial or radial arteries. The radial artery can be easily distinguished by the fingers, and seems to be filled with blood. There is evidently a pulsation in the anterior branch of the temporal artery, just as it is passing a little above the exterior canthus of the orbit; the left external carotid is beating with increased action, and appears larger than natural.

3 P.M.—Has taken a light dinner, and complains of a little headache; pulse has become tense, and is also increased in frequency; skin is considerably hotter than natural; tongue too indicates a febrile action; was bled to   viij. and directed to drink freely of a solution of the supertartrite of potass.

10 P.M.—Since the last report he has become more comfortable; complains of no pain, and says he lies perfectly easy; pulse increased in frequency to 78, but of the natural soft feel; the right side of the face has been at times a little cooler than the left, and is so at the present time; it is, however, not so much so as to be perceptible to the patient; temperature of the right arm natural: that of the left, and the whole body, is above the natural standard, but it is moist; tongue is clean: having had no evacuation from his bowels since the operation, is directed to take a saline cathartic, in divided doses.

1 A.M.—Complains of nothing; has not slept any; cathartic has operated twice.

Third day, 5 A.M.—Has had no sleep in consequence of the operation of the medicine, it having produced free evacuations in the course of the night; skin not so moist, but of natural temperature; the two arms have equal warmth; pulse full, and rather more frequent than last evening: says his right elbow is a little painful, and the arm feels tired. The complete flexion of the arm at the elbow is prevented by a little rigidity of the extensor muscles.

9 A.M.—He is now comfortable, has slept a little, and feels refreshed; pulse is full, and rather more frequent than natural; skin natural and moist: the size of the tumor is considerably diminished; has taken a dish of chocolate and some rusk.

11½ A.M.—Patient still free from pain, or any uneasiness; medicine has operated seven times; skin not hotter than natural, and moist; tongue clean; the right facial and anterior temporal arteries communicate a distinct pulsation to the fingers: having slept but little during the last night, directed him to take an anodyne of Tinct. Opii.gtt.xxx and to have the room made dark, and kept quiet, in order to procure him some sleep: let him have sago or panada as often as he inclines to take nourishment.

4 P.M.—Has slept the last two hours, and is still sleeping; respiration free and easy; nothing the least unnatural in his appearance.

10 P.M.—He has slept four hours, and is much refreshed; is free from pain, except a little in the elbow; pulse small and soft, beating 105 strokes in a minute; tongue clean; feels a little soreness in the wound when swallowing; has taken a considerable quantity of sago and panada; his appetite is good; temperature natural and uniform in both arms.

12 P.M.—Patient has slept the greater part of the time; is free from pain, and perfectly comfortable; skin moist and natural; pulse soft, small, and frequent.

Fourth day, 6 o'clock A.M.—Patient has passed a good night; says his right elbow gives him some uneasiness, but complains of nothing else; tongue is clean; skin moist and natural; can move the right arm with considerable ease; says he takes as much light nourishment as he has been accustomed to for some time past: no unfavourable symptom has yet made its appearance.

11 A.M.—Symptoms continue much the same; tongue slightly furred; pulse comparatively small and soft, beats 105, and regular; respiration has been uniformly natural since the operation; suppuration has begun to appear through the dressings, and is attended with a little foetor; let them be covered with a yeast pultice; it is thought that a faint pulsation or undulation is at intervals felt in the radial artery of the right arm: the left external carotid continues its increased action.

6 P.M.—No change is observable in the patient's symptoms; he still continues comfortable, and complains of nothing.

Fifth day, 11½ o'clock A.M.—The wound was dressed to-day: on removing the poultice the dressings were soft and easily came away; the suppuration was considerable, and of a healthy appearance; it was found that the extremities of the two incisions were united as far as the sutures, each about one inch in extent; one suture at the angle of the wound was removed; the wound was dressed with dry lint, gently pressed into it; adhesive straps and a compress; his pulse beats 110, is fuller and stronger than yesterday.

6 P.M.—Patient is very comfortable, subject to no pain or unnatural sensation; pulse still 110, but softer.

Sixth day, 6 A.M.—Patient sleeps; respiration not attended with the least difficulty; skin moist and natural.

9 A.M.—He has rested well during the night, and is perfectly free from pain; pulse 110, and soft; skin moist; tongue clean: having had no alvine evacuation since the 13th, directed to take of sulphate of soda j, in divided doses.

11 A.M.—The dressings were again removed, and the discharge seemed more considerable than at the former dressing; the sides of the wound are granulating, and appear perfectly healthy; on the ends of the muscles that were divided in the operation, there are small sloughs which are beginning to separate, leaving a healthy surface underneath; wound was dressed with lint spread with Ung.Res.Flav.[5] and adhesive straps: pulsation is now perfectly distinct in the branches of the right external carotid artery: complains a little of the back part of his head, which he says is sore from lying; in other respects is comfortable.

6 P.M.—Has no pain, and is in every respect much as usual; tongue clean; skin natural; says he feels "no weaker than before the operation."

Seventh day, 6 A.M.–He has passed a comfortable night, and is free from pain or any uneasiness; pulse regular and soft, and beats 105 in a minute; skin moist, and of natural temperature.

11 A.M.—The wound was again dressed: suppuration considerable and healthy; some of the small sloughs came away, leaving a healthy and florid surface beneath: sprinkled the wound with powdered carbon, then filled it lightly with lint, and over this applied the yeast poultice, which was secured with adhesive straps: temperature of the two arms is the same, cathartic having produced no effect. *Habeat enema purgans statim.*

9 P.M.—Symptoms have not varied materially: the enema has pro-

---

5. Unguentum Resinae Flava or ointment of yellow resin, a mildly stimulating ointment.

duced a copious evacuation: says he feels more comfortable, and desires to sit up in bed, which was allowed, taking care to have him raised up very cautiously, in order to prevent any exertion being made with the right arm and shoulder.

Eighth day, 6 A.M.—Patient has rested well during the night; says he feels some pain on swallowing, and that when the attempt is made, it gives rise to a fit of coughing, which fatigues him; it also occasions some soreness in the wound: pulse still soft, and less frequent than yesterday: he takes a reasonable quantity of light food every day:— Directed a cetaceous mixture for his cough, and is permitted to sit up for a short time, if he feels disposed.

11 A.M.—Pulsation of the radial artery of the right arm to be felt occasionally pretty distinct; cough has become more troublesome; pulse 100; skin natural and moist. The dressings were again removed, and the suppuration is more profuse, apparently healthy, though attended with considerable foetor; appearance of the wound every way favourable; small portions of the sloughs are removed at each dressing, and the sides of the wound look perfectly healthy; the same dressing to be continued.

9 P.M.—Complains only of his cough, which troubles him frequently; can move his arm with much more facility, and has no pain in it; circulation as before, and the temperature uniform and natural. The wound was dressed this evening in consequence of the foetor being unpleasant to the patient; continue the dressings.

Ninth day, 7 A.M.—Patient was found sitting up in bed, supported by a bed-chair, having passed a good night; is in good spirits, and expresses his gratitude for the relief afforded by the operation; says he can move the arm with greater ease, and it gives him no pain; pulse 105, regular and soft; skin natural; every symptom as favourable as could be wished.

10 A.M.—Pulse less frequent, regular and soft; temperature perfectly natural; wound has a more favourable appearance, discharges less in quantity, and it possesses less foetor; dressed the wound as yesterday; tumour has diminished two thirds, is soft, and less florid. The apex of the tumour is now below the clavicle.

6 P.M.—Patient still in every respect as comfortable as at the last report.

9 P.M.—Pulse 110, regular and soft: the dressings were removed this evening; the wound is much contracted in size, and is perfectly healthy, except a small slough which still remains in the deepest part of the wound; granulations are shooting up rapidly from the sides.—When preparing to renew the dressings, an unexpected and an unaccountable

hemorrhage took place, which suddenly filled the cavity of the wound. The rapidity with which the blood flowed, and the size of the stream, gave rise to fearful apprehensions for the man's safety: dry lint was immediately placed in the wound, and as much pressure made as the patient could conveniently bear, which quickly stopped it. After continuing the pressure for a short time, the lint was removed, when no hemorrhage recurring, the usual dressings were repeated: the patient experienced no ill effects from the bleeding, nor did he seem to be much agitated. At 10 o'clock P.M., has no pain, nor has he has yet had any sleep.

Tenth day, 7 A.M.—Has passed a comfortable night, except that he has been frequently disturbed by his cough: tongue clean; skin moist; pulse soft, and has much less strength than before.

11 A.M.—The dressings were again removed, and the wound made clean; its appearance is in every respect favourable; does not appear to have been the least injured by the hemorrhage: the dressings were renewed as before: he is directed to take half an ounce of the cold infusion of cinchona every hour, and to drink occasionally of ale when thirsty: has had an evacuation from his bowels today.

6 P.M.—Symptoms much as before; complains a little of his elbow, and a numbness in his hand, to relieve which he is directed to have the arm and hand rubbed well, and wrapped in wadding.

Eleventh day, 6 A.M.—Patient has rested well during the night; cough has not been so troublesome; says he has no pain, and feels perfectly comfortable; pulse better than yesterday; other symptoms as before.

11 A.M.—The wound is dressed daily at this hour; its appearance is still very favourable, although there is still some foetor in the suppuration: the wound has contracted perhaps one third: the tumour is also considerably diminished, and softer than before; pulsation in the right temporal and radial arteries as before: the same dressings to be continued.

6 P.M.—No change in the patient's general symptoms: pulse soft, and rather more frequent; appetite is as good as usual.

9 P.M.—Appearances have not varied.

Twelfth day, 6 A.M.—Our patient has visited as usual this morning, but there is no evident change in any of his symptoms; says he now rests well at night.

11 A.M.—To-day, when the dressings were removed, that portion of the slough which occupied the bottom of the wound (apparently a portion of the sheath of the vessels) came away; every part of the wound now, where its surface can be seen, has a healthy look: the most de-

pending part is obscured by a quantity of pus, which cannot be wholly removed by lint, and it is not thought safe to permit the patient to lie in such a position as will allow it to be discharged: with the slough came away the ligature which had been applied to an artery under the lower portion of the sterno-thyroid muscle; it was followed by no hemorrhage: the wound was now dressed with pledgets of lint, spread with Ung. Resinae Flavae and adhesive straps. He remains much as yesterday, has drank freely of ale; pulse rather stronger than yesterday.

Thirteenth day, 7 A.M.—No perceptible change in his symptoms; complains of no pain, and says he feels very comfortable; cough has given him very little trouble for the last two days; he is evidently considerably weaker than before the operation, but is not sensible of it himself.

11 A.M.—The wound was again exposed; it is not as florid as yesterday, and there is a greater secretion of pus; the cavity of the wound was filled with dry lint only; the pus appears well formed, and has very little foetor.

The same dressings were repeated in the evening; there is still a quantity of pus at the bottom of the wound, which rises and falls at each inspiration and expiration: it continues to contract above, leaving us uncertain of its extent beneath; during the last three days, the patient has sat up for several hours each day.

9 P.M.—Pulse and skin perfectly natural; has had a natural evacuation from his bowels to-day; continues the infusion of bark as prescribed before.

Wound was again dressed, and is as healthy as usual; suppuration just sufficient to moisten the lint: the same dressings to be continued.

Fourteenth day, 7 A.M.—Patient has slept well during the night, and is as well as usual; complains of soreness of the ulcer which he has had for some time between his shoulders; it is improving in its appearance, and is directed to be dressed as usual with Ung. Resinae Flavae. The erysipelatous blush which surrounded it, is not as florid as heretofore: it is beginning to granulate, and assume a healthy appearance: in other respects he is perfectly comfortable: he is now able to raise the right arm to his lips, which he has not done since the fourth day after the accident by which his shoulder was injured; says too that he is getting stronger, and that he walked across the floor this morning without any assistance.

11 A.M.—On removing the dressing, the granulations appear perfectly florid and healthy: the bottom of the wound is not visible, owing to the small quantity of matter which collects there, and from its depth cannot be easily removed, and perhaps not altogether safely: the posi-

tion of the patient in bed must necessarily make the bottom of the wound the lowest: when he coughs or swallows a small quantity of fluid pus at the bottom of the wound is seen to rise and fall; from the general appearance however of the wound, the man's feelings, and many other circumstances, it is not probable that there is any considerable quantity: the large ligature lying very loose in the wound, was taken hold of, merely however to see if it was separated; no force was used: pulsation of the right radial artery more distinct than heretofore: countenance of our patient is improving; says he feels more comfortable than before the operation: he can now straighten his arm, and raise it to his mouth with facility: as yet he has not recovered his strength, but is improving daily; has been sitting up all day: directed him when lying down, to assume a more recumbent posture; continue the sulphuric acid and infusion of cinchona, as before: complains of the ale being too strong; let it be diluted and made pleasant with sugar and nutmeg.

9 P.M.—The large ligature since the operation, has been confined upon the upper part of the sternum by a piece of adhesive plaster, to prevent any accident during the dressings. Upon dressing the wound this evening, the large ligature, as it lay in the wound, appearing to be loose, was again taken hold of with the forceps, and found floating upon the pus, being completely separated from the artery below. The ligature was drawn so firmly upon the artery, that the noose was only large enough to admit the rounded end of a common probe. The wound looks healthy, and is contracting rapidly; it is now perhaps not more than one third of its original size. Suppuration is now only sufficient to moisten the lint through.

Fifteenth day, 12 o'clock.—The patient is comfortable in every respect; pulse and skin perfectly natural; is sitting up in bed, and occasionally amusing himself with a book; not the least symptom about him indicating indisposition: wound is healthy, and continues to improve in appearance. The right arm at intervals gives him a sensation of numbness,–no more, however, than can be accounted for from the uniform position in which the arm rests, and no doubt a more languid circulation, as it readily removed by a little friction and motion of the arm. His appetite improves, and he expresses a desire to walk about the room. The bark and sulphuric acid to be continued.

9 P.M.—In the afternoon he was removed down stairs, from the private room in which he was placed immediately after the operation, to the ward in which he formerly lay, and appeared highly gratified with the idea of again seeing his friends, whom he had left with very little hope of ever returning to. The wound, upon being dressed, did not appear to have undergone any perceptible change.

Sixteenth day, 11 A.M.—Our patient's strength is improving. To-day he made an effort, and with success, to visit his friends in Ward No. 7, where he lay previous to his being transferred to the surgical department, and returned, without having any support; pulse as strong as before the operation, and in every respect natural; appetite better than before the operation; cough a little troublesome, but less so than for several days previous; wound dressed with dry lint.

9 P.M.—Dressings removed; patient as before; suppuration small in quantity, and appears to be well-formed pus, and is not attended with the least foetor.

Seventeenth day, 11 o'clock.—The ends of the divided muscles are nearly in contact, and the surfaces of the wound are rapidly granulating, and in every respect looks well: patient's health continues to improve; he walks about the room with perfect ease, and into several wards in the same story; the ability to move the arm increases; pulse and skin natural. The dressings were removed at 4 P.M., and also at 10 P.M.

Eighteenth day.—The patient's strength continues to improve; every symptom remains highly flattering; cough less troublesome. The dressings were again removed to-day three times.

Twentieth day.—To-day he passed down two pair of stairs, and walked several times across the yard, and was highly delighted with his performance, and felt not the least inconvenience from it; sleeps uniformly well during the night, and takes more food during the day than he did previous to the operation; continues the infusion of cinchona and sulph. acid as before, and directed to use dry lint as the dressing.

Twenty-first day.—Dressed the wound three times again to-day; it is nearly closed at the bottom; the power of motion in the right arm continues to increase; he can move it with as much facility as the left, though not to the same extent: his strength is daily improving, and the operation is considered by all to have been completely successful: size of the tumour continues the same, no diminution of it having been perceived for the last week: the most prominent part of the tumour is yet below the clavicle, that above rises to about the height of the clavicle, which gives a little convexity to the place between the clavicle and trapezius muscle.

Twenty-second day.—Continues to improve in every respect; dressings renewed as often as yesterday; owing to the weather he has not left his ward to-day; pulse full and strong; temperature of both arms the same.

Twenty-third day.—A few minutes before the hour of visiting to-day, a message was brought that the patient was bleeding from the wound. The dressings were immediately torn off, and dry lint crowded into the wound, and slight pressure applied for a few minutes, when the hemorrhage ceased. The patient lost at this time, perhaps, about 24 ounces of blood, and was very much prostrated. Pulsation ceased in the radial artery of the left arm, and the countenance, gasping, and convulsive throes of the patient, threatened immediate dissolution; all present apprehended the instant death of the patient. The first impression was, that the trunk of the arteria innominata had given way. The conjecture afterwards was, that the subclavian artery, from the diseased state of it, had not united by adhesion, and that the fluid blood from the tumour had regurgitated through its ulcerated coats. This appeared to be the most probable, both from the suddenness with which the blood ceased flowing, and the cause the patient assigned for the hemorrhage. He says that he felt weary of lying on his left side and back; that he had just turned on the right, which he had not done before since the operation, agreeable to my request. At the instant of turning over, something arrested his attention, which caused him to turn his head to the opposite side suddenly, and he felt the gush of blood from the wound.

He was directed some wine and water frequently, which soon revived the circulation. The wound was dressed with dry lint and a compress. Pulse as frequent as natural, but very small and soft: he appears very languid, and complains of a numbness and painful sensation in his hands; says also that his back aches. During the last twenty-four hours he has taken a pint and a half of Madeira wine; he also took occasionally some egg and wine, which was immediately rejected from the stomach.

9 P.M.—Patient has lost his appetite, and appears considerably depressed; circulation very languid in the right arm; temperature of it is a little less than the left: directed a hot brick to be wrapped in flannel, and placed close to the arm. For a profuse perspiration which he has been in for the last three hours, he was ordered to be bathed with cold rum.

Twenty-fourth day, 6 A.M.—Slept the greater part of the night, and feels comfortable; is still languid, and has no disposition to eat any thing; says he feels sick, and once last evening vomited after drinking some wine and water.

Wound looks exceedingly pale, and the discharge is thin and foetid, for which the carbon and yeast dressings were applied. He has vomited several times to-day, and has some considerable difficulty in swallowing, and complains of a soreness in the wound upon pressure.

9 P.M.—Dressings removed; wound very pale; right arm of the natural temperature; feels occasionally a little numbness in the hand; has

taken very little nourishment during the day; pulse natural as to frequency, but small and feeble; a few minutes after dressing the wound, information was brought that hemorrhage had ensued, and before it could be commanded, he probably lost four ounces of blood. For his restlesness and pain in the bones he was ordered two grains of opium.

Twenty-fifth day.—Has rested well during the night, and is perhaps a little better this morning. The repeated hemorrhages have debilitated him exceedingly, and from the irritable state of the stomach he can take only a very little nourishment. In the morning he was directed the effervescing draught to be repeated every two hours; this allayed the irritability of his stomach, and enabled him to take a little breakfast.

His countenance has altered since the first bleeding surprisingly, his eyes are now heavy, and for the most part fixed; his cheeks are sunken, and a universal pallor has spread itself over his countenance; and from every appearance, a short time will terminate his existence. He has not vomited since early in the morning; is advised to take a little soup, and to drink freely of wine and water; dressings were renewed at 3 o'clock P.M. shortly after which the patient again bled, but not to exceed, however, an ounce. He was dressed with dry lint as usual.

11 P.M.—Patient has not as yet had any sound sleep, is restless and apparently distressed, although he says he feels no pain; breathing is attended with some difficulty; his hands and legs are continually in motion; pulse small and feeble.

Twenty-sixth day, 6 A.M.—Patient has not rested well; is occasionally falling into little slumbers, but is awakened by the least motion: Pulse small and feeble; respiration somewhat laboured; appears to be sinking, seems disinclined to take any thing; legs and arms constantly in motion.

11 A.M.—More feeble than before; has been forced to take a little chocolate; is evidently sinking; wound was dressed, but there was no secretion of pus in it; countenance of the patient foretells his approaching dissolution.

6 P.M.—Is extremely low; respiration very much laboured; is not able to articulate: for the last three hours there has not been such continued throwing of the legs and arms about the bed: he lays in a state of insensibility; *temperature of the two arms the same to the last.*—My pupil, Abraham J. Duryee,[6] the House Surgeon (to whom I am indebt-

---

6. Abraham Jacob Duryea (c. 1800–1822) was a promising young man who died prematurely. He had both a B.A. and an M.A. degree from Yale and

ed for the correct reports, and the most unwearied attention to this case, and whose ingenious application of means for the recovery of many of my patients, will long be held by them in grateful remembrance) having for a few minutes left the patient, he was sent for immediately, as there was another bleeding from the wound, by which he lost probably eight ounces of blood: during the whole time he did not manifest the least appearance of consciousness, nor was the least motion perceptible, except that necessary for respiration and circulation: the hemorrhage was stopped with lint, after removing the former dressings; respiration is now performed with the utmost difficulty, and the patient appears as if every respiration would be the last; he expired at half past six in the afternoon: the temperature of the right arm after death, appeared by the touch to be the same as the left; it was as natural and uniform as other parts of the body.

EXAMINATION OF THE BODY

About eighteen hours after death, I opened his body; there was considerable emaciation, and the surface of the wound was of a dark brown colour, and foetid; the wound was perhaps about one third of its original size; it had been enlarged by the pressure of lint into it, and other means to arrest from time to time the hemorrhage: the ulcer between his shoulders was ill-conditioned.

For the purpose of examining the condition of the aorta, where the arteria innominata is given off, as also the origin of the latter vessel, as well as the state of the pleura at the part about which the ligature had been applied around the artery, the chest was opened in the following manner: after removing the integuments and muscles from the fore part of the chest, the sternum was carefully sawed through about an inch from its upper extremity, and raised by sawing through the ribs below the junction of the cartilages; this removed so much of the front part of the chest as to facilitate and expose fully to view the subsequent steps of the dissection; by thus leaving the clavicles attached, every part connected with the ulcer and great vessels could be seen and examined in situ.

The arch of the aorta and origin of the innominate being fairly exposed, not a vestige of inflammation or its consequences could be discovered, either upon them, the lungs, or the pleura, at any part. An

---

then received his M.D. from New York's College of Physicians and Surgeons in 1819.

incision was next made longitudinally into the aorta opposite the origin of the innominata, and upon introducing a probe cautiously up the latter vessel, it was seen to pass into the cavity of the ulcer; the innominata was then laid open with a pair of scissors into the ulcer; the internal coat of this vessel was smooth and natural about its origin, but for half an inch below where the ligature had cut through the artery, it showed appearances of inflammation, and there was a coagulum adhering with considerable firmness to one of its sides; showing that nature had made an effort to plug up the extremity of so large a vessel, after the adhesion, which no doubt had been effected by the ligature, was swept away by the destructive process of ulceration. The upper extremity of this vessel was considerably diminished in its diameter by the thickened state of its coats, occasioned by the surrounding inflammation. The innominata about half an inch from the aorta, and a little to the left side, gave off an anomalous artery large enough to admit a small size crow-quill.

The ulcer at the bottom was more than twice the size of the wound in the neck; it extended laterally towards the trachea and under the clavicle towards the tumour. The tripod of great vessels, consisting of the innominata, subclavian, and carotid arteries, to the extent of nearly an inch, was dissolved and carried away by the ulceration. The extremities of the two latter vessels were found also to open into the cavity of the ulcer. The upper surface of the pleura was very much thickened by the deposit of newly organized matter, for the safety and protection of the cavity of the thorax. Indeed, instead of having increased the danger of penetrating this membrane, the adhesive inflammation which proceeded the ulcerative, seemed, by the consolidation of cellular membrane, and the addition of new substance, to have more securely and effectually shielded it from danger.

The internal surface of the carotid artery was lined with a coagulum of blood, more than twice the thickness of its coats, and extending above the division into internal and external, so as almost to give them a solid appearance, insomuch that a probe could barely be introduced. The subclavian artery, internally and externally to the disease, was pervious. The brachial and other arteries of the right arm were of their common diameter, and in every respect natural. The external thoracic or mammary arteries, as they went off from the subclavian, were larger than natural: the right internal mammary was pervious, and of the usual appearance. Upon opening into the tumour, which now gave (from its small size) no deformity to the shoulder, the clavicle was involved in it, and found carious, and entirely disunited about the middle. A number of lymphatic glands under the clavicles, and particularly the left, were considerably enlarged and, when cut into, very soft, and evidently in a state of scrophulous suppuration. No other morbid appearances were observed.

Several very important facts are established by this operation—facts which no surgical operation has ever before confirmed. It proves very conclusively, that the heart, the brain, and the right arm, were not the least injured by it, in any of their functions. To tie so large a vessel, so near the heart, might very reasonably be expected to occasion some immediate derangement in the actions of that organ: but it was neither increased or diminished in its contractions, nor did it give rise to the least visible change in his respiration. All this could not have been anticipated. I apprehend there are no ingenuous surgeons, who would not have expected quite a contrary result. For my own part, I must confess that this was to me an anxious moment, when I drew the ligature upon this artery. Indeed, so apprehensive was I that some serious, if not almost immediately fatal consequences, would follow, from arresting so large a proportion of the whole mass of blood suddenly, that I drew the ligature very little at first. But when no change took place in the actions of the heart, or respiration, I felt a confidence in completely intercepting the whole current of blood through this great vessel.

The brain in no operation has been deprived of so large a quantity of blood as in this, and yet it suffered no inconvenience: from the effect of experiments however upon animals, I entertained no fear as to the consequences of my operation upon this organ.

The right arm, as the report of the case from day to day will show, was in no want of a sufficient supply of blood for the purposes of its economy. That circulation went on to a degree adequate to its wants, the natural warmth and function of the skin fully prove; and although at no time could all be satisfied that a pulsation was perceptible in the radial artery, yet many at times were of the opinion, that an occasional undulatory motion was very evident: every one was confident of the distended and elastic feel of this artery, and could plainly see, from pressing on the distended veins upon the back of the hand, that a free circulation of blood was going on: but independent of these evidences, the natural warmth and free perspiration would alone be sufficient to establish the fact.

The route of circulation to the right arm was somewhat different, at first, from what took place after the ulceration had extended. The inosculation of the epigastric and internal mammary must have thrown a considerable retrograde current of blood through the latter vessel into the subclavian directly, and which in all probability passed on into the arm: after the ulceration had extended, this communication was cut off by the destruction of the subclavian to some distance. It was now that the principal supply of blood to the arm must have been derived from the free communication of the intercostals with the thoracic arteries. From the large size of these, as found in the dissection, I apprehend they must have afforded the principal channels through which the blood was conveyed to the arm after the operation: the anastomoses of the infra-scapular and other arteries of the axilla, more or less with small branches of the intercostals, as also the occipital, with small ascending branches from the subclavian, may have given some trifling assistance.

The ulceration which went on so insidiously at the bottom of the wound, was the sole cause of the death of my patient. While the upper part of the wound put on a favourable appearance, and seemed healing, mischief was extending below. The separation of the ligature on the fourteenth day, spontaneously, without being followed by any hemorrhage for a number of days, and not until ulceration had extended, conclusively proves to my mind, that all the purposes of the ligature were completely answered—that adhesion was fully effected. Had it not been for the ulcerative inflammation, no doubt will be entertained, I think, by surgeons, but that my patient would have recovered. From occupation, his constitution was indeed very old, and with an ill-conditioned habit, every thing favoured the process of ulceration. The position of the wound may be said by some to favour this process, but in a sound healthy habit it would only retard the wound in its recovery, but would never promote ulceration.

The practicability and propriety of the operation appear to me to be satisfactorily established by the case: and althought I feel a regret, that none know who have not performed surgical operations, in the fatal termination of it, and especially after the high and just expectations of recovery which it exhibited; yet I am happy in the reflection, as it is the only time it has ever been performed, that it is the bearer of a message to Surgery, containing new and important results.

Case Reports:
From Injuries of
the Head

BENJAMIN WINSLOW DUDLEY, M.D. (1785–1870)

The following case reports were excerpted from the first article of the first volume of the Transylvania Journal of Medicine, *a periodical that made its appearance on our western frontier in 1823. Benjamin Winslow Dudley, the author of this paper, was an unusually competent surgeon and teacher of Lexington, Kentucky, and was for many years the foremost practitioner of his specialty in the western United States. These cases represent an early series of patients for whom craniotomy was performed for the relief of epileptiform seizures (another case was reported at a later date). As such they are a pioneer (and often overlooked) contribution to neurosurgery. This article was the first of a number that appeared under Dudley's name in the* Transylvania Journal of Medicine *on surgical subjects. Most of these contributions demonstrated a conservative surgical philosophy that was both unique and premature for its time.*

Benjamin Winslow Dudley was born in Virginia on April 12, 1785, but moved with his family to Kentucky while he was still an infant. He studied as a pupil under Dr. Frederick Ridgely (1757 – 1824), a leading practitioner of Lexington, and then took his degree in medicine at the University of Pennsylvania in 1804. Dudley practiced for a time in Lexington and then was able to travel to Europe to complete his training as a surgeon. He returned to the United States in 1814. Dudley became the best-known surgeon to practice on this country's western

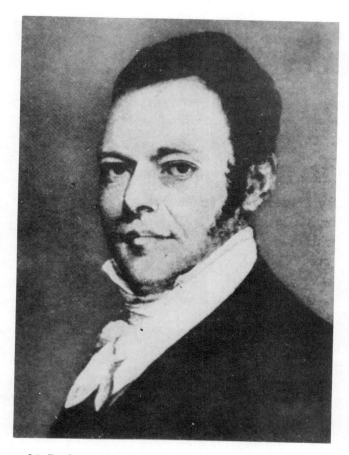

Figure 26. Benjamin Winslow Dudley (1785–1870). (Courtesy New York Academy of Medicine.)

frontier. He contributed greatly to medical education in the expanding midwest and was the heart and soul of the Transylvania Medical School, a flourishing institution that expired with Dudley's death. Dudley was best known as a lithotomist but was thoroughly competent in the entire field of surgery. His practice was restricted to his own specialty, a decided rarity in that day. He died on his estate outside Lexington, Kentucky, on January 20, 1870.

The lengthy paper from which the following case reports were excerpted appeared in the Transylvania Journal of Medicine *(1:7, 1823).*

Case Reports: From Injuries of the Head

In the month of September, 1818, Mr. K., a carpenter of this town, called to consult me on account of a severe pain in the superior and posterior part of the cranium which had afflicted him for nine months. A succession of tumors had at various periods appeared about the seat of the pain. Upon an examination, in place of tumors, two very sensible depressions were discovered on the surface of the skull, attended by extraordinary sensibility in the integuments of the parts. About Christmas all the symptoms became aggravated and severe epileptic convulsions ensued. His convulsions were so frequent and violent in the latter part of winter that it was apprehended he would speedily fall victim to his disease. During the progress of his case he had used large quantities of mercury, both in the form of unguent and of pills, and he was induced to believe that the mercurial unguent had an especial influence in aggravating his convulsions.

In the early part of the winter, I urged the propriety of trephining the cranium,[1] under an impression that a morbid growth on the inner surface of the skull was now aggravating, even if it had not caused his malady. In April he determined as previously advised to submit to an operation. During the months of February, March, and the beginning of April, he was constantly confined with a severe affection of his head attended by violent epileptic fits every five or six days.

---

1. Trephination (or trepanation) was one of the first operations ever performed, and skulls bearing the marks of healed trephine wounds have been found dating back to the neolithic age. The operation apparently has been used continuously since; deterioration after head injury has always been an indication for trephination. Excellent results frequently followed the removal or elevation of depressed bone fragments or the evacuation of clot or fluid. Trephination, in the days before antisepsis, was one of the most important procedures in the surgeon's armamentarium.

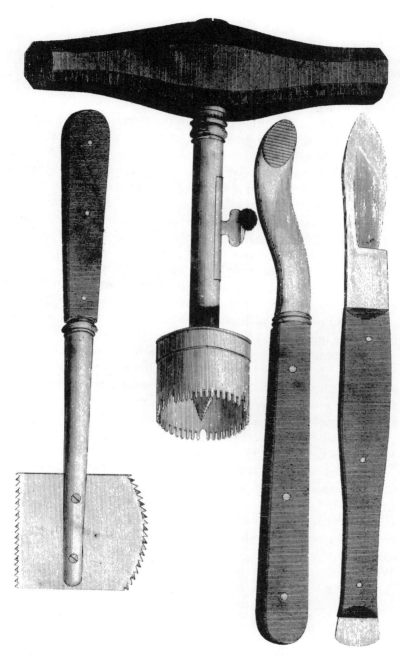

Figure 27. Instruments for trephination. An illustration from Dorsey's *Elements of Surgery* (Philadelphia: W. Brown, printer, 2:180, 1813) showing the instruments used in trephination. These are, from left to right, Hey's saw, trephine, elevator, and scalpel.

The trephine was used on the 16th day of April, two circular pieces
of bone being removed, corresponding with and including those portions which by previous examination seemed to be depressed. The pericranium was remarkably thickened and morbidly sensitive. The bone
was porous and admitted of large processes of this membrane and of
blood vessels to pass directly to the dura mater. The bone removed by
means of the trephine was immediately in the direction of the longitudinal sinus, while there was great difficulty in breaking up the con-
nexions between it and the dura mater.

After the operation was completed I was astonished on turning
my attention to the dura mater, to discover a copious secretion of fluid
which separated that membrane from the surface of the brain more
than half an inch; while that organ in place of giving to the finger a
sense of pulsation, felt as hard and as unyielding as a board. The patient being dressed in the usual way, was put to bed and kept quiet until
the fifth day, when from the establishment of free suppuration the bandages were removed. It was now ascertained on examination that the
fluid beneath the dura mater was absorbed. The brain had regained its
proper level and pulsated with unusual vigour: no convulsion had occurred since the operation. The dressings being renewed, he was ordered a mercurial course of treatment with a view to correct the secretions
and to promote the healthy action of the absorbents. At the expiration
of three months he was perfectly restored to health, having experienced
only two slight attacks of epilepsy during his recovery, while his head,
which had for many months given him excessive pain, caused but little
inconvenience after the operation.

From an occasional intercourse with this patient for many months
after all professional attendance and advice were suspended, I am prepared to pronounce on the cure as radical.[2]

In the spring of 1825, W. T., a young gentleman twenty-one years
of age, in company with his mother, came to this place from South
Carolina; and from the mother was received the following history of
her son's case.

When five years of age, he received a severe blow accidentally on
the superior and middle portion of the left parietal bone. Being at
school, he was able to go home on foot without giving any particular

---

2. For "radical" read "complete"; the radical cure of a hernia, as an example, implied not only that it was reduced but the hernia itself was cured. The
use of "radical" in surgical terminology has undergone a change during recent
years to mean "extended."

manifestations calculated to excite alarm. On the ninth day he became suddenly apoplectic, and paralysis on one side ensued.

The paralytic affection gradually disappeared, so as to leave him in the enjoyment of his faculties, as well corporeal as intellectual, at the expiration of two months; but from that period he became the subject of severe pain in his head, and especially about the seat of the injury he had previously sustained. From this time his constitution became exceedingly delicate and excitable, with the disinclination for excerise, and liability to faintness after the slightest exertions: finally about his fourteenth year, nine years after the reception of the injury, he became the subject of epileptic convulsions. These had ever since continued to recur at irregular intervals of two, three, or four weeks, varying with the occasional causes which for a time invited or retarded their appearance.

He had been but a short time the subject of epilepsy, until a most manifest improvement in his constitution took place.

His personal appearance and constitutional vigour being much changed for the better, his former excitable habit, with his liability to faint after every slight exertion, now left him. But these flattering symptoms were soon followed by a perceptible injury of his intellect, insomuch that it became useless to confine him longer to his studies in school.

The physicians of his vicinity who were consulted, differed in opinion concerning the cause and seat of his malady, as did most of those in the southern states, to whom application was made for professional assistance. The father of the young man had by letter consulted professors Physick and Chapman,[3] who discouraged any effort at relief by an operation, because of the protracted character of the case, while a rigid regard to abstemious living was advised as necessary to render the convulsions more mild in character.

After receiving this history of the situation of the patient from the mother, upon turning to himself with a view to additional information, I observed a stammer in every attempt at enunciation; while his memory had become so entirely treacherous, an event which had transpired within two days, his recollection being good however, in relation to circumstances of his childhood. For most particulars in relation to his

---

3. Nathaniel Chapman (1780–1853) graduated from the University of Pennsylvania in 1801. He became one of Philadelphia's leading physicians and succeeded Benjamin Rush as professor of medicine at the University of Pennsylvania. Chapman held this post for 30 years. He was also a cofounder of the *American Journal of the Medical Sciences,* a journal that thrives today.

daily history, even in reference to the operation of a dose of medicine, it was necessary to consult his mother.

A cicatrix on the side of the scalp pointed out the seat of the original injury. Under all these discouraging circumstances, after a few days preparation, the operation was resorted to on the 10th of May, 1825, to relieve him of an injury, the consequences of which had been accumulating upon him for sixteen years. A small depression of bone appearing manifest, corresponding with the original site of the injury, indicated the point upon which to apply the trephine. The crown of the instrument was made to embrace the depressed bone, which when removed, presented a process projecting from its inner surface about one inch in length, of the size of a small quill at its base, the extremity tipped with soft cartilage. This spiculum of bone had penetrated the dura mater, and communicated with a large preternatural sinus, from whence issued a stream of blood as thick as a man's little finger, which continued to flow from the instant the bone was removed, until from the quantity lost, it was judged proper to check it by means of pressure.

The dura mater was diseased, presenting a dark blue appearance over a space nearly as large as the opening in the cranium made by the trephine; while the sinus beneath appeared to be, from an examination made by the little finger, more than an inch in depth, and of equal width.

The disposition to hemorrhage was checked in a few minutes by means of pressure with the thumb, and being now satisfied that the trephine was not further necessary, it was proposed to cleanse and dress the wound. Before the dressings were applied, an alarming convulsion came on, during the continuance of which, a stream of blood issued through the opening in the dura mater, that projected three or four feet. A second and third convulsion ensued, with like discharge of blood from the opening of the dura mater, before the patient could be placed in bed. For six or eight hours after the operation, he remained in an insensible state, and then his natural feelings and reason returned.

It was now supposed, whatever might be the termination of the case, the cause originally productive of the disease was removed. From bloody water, the discharge from the wound changed in the course of twelve hours to a colourless serum, and for three days and nights in succession, it was so copious as to make it necessary to change towels, pillows, bolsters and sheets, two or three times during the day. Those young gentlemen who assisted in dressing and attending to the case, insisted that the entire amount of serum discharged, could not be less than two gallons. On the morning of the fourth day, the dressings were dry, and in some few hours after, suppuration became manifest. The wound was now dressed with adhesive plaster, which was renewed daily for about thirty days, when it was healed.

The patient had no convulsion after the day on which the operation was performed; a manifest improvement in his memory became perceptible in a few days to all around him. His stammer, which appeared to proceed from an indistinct recollection of things, very suddenly vanished, his eye which had been half closed, heavy, and inanimate, was now sprightly and intelligent. In ten days he left his room, and at the end of six weeks, he returned home in the enjoyment of perfect health; travelling a distance of five hundred miles in the month of July, in ten or twelve days.

A few months after this young gentleman returned home, I was informed that by excess in eating and drinking, together with severe exercise in dancing, a slight epileptic attack was produced.

He is, however, as I have been very lately informed, through a letter received from an individual affected as he formerly was, now in the enjoyment of uninterrupted health.

Gofourth, a young man of Jessamine county, Kentucky, aged twenty-three years, when five years old, received a kick from a horse, which fractured and depressed a portion of the right parietal bone. The immediate symptoms were not particularly alarming, notwithstanding a wound also in the scalp, nor was there any extraordinary defect either in general health or constitutional development, until about the fifteenth year of his age, when, without any assignable cause, he had for the first time an epileptic convulsion.

From that time he continued to be the subject of epilepsy every second, third, and sometimes fourth week, according as the exciting causes acted with more or less intensity. The continuance of epilepsy for eight years, had reduced his constitutional vigour, and rendered his system morbidly excitable. The condition of his mind was still more deplorable, his memory having undergone almost a total extinction. In the latter part of February eighteen hundred and twenty-six, after spending a few days in preparing the system, the operation was performed in the amphitheatre, in the presence of all the class.

The external incision being made, the trephine was applied in such a manner as to cover the larger portion of the depressed bone. In two or three turns of the instrument, the cranium was penetrated in one point of the circle; and through this opening, which could have been closed with the small end of a surgeon's probe, transparent colourless serum flowed during the balance of the operation.

The circular piece of bone being removed, the dura mater was found defective to the extent of a twelve-and-a-half cent piece of silver, which exposed a sinus reaching down to the petrous bone, near the base of the scull. A spinous process projected from the inner table of the bone about half an inch long, its base being of equal dimensions. A small portion of the spinous process was not included by the trephine; this was removed by means of a strong pair of forceps. The sinus in which the serum was collected, was large enough to receive a hen's egg. The patient had two light attacks of epilepsy on the second and third days after the operation; but on the fourth, suppuration was established, the dressings were renewed, and he began to give assurances of a successful issue by a more sprightly and animated countenance. Each successive dressing was accompanied by new evidences of intellectual and corporeal improvement; and at the end of the fourth week, the wound having cicatrised, the patient returned home in the enjoyment of perfect health. Early in the spring season, he accepted a situation as fireman on board a steam-boat trading between Louisville and New Orleans, where he continued until August, when the waters of the Ohio were too low for navigation. Being discharged from this laborious and hazardous occupation, he passed through this place on his return home, and reported himself to me as having enjoyed good health, with an exemption from his former malady.

Obrien, a man of middle age, came to this place in the summer of 1826, and gave the following history of his case. About four years previous to that time, while engaged in raising a house near Cleveland, Ohio, he received by accident, a blow on the side of his head, which deprived him of motion and of the use of his intellect for several weeks. He had scarcely recovered from the immediate effects of the injury, when he was attacked by severe convulsions, while he was never free from pain in his head, jaws, neck, chest, sides, and abdomen. Upon examination, I found most of the muscles of his system in a state of morbid contraction. The organs of speech were exerted with great difficulty and his enunciation was very indistinct.

His senses of taste and smell were nearly destroyed–the fragrance of the rose and the offensiveness of the thorn-apple, were alike to him. His fingers were constantly in a state of semiflexion, while the abdomen was habitually and painfully tumid. I have never seen a patient under any circumstances, who appeared to be the subject of such unceasing agony. For weeks in succession, his convulsions recurred daily, producing most terrific contortions of his entire system. A large cicatrix, with apparent depression, extended in the direction from behind the external canthus of the right eye, to the central portion of the parietal bone of the same side.

After a few days delay with a view to preparation, the trephine was used; nor were there any very remarkable manifestations about the wound, except in the increased vascularity of the dura mater. But in the course of the same evening, after the operation, the patient expressed himself as being "unlocked" in all his limbs; while there was a most pleasing and perfect relief to the organs of speech. On the third day from the operation, suppuration having commenced, the wound was dressed; and thus far the patient gave the strongest manifestations of a speedy recovery, in the relief of all pain in his head, throat, chest and extremities, and in his faculty of deglutition and of speech. The rigidity of the muscles and the tumid condition of the abdomen had also nearly disappeared. About the sixth day from the operation, he experienced a light epileptic convulsion. The relief, however, which had been afforded, was followed by a ravenous appetite, and he was constantly inclined to commit excess in eating, both in the quality and quantity of his food. By the tenth day from the operation, he had so far recovered as to be enabled to take exercise in walking through the town, while he manifested great impatience in being controlled. From the tenth to about the twenty-fifth day after the operation, the patient had several light convulsions. He continued, however, to improve in his general health, and being impatient under farther restraint, withdrew himself secretly from my superintendence, and I have never heard of him since. This case, more than any other which has been under my charge, was attended by a highly deranged secretion of the liver, that rendered it necessary to use liberal and frequently repeated mercurial purgatives; and while the original causes of the affection may have been removed by the operation, I can readily conceive that the convulsions might be continued on account of the morbid condition of the liver. Under such circumstances, if now living, he may be the subject of disease that is under the control of medicine.

Froman, from the neighborhood of Bairdstown in this State, a man of middle age, received a blow on the posterior and superior portion of the left parietal bone, fifteen years ago, and came to this place for professional assistance in April 1827.

According to the best history given by his brother and himself of his case, a manifest defect of his memory was perceived in a few weeks after the accident was sustained; yet, it was two years before convulsions supervened, and these have continued to recur for the last thirteen years at very irregular periods, the patient sometimes having half a dozen a day, yet about every fifteen days, the convulsions are more sensibly severe. At present, he is in a state of fatuity. The tenuity of the integuments upon and immediately surrounding the cicatrix, on the site of the original wound, gave deceptive appearances of slight depression of the scull at this part. When the bone was laid bare, however, in the operation, there was no preternatural appearance, except in the close and morbid attachments of the pericranium. A circular portion of the scull being removed by the trephine, the dura mater presented a healthy appearance, as did the bone also. Perceiving no pulsation in the brain, I pressed my finger on the surface of the dura mater, and discovered a considerable collection of fluid beneath it, which, in the opinion of professor Short[4] and other gentlemen present, separated the brain from its investing membrane, not less than half an inch. On the fifth day from the operation, suppuration was established in the wound. The dressings being now removed, the brain was perceived at its proper level pulsating, while the whole of the fluid was absorbed. The progress of this case was extremely flattering for the first two weeks; after which, in consequence of indulging a craving appetite, and possibly because the operation was partial in its effects, the epileptic convulsions recurred, and thereby the benefits of the effort at relief are rendered extremely problematical. Some months after this patient returned home, I learned that his convulsions were less frequent and more mild in character, than they were previous to the operation.[5]

---

4. Charles Wilkins Short (1794-1863) graduated from the University of Pennsylvania in 1815. He became the dean and professor of materia medica (today's pharmacology) at the Transylvania School of Medicine. He was primarily a botanist, and several plants are named after him.

5. Guillaume de La Motte (1665-1737) of Paris trephined for epilepsy in 1705. His patient was only partially relieved. In 1804, Henry Cline (1750-1827), a pupil of John Hunter, attempted successfully to relieve a patient of the symptoms of epilepsy by trephination. Dudley's experience was the most extensive up to his time, and three out of five of his patients were relieved of their symptoms (another success was reported later). Other surgeons were not so fortunate. In 1852 Stephen Smith (1823-1922), a surgeon of New York, reviewed the literature and found a cure rate of only seven out of twenty-seven cases. As with many diseases in those days, the possibility of a cure made even such a great risk justifiable.

Wounded Intestines

AQUILA TOLAND, M.D. (dates unknown)

I encountered the following case report by chance while searching for something–anything–written by Samuel D. Gross (1805–84) that would be worth incorporating into this anthology. Gross was one of the most commanding figures in American surgery during the last century. He founded the prestigious American Surgical Association, was on the faculty of many medical schools, and ended his career as professor of surgery at Jefferson. He was a great teacher and a prodigious compiler, translator, and writer of texts; but, unfortunately, he was the author of nothing that I considered worth including here.

In 1843 Gross, then professor of surgery at the Louisville Medical Institute in Kentucky (later the Medical School of the University of Louisville), carried out a number of experiments on dogs similiar to those performed by Thomas Smith at the University of Pennsylvania 40 years earlier. A lengthy monograph on intestinal injuries, including his own experimental work, appeared first in four parts in the Western Journal of Medicine and Surgery *("Wounds of the Intestines," 7: 1, 81, 161, and 8: 1, 1843) and then in a text published in Louisville the same year* (An Experimental and Critical Inquiry into the Nature and Treatment of Wounds of the Intestine [*Louisville: Prentice & Weissinger, 1843*]). *In it he mentions the following article; and this is, apparently, the last notice ever taken of Aquila Toland, M.D. and his miraculous cure of a man with four wounds in his small intestine.*

Who was Aquila Toland? All that I have been able to learn about him is contained in the article that follows. Evidently he was a country doctor who practiced in London, Ohio, a few miles west of Columbus. Presumably he had previously learned medicine as an apprentice, for he had treated his patient during the summer of 1836 and he did not receive his M.D. "from the Medical Department of the Cincinnati College" until 1837. This paper was submitted as his inaugural (graduation) thesis. Samuel D. Gross was then the professor of pathological anatomy (pathology) at that school and would have been one of Toland's teachers. Quite possibly it was knowledge of the case that follows that led to Gross's interest in intestinal wounds. This appears to be one of the most severe intra-abdominal wounds ever reported up to that time in which the patient survived. Toland's case report shows a resourceful and capable country doctor at work, and it gives, with its decoction of slippery elm and squirrel broth, an unusual picture of rural surgery in America.

History of a case of Wounded Intestines and Omentum, Successfully Treated.

(Extracted from the inaugural thesis of Aquila Toland, M.D., of Madison County, Ohio, a graduate of the medical department of the Cincinnati College.)

On the 25th of August, 1836, I was called to visit W.B., aged twenty, an athletic young man, of a sanguine temperament, who in handling a scythe in a careless manner, with his foot upon the nib or handle and the point turned towards his body, leant forward, and his foot slipt from its position and forcibly brought the point of the instrument against the abdomen. It pierced the parieties an inch or so above and to the left of the umbilicus, in the line of the fibres of the rectus muscle, about midway between the linea alba and the linea semilunaris. There was a longitudinal wound inflicted through the parieties near five inches in length externally—internally the wound was about three inches and an half. The omentum was perforated, and the small intestines suffered four wounds. The first nearly divided the gut transversely, the second cut it rather more than half off in the same direction, the third made a longitudinal fissure of a about two inches in length, the fourth was mere puncture, but yet sufficient for the escape of the contents of the intestine. The accident occurred in a wild meadow about half a mile from the house, and he was hauled home upon a sled, in as easy a manner as posssible, an attendant being placed by his side for the purpose of supporting his bowels, which had largely protruded. The distance I had to ride was about eight miles, and when I arrived a large mass of the small intestines, together with a portion of the colon and omentum were found in a pile, covered with blood and their own extravasated contents, which had been very abundantly poured out upon them. Nothing had been done for his relief, save only that his friends had taken the precaution to cover his bowels with some linen cloths, to keep them warm and screen them as they supposed from the effects of the atmosphere. In this situation they had lain out near four hours. The omentum being wounded, had thrown out a considerable quantity of blood, and this as well as their own contents which had also been poured out, had dried upon their peritoneal covering. There was a frequent wiry pulse, constant nausea and vomiting, the surface and extremities were colder than usual, and bathed in a clammy perspiration; in short, all the symptoms of strangulated hernia were present and, indeed, there *was* strangulation, for the abdominal muscles, from being divided chiefly in the longitudinal direction of their fibres, had closed upon the protruded mass, more particularly upon the neck of the mesenteric portion of it. From the jejunum which had four perforations, and was at least partially strangulated, there was a constant escape of gaseous and foecal contents. The lips or edges of the wounds in the intestines, presented an everted appearance. This eversion was produced by the elongation of the mucus membrane, which completely covered the cut edges of the peritoneal and muscular coats; in the longitudinal cut the eversion was less apparent.

The accident occurred soon after dinner, and as he had vomited much, what he had eaten was of course ejected; and in consultation with Dr. Wilson,[1] who assisted me in the operation, we came to the conclusion to make soft gentle pressure upon the bowels, in such manner as thoroughly to empty them of their contents, and thereby moderate the symptoms of strangulation, as well as obviate a cause of aggravation to the subsequent inflammation. We, then, by the application of tepid milk and water, cleansed the surface of the bowels from the dried blood and foecal substances, and proceeded to bring the lips of the wounds in the intestines together, by suture. This was done without including the mucous coat. The ligatures used were broad, and composed of very fine flax thread slackly twisted. The lips of the transverse wound, which had so nearly divided the gut, were brought together, and retained in their proper position, by the glover's suture—that is, the

---

1. Dr. Wilson has not been further identified.

ligature was armed at each end, and with a needle of small size, and the points of the needles were carefully entered at each side, on the inner edge of the wound between the mucous and muscular coats, and passed alternately from side to side, the former being pushed back, and not included in the ligature. All the other wounds were brought together by the interrupted suture, the needle being entered as above described.

The next indication, which was to return the bowels into their proper cavity, was now attempted, but found to be impracticable by gentle means, until the wound in the inner parieties which as before observed, was shorter than that externally, was enlarged and this I readily accomplished by a blunt pointed bistory. I have, however, neglected to remark, that the lower and most depending portion of the wound, was abruptly transverse, inclining to the left, in the direction of the superior, anterior, spinous process of the ilium. It was this portion which was enlarged. The edges of the longitudinal wound were then brought into apposition, and retained by the quilled suture. The transverse portion of the wound was left open, with a view to permit the escape of any extravasated matter, which might already exist in the peritoneal cavity, be produced by effusion or suppuration.

Immediately upon the return of the bowels, the patient expressed himself relieved. The nausea and vomiting, which had been so urgent, and which were greatly aggravated during the operation, now abated; there was an increase in the volume of the pulse, and its frequency was diminished. The surface of the body, which had been bathed in a profuse cold clammy perspiration, now appeared gradually to regain its activity and his extremities became warm. Previous to the commencement of the operation, opium both in the solid and liquid form, had been administered, but had been speedily rejected; one grain and an half of pulverized opium was now given and retained, which apppeared to have a tranquilizing effect. Mucilaginous drinks composed of the recent bark of the elm (Ulmus Americana) in cold water, were directed for his common drink,[2] and cold injections of the same substance were ordered to be thrown into the rectum every three hours. It was now about sun down, and I left him for the night.

August 26th. This morning about 10 o'clock, I visited him. He had

---

2. Toland's taxonomy was incorrect: the slippery or red elm (*Ulmus rubra*) is a smaller and separate species than the stately white elm (*Ulmus americana*). The dried, finely ground, slippery inner bark of the former was a very important medicinal in the days before antibiotics. It was used to treat a number of conditions, including diarrheas and particularly sore throat (and by extension, febrile illnesses in general). The *United States Dispensatory*, 11th ed. (Philadelphia: Wood & Bache, 1858) notes that the mucilaginous

passed a bad night; experienced several severe chills, and now had a violent fever; his pulse was frequent and rather tense, the tongue dry, red at the tip and round the edges, with a streak of brown fur along the middle; the skin was dry, the urine rather scanty and high colored.

He complained of some headache, had drunk largely of the cold elm bark water, but was still thirsty, and there was an uneasy sense of tension and fullness, in the abdomen. I immediately opened a vein, and drew about twenty ounces of blood in a full stream, which produced a decided impression upon the pulse, attended with slight syncope, and was followed by a copious perspiration. I gave him no medicine, but directed the mucilage to be continued for his common drink, cold injections[3] of the same to be administered every three hours; and left particular directions, that he be allowed no other nourishment during my absence.

27th, 10 o'clock. He had been more comfortable, obtained some refreshing sleep through the night, there was not much fever, his tongue was moist, and there was rather less thirst, but he still called, frequently, for the elm water. He remarked, that the cold ejections were in the highest degree refreshing, and desired me to permit them to be used more frequently. There had been no alvine discharge, there was a great fulness and tension in the hypogastriac region, and upon introducing a blunt pointed probe into the transverse wound, which had been left open, I discovered that a portion of omentum had insinuated itself into the wound and closed the aperture. When this was pushed back, a copious discharge of purulent matter mixed with blood issued from the wound, which speedily relaxed the distention, and relieved the oppression. The mucilaginous drink and injections were directed to be continued, and no other nourishment was allowed.

28th. He had been pretty comfortable through the night, had some refreshing sleep and but little fever, his pulse was yet a little too frequent, there had been several copious discharges from the wound; and he now for the first time, expressed a desire for some nourishment, but I directed only a tea spoonful of gum arabic with the same quantity of sugar, dissolved in cold elm water, to be given every three hours by way of diet—the other treatment to be continued.

---

extract is highly nutritious and quite capable of sustaining life. Slippery elm bark was also widely—and apparently effectively—used in surgery as a wound dressing (James Thacher, *The American New Dispensatory,* Boston: T. B. Wait, 1810).

3. "Injection" refers to rectal administration rather than percutaneous, as we use the term today.

29th. He was doing well; had but little fever, and the wound still discharged freely, whenever the omentum was pushed back, and this was directed to be done frequently in my absence. I still limited him to the same quantity of gum arabic,[4] and the same quantity of sugar as before, and directed the former treatment to be continued.

30th. Every thing going well, the wound still discharging freely when opened, and no change made in the treatment.

31st. No fever. There has been a free discharge from his bowels, for the first time since the accident. The dejection was dark and offensive, his appetite was excellent, and I now directed, at his own urgent request, that he be allowed a pint of squirrel broth in broken doses, at regular intervals, in addition to his former allowance, the other treatment as before to be continued.

Sept. 1. He was worse; had slept but little, his pulse was considerably accelerated; and his tongue rather dry, the thirst had increased, and his appetite failed; the wound still continued to discharge freely, and threw out purulent matter of little consistence, colored with blood. I prohibited the broth and desired him to confine himself to the gum and sugar as before, the other treatment being continued.

2d. There was an abatement of fever, no thirst, and his appetite had returned, there had been another alvine discharge.

3d. No fever or distention of the abdomen, his appetite fine, and rather hard to control—the treatment and diet continued.

4th. Symptoms all favorable; very hungry; there was but little discharge from the wound, which was now nearly closed by adhesion withe the omentum. I now allowed him an ounce of the gum arabic with the same quantity of sugar, and continued the treatment as before directed.

5th. The wound nearly closed; but little discharge and no sense of fullness; all the other symptoms favorable; his appetite was very urgent, and he complained of starvation. I now increased his allowance of gum and sugar, and applying a broad bandage round his abdomen, permitted him to exercise a little, by walking his room when he chose; for he had been confined to the recumbent position ever since the occurrence of the accident.

6th. He had been using some exercise; his only complaint was the want of food; his bowels were in a good condition. I allowed him

---

4. Gum arabic is the dried sap of the acacia tree. Its medical and nutritive properties were considered to be identical to those listed above for slippery elm.

as much of the gum and sugar as he chose, and the cold injections were discontinued.

7th. Did not visit him. 8th. Found him quite well, walking about, but still very hungry; there was no inconvenience whatever experienced in the abdomen, and the rigid abstinence to which he had been subjected for fourteen days, was commuted for a more generous diet of mush and milk.

The wound was now nearly cicatrised; there was no inconvenience experienced in the region where it was inflicted, and his bowels were regular, and my attendance was no longer necessary. Some weeks afterwards I saw him in excellent health, in which condition, as I am informed, he still continues....

February, 1837.

[The last four pages of Dr. Toland's article have been omitted. In them he rambles on about the virtues of the mucilage extracted from the inner bark of the slippery elm tree and the importance of providing drainage "when effusion takes place into the peritoneal cavity" (certainly lifesaving for this patient) and then speculates on the possible value of abdominal section for a number of pathologic conditions, including strangulated hernia and volvulus. He can reasonably be excused for writing in this fashion some years before the coming of anesthesia and clean surgery: his patient's recovery had provided him with a glimpse of the future.]

Case Reports of the Massachusetts General Hospital Before 1846

HENRY H. A. BEACH, M.D. (1844–1910)

The following case reports were collected from the surgical records of the Massachusetts General Hospital by Dr. Henry Beach and were published during the observance of the fiftieth anniversary of the first public demonstration of ether anesthesia. These cases present representative operations performed during the preanesthetic era. Few persons now living can imagine the pain experienced by the patients who were the subjects of these reports. This aspect of surgery is often forgotten as one reads of surgical tours de force carried out in the days before anesthesia became available. The terrible suffering that was an inevitable part of surgery mercifully disappeared, almost overnight, after the demonstration of the anesthetic properties of sulfuric ether in 1846.

Dr. Henry Beach graduated from Harvard Medical School in 1865 and became a house pupil at the Massachusetts General Hospital. He later became a surgeon on the hospital staff. His paper on the case reports of the Massachusetts General Hospital is included here in a somewhat abridged form. It appeared in the Boston Medical and Surgical Journal *(136:11) in 1897.*

Excerpts from the Surgical Records of the Massachusetts General Hospital Before 1846

An eye-witness of many a bloody struggle between operators, patients and assistants in and out of hospitals, has characterized the fearful scenes that commonly occurred before the days of anesthesia, as fights exhausting alike to all concerned, but to which suffering humanity willingly turned for the relief of deformity, pain and the saving of life.

The grim associations of the old operating-theatre have been dispersed by what Sir Joseph Lister calls "the priceless blessing to mankind from America."

Present generations have appeared with the birthright of anesthesia, sunshine and air. Few living witnesses can paint for them a perspective of surgery without anesthesia, describe the wonder and astonishment it produced, or its power in developing the science and art of surgery.

A short review of the earlier records may supply facts that will revive the atmosphere of the period and convey some idea of the relief that ether brought, alike to patient and surgeon—whose great and stern duty it was to be self-forgetful, strong and faithful while inflicting the worst tortures upon suffering men, women and children.

The first surgical record of the Massachusetts General Hospital was a folio volume of 247 pages. It was sufficiently large to contain the histories of surgical patients admitted in the years 1821, 1822 and 1823. At the present time, six volumes of very nearly the same size are used in making the records of eight or nine months. The operations to be described were selected with care after an examination of every record of surgical cases admitted between the establishment of the hospital and the year 1846.

The first history recorded is that of a seaman who had been afflicted with hemorrhoids for eleven years. His many voyages to India, China, the West Indies and America in that time were complicated with much pain, tenesmus, bleeding, debility, difficulty in walking, and at times complete disability. Purgative medicines were continually necessary for his comfort.

An examination was made in order to ascertain the cause of his complaint. A stricture was found to exist in the rectum two or three inches from the verge of the anus, which with great difficulty would admit the tip of the forefinger. Several tubercles were found around the anus. Three of them were removed, first passing a curved needle with a large ligature through them and drawing them out in order to extirpate them at their bases with a knife. Very little blood was lost. Light dressing. Five days after, hemorrhage of a pint of blood, checked by cold applications and injections of a solution of sulphate of copper. Bougies were passed to dilate the stricture, as the wounds gradually healed.

Patient discharged cured.

The second patient was a young man who had suffered intolerably for a year with symptoms of stone in the bladder.[1] They had followed the introduction of a bean into the bladder with the intention of dilating an obstructed urethra. The obstruction had followed a slight injury of the urethra received from a fall. The record is illustrative of the care taken in preparing for an operation and exemplifies the surgical therapeutica of the times.

On the 8th of October a convention of the consulting staff (seven in number) was held, but the stone was not felt and the operation was postponed. In the following week, after an injection of the bowels, the sound was passed and heard to strike distinctly upon a stone. The operation was decided upon for October 18th at 12 o'clock.

MEMORANDUM OF ARTICLES, ETC., TO BE IN READINESS FOR THE OPERATION

A heavy table; table for dressings; pillows, blankets and sheets; binders, sponges, lint compresses and bandages, towels, oil, ice, syringe, ligatures, warm and cold water, wine and water, warm barley-water, basins, blood-catcher, coat.

INSTRUMENTS

Staff-knife, pointed knife, Cooper's knife, probe, pointed bistoury, gorget, forceps, scoop, sound, needles, tenaculum, canula, needles and forceps.

---

1. This patient, the second to be operated on in the Massachusetts General Hospital, was a young man named Elisha Goodnow. He entered the hospital in September, 1821, as a patient of John Collins Warren (q.v.). Goodnow survived his surgery for bladder stone, and in later life became a wealthy merchant in Boston. He died in 1851 and left the greater part of his estate for the founding of a city hospital. The ultimate result of Goodnow's beneficence was the Boston City Hospital (1864). Undoubtedly his experience as a youth impressed him with the need for good hospital facilities.

PREPARATION

The patient, well-purged the day before, early in the morning of the operation should have a good injection. After this has operated, a string must be tied on the penis four hours before the operation to retain the urine. The hair must have been well-shaved. Laudanum injected. 120 drops to the cup.

ARRANGEMENT OF PATIENT

Assistant adjusts head, secures the feet. Two at shoulders. Staff introduced. Assistant holds it straight; then to the right; then carries the handle down; retains it until ordered, touching the stone.

OPERATION

Tighten skin, take knife. Incision of four inches deep above. Cut transversus, avoid rectum, feel bulb, touch staff, lay bare staff. Introduce probe-knife flat, and push into bladder. Observe urine. Cut gently towards ischium, following knife with the forefinger into the bladder. Enlarge if necessary. Scoop or forceps introduced. Staff withdrawn, first touch stone. Carry forceps along staff to stone, finger in the wound, finger in the rectum. Search stone, low down. Withdraw downward. Dressing, lint in wound. Patient untied.

The stone was small, and broke during its extraction; the remainder was removed with difficulty with a scoop, and the bladder syringed out with warm water. The latter gave great pain, and did not appear to remove any fragments of stone. The patient expressed great pain in every part of the operation as he had done in sounding. One hundred and eighty drops of laudanum were given to relieve pain at intervals after the operation.

October 19th (the following day). Complains of severe pain in the bowels and hypogastric region. Slight flush on the cheeks. Sixteen ounces of blood taken from the arm. Tartrate of soda and potash, half an ounce every three hours until a discharge from the bowels occurs. At 5 P.M., a small discharge. No flush on the face. Skin warm. No opiate.

Hyd. submur .... gr. xii
Pulv. opii .... gr. iii
Ft pil, no. xii. Take one every three hours.

October 20th. Much better. No flush on the face. Slept well. Had three discharges from bowels.

Tartrate of soda and potash .... ℥ss at once.
                        Pills as before.

Evening: Skin warm. An injection of one pint of gruel with a table-spoonful of salt wine-glass of molasses and sweet-oil. Suffered from great pain after the injection. In fifteen minutes one-half came away; pain continued but not so violent.

October 21st. Had three discharges during the night. Evening:

Tartrate of soda and potash .... ℥ss

October 22d. A little sallow in the face. Pulse 77, quick, but not hard. Suppuration going on well in the wound. Evening, pulse 80, a little hard.

Tartrate of soda and potash .... ℥ss
                        Pills as before.

October 23d. No evacuation from the bowels.

Tartrate of soda and potash .... ℥ss
                        Immediately.
At 1 P.M., as before, gums sore. Omit pills.

Tartrate of soda and potash .... ℥ss

At 7 P.M., considerable pain and movement of the bowels. One small discharge. Fomentations applied.

Tartrate of soda and potash .... ℥ss
                        Immediately.

At 8 P.M., medicine not operated. Complains of wind in bowels, with pain. Pulse 90, a little hard and more full.

Tartrate of soda and potash .... ℥ss

Midnight: Great pain in the bowels; very restless; pain in the wound. Pulse 100. Take twelve ounces of blood from the arm. Fulness of pulse subsides. Pain continues. Forty drops of laudanum.

October 24th. Medicine operated four times toward morning. Considerable pain all night. Slept half an hour. Pulse 92. No pill this

A.M. Take one tonight. At 5 P.M., pulse as before. Tongue moist. Pain and soreness in the bowels.

> Vini antimonii 3i
> Spt. nit. eth.
> Camph. tr. opii ^{aa} .... 3ss M.
>   Thirty drops every two hours until asleep.

Wounds look better. Hot fomentations, with tansy and wormwood.

October 25th. Took drops twice. Bowels easier. Sleeps considerably. Pulse 120, more hard. White fur on tongue; edges well defined. Mercurial fetor in the breath. Wound looks well; edges not much swollen; good granulations shooting up. Urine passes freely from wound.

> Olei ricini .... ℥ss
> Essent. menth. pip. .... gtt. x
>   Every three hours until it operates.

October 26th. Mouth and throat very sore. Oil operated twice. Pulse 120, hard. Tongue as before.

Evening: More pain in bowels. Hot fomentations. Abdomen rather tense. Skin hot and sweating. Cold chills. Pulse as before. Brown fur on tongue. Very thirsty. Blister to abdomen. Ol. ricini half an ounce.

October 27th. Blister on four and one-half hours. Five discharges in the night. Wound inclined to heal.

October 28th. Countenance better. No pain in bowels. Pulse 120, less full. Tongue moist. Mouth and throat more inflamed.

> Olei ricini .... ℥ss

October 29th. Slept well. No pain but in mouth and fauces. Pulse 108, not hard. No discharge from bowels.

> Pulv. rhei 3i
> Aq. bul. 3ii
> Aq. cinnan. .... 3i M.

October 30th. Pulse 92. No pain in bowels.

October 31st. Discharge of urine by urethra. No movement of bowels.

> Olei ricini .... ℥ss

November 1st. Pulse 112. Wound diminishing. Suppuration healthy. Medicine operated twice.

November 2d. Good night. No movement of bowels.

Olei ricini . . . . ℥ss

November 3d. Two operations from oil. Face and throat still painful. Little salivation.

November 4th. One discharge from bowels. Pulse 90. Pains as
yesterday.

November 5th. Pulse 88. Considerable wind in the bowels last
night.

Olei ricini 3ii
Comp. tr. senna 3i
Essent. menth. pip. . . . . gtt. x M.

November 6th. Face sore without pain. Pulse 82. Good night.
Medicine operated twice yesterday.

November 7th. Face better. Pulse 86. Appetite improving.

November 8th. No discharge from bowels. Symptoms same.

November 9th. Disposition to diarrhea. Pulse 85.

November 10th. Pulse 76. One stool yesterday and one in the night.
Urine passes freely through the urethra.

During the following six weeks his progress had the usual inter-
ruptions of no movement, cathartics, movements, diarrhea, the wound
in the meantime becoming firmly healed. He left the hospital well.[2]

The next case of interest was one of popliteal aneurism. The preparation for operation consisted of a bath, clearing the bowels for a few
days, opium to relieve pain, and eight ounces of blood from the left arm
three days before the time appointed. Two hours before the operation
the patient (a woman) took six grains of opium; and as the muscles
were relaxed so that their course could not be determined, the place for

---

2. The postoperative care that this patient received was standard for
the era. The various medicines given Elisha Goodnow, in order of their
administration, were powdered opium mixed with calomel (mercurous
chloride); the latter functioned as a purge. The rationale for mixing these
two drugs may have been to offset the constipating effect of the opiate with a
cathartic. Next, a milder cathartic, sodium and potassium tartrate salts,
was administered. On the evening of the second postoperative day, a nutrient
enema was given. Understandably, this was painful.

By October 24th the purgatives were producing the desired results.
That evening antimony wine (antimony tartrate in sherry), a diaphoretic, was

making the incision was settled by carrying a line from the point of the inguinal artery in the groin down to the inner edge of the patella. Another line was carried from the anterior superior spinous process of ilium to the back part of the internal condyle. One inch and a half below the point of meeting of these two lines, the incision began, and was extended upward nearly three inches toward the inguinal artery (left side). The usual dissection for tying the femoral artery was made and afterward closed. A flannel bandage was applied, and forty drops of laudanum given. The wound was healed by first intention above and below the ligature. She left the hospital cured of her aneurism.

The operation for fistula ani was commonly done with giving opium or spirit.

C. B., an officer of the frigate *Constitution*, entered the hospital October 25, 1821, with urethritis; and he left it, cured, on November 9th.

C. L., male, adult, was admitted December 7, 1821, with dislocation of the left femur. The accident occurred in September, when he was thrown from a horse, and while lying on his back received the body of the horse across his thigh. His physician recognized the dislocation. The leg remained fixed in an oblique position with respect to his body; he had not the least command of it, and was in considerable pain.

The physician immediately undertook the reduction, and after about ten minutes of considerable force told him that it was reduced. The patient experienced no alleviation of his pain, neither had he the power of motion in the limb; it still remained in the same position. Not satisfied, he sent for another physician who arrived in four hours, and he declared the dislocation to be still unreduced. He immediately bled the patient about twelve ounces, and then undertook the reduction. After trying a short time, he told the patient that it was then reduced, and the patient agreed that it was. The leg could be brought nearer the other; but still there was a tendency to the oblique position—a constant

---

administered along with an anodyne consisting of paregoric mixed with ethyl nitrate and alcohol. The following day the patient was started on castor oil mixed with a tincture of oil of peppermint. This had the desired effect. By October 26th he was showing the effects of his wound infection. A blistering poultice, probably of cantharides, was used. His sore mouth and throat may have been caused by the mercury he had been given several days earlier.

His physicians continued to worry about his bowels. They followed castor oil with powdered rhubarb, then more castor oil; then composite tincture of senna (which also contained jalap, still another cathartic) was added. He was finally discharged, nine weeks after his surgery.

inclination outward. A bandage was put about the knees to keep the thighs together. This physician then left him. He felt some relieved, and was able to sleep some that night. The next day he was again bled about a pint, and took some purgative medicine. He was then seen by the physician who first examined him, and told that the bone was broken in the neck. The patient lay on his back for fourteen days after, and then began to walk with crutches. The second physician examined him again after eight days, and told him that he was doing well. He came again in about ten days and said the same, although the patient had then no command over his leg.

About two months from the time of the accident, on visiting him his physician ascertained that the affected leg was longer than the sound one; he then told him that the thigh was not reduced. No efforts had since been made for its reduction. His health otherwise was good. Upon examination it was ascertained that the femur was dislocated and the direction as far as could be ascertained was downwards and backwards, in consequence of which the affected limb was longer than the sound one. The head of the bone was distinctly felt through the inferior border of the gluteus muscle. Considering the time that had elapsed since the accident and the difficulty of reduction of dislocations in this direction even when recent, it was thought advisable not to undertake an operation; but the patient being very anxious to have a trial made, and still desiring it after it was stated to him that there was hardly a possibility of succeeding, it was thought justifiable to attempt the reduction of the bone. On the day of the admission of the patient he was ordered to take

Magnesae sulph. . . . . ℥i
Fol. sennae . . . . ℥ss

and to live light; next day a warm bath was ordered. At two o'clock he began taking tart. antim., gr. i, every ten minutes, until the operation. He took five grains, when vomiting was induced. At three o'clock was bled to sixteen ounces, but no faintness was produced.[3] The operation was immediately proceeded with, and after continuing it about an hour the case was abandoned as hopeless.

December 10th. Discharged by request.

---

3. Bleeding was frequently used as a form of anesthesia, especially for the reduction of dislocations. Phlebotomy was carried out with the patient in an upright position and continued until syncope ensued. Then, quickly, while the patient was both unconscious and relaxed, reduction was attempted.

This case became celebrated through the suit of the patient against the two physicians who first attended him, for damages, contrary to the advice of Dr. Warren.[4] In the testimony given Dr. Warren maintained the fact of dislocation, and in that view of the case he was supported by the consulting surgeons of the hospital. The juries disagreed, and the patient lived with a shortened and partly-flexed leg until thirty-seven years afterward, when at his death, Dr. J. Mason Warren[5] was notified by his friends that an examination was desired. At Dr. Warren's request, Dr. H. K. Oliver[6] went to Ellsworth, Me., and removed the pelvis with the upper part of the femur of each side, and brought the mass to Boston for a careful dissection of the parts. In the course of the dissection Dr. Warren's diagnosis of dislocation was verified; and after the bones had been macerated they were mounted and deposited in the museum of the Harvard Medical School.[7] An interesting account of the case and the dissection of the specimen, with a plate illustrating the latter, may be found on page 372 of "Surgical Observations, with Cases," by J. Mason Warren, M.D.

In a case of gangrene of the foot and leg following a compound fracture of both bones of the leg, the following preparations were made before amputating the limb: "The patient was gently purged with tincture of rhubarb the day before, supported by some wine and water and good broth. Laudanum, if necessary. Forty minutes before operation

---

4. John Collins Warren (1778–1856), professor of surgery at Harvard Medical School. See page 174 and footnote 10, page 189.

5. Jonathan Mason Warren (1811–1867) was John Collins Warren's son. He graduated with an M.D. from Harvard in 1832. A staff surgeon of the Massachusetts General Hospital, J. M. Warren was best known as a pioneer in plastic and reconstructive surgery.

6. Henry Kemble Oliver (1830–1919), M.D., Harvard, 1855. Oliver was a visiting physician at the Massachusetts General Hospital and later became the first instructor in laryngology at Harvard.

7. This became one of the most famous medicolegal cases in New England's history. The patient, Charles Lowell, apparently was a contentious malcontent. He eventually (despite J. C. Warren's advice to the contrary) sued the two Maine physicians who had first treated him. Warren reluctantly testified that the dislocation had not been reduced by the defendants. Nathan Smith (q.v.) appeared for the defending physicians and stated that the injury was not a dislocation but was a fracture and that reduction could not have been accomplished. A hung jury resulted and the defendants were thus freed of obligation. Despite Beach's comments above, examination of the specimen reveals that both expert witnesses were correct—a dislocation was indeed present, as was a fracture of the acetabulum that would probably have prevented reduction. (O. S. Hayward, *New England Journal of Medicine*, 261: 489, 1959).

a strong dose of laudanum was given before being carried to the operating-theatre at ten o'clock with dressings on except pillows and cradle. Laid on table, with his hands raised and held by two persons; knees six inches below the edge of table; each leg supported by an assistant."

A woman of forty-nine entered, with a tumor of the breast, April 24th. All things being ready, operation commenced by making a semilunar incision from the axilla to the sternum, and a similar one from the same point above the nipple. The tumor was dissected out with about one-third of the breast, beginning at the sternal part and advancing toward the axilla. Several glands there were enlarged and indurated. They were taken out (a foreshadowing of the modern operation).

Compound fracture of both patellae. The injury was caused by the kick of a horse. A loose portion of the right bone removed. Both knees became much swollen. Had been bled freely. Alkaline cathartic. Calomel and opium every three hours. Leeches to the joints. Gruel and tea. No solid food. Apply a wash to the joints of plumbi acet. Profuse suppuration of the right joint followed. Discharged well, in two and one-half months, with good union.

In the description of the excision of a considerable tumor of the lower jaw from a man about thirty-four years old, the record states that the operation was performed and the wound dressed in forty-five minutes—rather tedious to the patient from the proximity of the tumor to an important artery and other parts of consequence. It was borne, on the whole, with a good deal of fortitude. During the operation the patient occasionally took wine and water to drink.

For the removal of piles in another case, a springhook was now passed through the largest tumor and drawn downwards, which exposed its full extent. The tumor was then removed by a single excision with a scalpel, and with the loss of a small quantity of blood. The others were treated in the same way. The patient was allowed a little wine and water for faintness.

During an operation for fistula in ano upon a young man, the integuments and a portion of the cellular substance was divided for the space of half an inch towards the anus and through the whole depth of the ulcer. No obstacle now presenting, the patient being secured upon the bed by five assistants, one at each lower and upper extremity and one at the head and one on each side to assist in extending the parts, an attempt was made to thrust the bistoury through the coats of the rectum; but such was the resistance and the danger of breaking the instruments that a further attempt was useless. A careful dissection was, however, made. The patient during the operation complained of great pain, but bore it well.

The large variety of operations undertaken at the hospital included a number for cataract, from one of which the notes are as follows:

A woman of seventy-five years entered the hospital November 4th. From then until the 27th, when the operation was performed, she was purged and dieted. The eyelids, which were somewhat irritated, were treated, and the pupils kept well dilated by the external application of a preparation of belladonna. The operation was done by breaking up the cataracts with a needle and pushing the fragments into the anterior chamber. This was accomplished without much pain to the patient. Later, as the right eye did not clear up satisfactorily, the operation was repeated, and the cataract, which was very firm, depressed into the vitreous. A successful result occurred.

In another case, during the removal of some carious bone from a rib, the patient was given eighty drops of laudanum forty-five minutes previously. Being fixed upon the table and secured, by three assistants, the bone was exposed and the carious portion removed by chisel and forceps. The operation was borne with a good deal of fortitude.

Large fatty tumor of abdomen. The patient, a young woman, was given forty drops of laudanum half an hour before operating. The incision required was twelve inches, and she was held by three assistants. For most of the time during the operation was very uneasy and complained of great thirst and exhibited some signs of delirium. After being removed to her bed she became more tranquil.

In a case of aneurism, during the dissection necessary to expose the iliac artery (the patient having previously taken an opiate), when the time arrived to open the sheath of the vessel "the patient was directed to keep himself perfectly still at the moment when a division of the sheath was made over the artery in order to lay bare the coats of the artery and to separate it so as to pass the aneurismal needle completely around it and under its sheath, after which, the ligature was tied with a double knot. The patient endured the operation with considerable firmness."

An early employment of surface thermometry occurs in the subsequent treatment of the case when the following entry is made:

"February 20, 1823. Temperature of the limbs by the thermometer as follows; right limb, just below groin inside, 98°, at sole of foot, 96°; left limb (sound), inside of thigh, 97°, at sole of foot, 94°."[8]

---

8. Clinical thermometry was not as new as Dr. Beach suggests. It was used as early as 1626 by Sanctorius (1561–1636) in Italy to study disease. John Syng Dorsey (q.v.) of Philadelphia used it in 1811 in the same manner as used here (see page 72).

The ligature came away on the nineteenth day, there having been abundant suppuration.

March 18th. Limbs both alike as to strength and temperature. Discharged cured.

Nerve section. The case was one of severe neuralgia of the fifth pair. After the facial nerve had been severed at the point where it emerges from the skull, there was so much suffering that another operation was undertaken.

February 26, 1823. The patient having taken three grains of opium was seated in a convenient chair and an incision made beginning just below the zygomatic process of the os temporis and over the body of the inferior maxillary bone on the right side.

The first incision through the integuments and subjacent cellular membrane exposed the anterior portion of the parotid gland and the fibres of the masseter muscle. The dissection was then continued through the glands dividing the duct and thence carried through the muscle to the bone without dividing any considerable artery except one which was secured by a ligature. The great facial artery was exposed in the upper part of the wound. The bone being laid bare of the muscles which covered the spot opposite to the foramen for the passage of the inferior maxillary nerve into the bone, the raspatory was applied, and the periosteum removed. The trephine was next applied, and the bone perforated just opposite to the foramen, as was shown by a furrow or notch in that portion of the bone which was removed, bringing with it a portion of the nerve with one of its branches. The remaining part of the nerve was then drawn out by the forceps and cut off at the foramen, and the other end divided, making the piece removed about half an inch long and something more. The dividend ends of the parotid duct were brought together by a suture. The patient walked to his room pretty well satisfied that the desired relief was obtained. Discharged cured.

Necrosis of the tibia. The necessity of a protracted operation without anesthesia is well illustrated by the next case described.

The patient (a man) was placed upon the table and held by assistants. Surgeon first made an examination with probe, learned the extent of the dead bone and the firmness and strength of the living bone. He then commenced the operation by making a longitudinal incision through the integuments of about four inches, which he afterwards crossed with another of two inches, and then carefully dissected up the integuments and exposed the bone, which proved to be thick and firm. The sequestrum was completely encased, excepting the orifices where the matter escaped. To effect the removal of this, the raspatory was applied to the external surface of the bone. The trephine was then used and the chisel and gouge until a portion of the living bone was taken out and a part of the dead bone laid bare. A probe was again passed in, a further examination made, and the cavity ascertained to be well filled with the old bone. The operator proceeded to the removal of more of the new-formed bone using one of Hey's saws, gouge, chisel, etc., as particular circumstances required. At the same time incisions through the integuments were carried further, others made cross-wise and the flaps dissected up.

Though a good part of the sequestrum was now exhibited, it was found necessary to divide it before it could be taken out. It was accordingly done with Hey's saw,[9] and two portions of the bone extracted without any difficulty. In consequence of the ragged edges of the dead bone being strongly interlocked in those of the new-formed bone, successive portions of the sound bone were again and again removed by the same instruments until the whole sequestrum was extracted and the operation completed. The dead portion of the bone was found to extend nearly the whole length of the tibia, and the newly-formed bone sufficient for the strength of the limb.

The patient was conveyed to his bed much exhausted. During the operation his strength was supported with wine. The operation continued about two hours, and was borne by the patient with great fortitude.

Some of the difficulties in operating for cataract are shown by the next case, which was that of a child.

April 26th. The usual preparation being made, seats adjusted and the child held by a female sitting in a chair, the speculum was applied, and the surgeon passed the needle into the eye, puncturing and dividing the cataract. During the operation the child made much resistance, with cries. The upper eyelid was inverted, which together with the tears almost entirely obstructed the site of the operation. Occasionally the opaque spot appeared to view, and was very well lacerated. Small compresses of lint were applied with bandages around the head and in a short time, the child was perfectly quiet.

The following quotation is made from the description of another case of double cataract: "Depressing the cataract was somewhat embarrassed from the circumstance that the patient, a woman of sixty-five, during the operation sunk a little forward in the chair,

---

9. "Hey's saw" was devised by William Hey (1736–1819), surgeon of Leeds, England. Itw was a small, hatchet-shaped instrument used for enlarging bone defects (see Fig. 27).

which of course depressed the head and altered its position in such a way that the operator was obliged to raise his head, which gave only an imperfect support to his elbow and proved rather inconvenient. The operation for depression was performed on the right eye with the left hand of the operator."

In another double cataract operation the "patient suffered considerably during the operation upon the left eye, very little in that of the right."

Dr. Warren's biographer tells us that not an eye was lost by cataract operations.

Shoulder-joint dislocation. The patient was a man sixty-two years old, and the dislocation had existed eight weeks. It was subcoracoid. Magnesiae sulph. sol., qs. Warm bath.

"Tomorrow at 10 let him be bled in the erect position so as to faint. At 11 take 1 grain of tartarized antimony every fifteen minutes until nauseated. Operation at 12.

"Patient placed upon a stool. Pulleys and straps applied. Padded belt under the axilla, and secured to opposite wall. Extension then made by pulleys attached to a strap buckled at the arm, the latter at right angle with the body. The muscles became relaxed very considerably, and an effort was made, by bringing the arm forward and upward to replace the bone, but ineffectually.

"Extension was next made nearly in front of the patient, downward, and a powerful, but gradual, extension made, but without reducing the bone. The patient suffered much pain from the severity of the process, but did not refuse a further trial. Accordingly he was directed to lie on his back. The bite was passed under the axilla and secured firmly to the floor by the cord used for counter-extension, then extension was made on the arm nearly in the natural direction of the limb, the body of the patient being in line with that of the extending force. This position was very favorable for reduction, and the bone had apparently got into its place, for a hollow on the outside of the shoulder was filled up, and the head of the bone, by the pressure of the belt in the axilla, was carried toward the socket. At this time the extension was relaxed, the arm brought forward and upward over the body, but without effecting the desired object. Is thirsty. Wishes for brandy and is given two glasses. Eloped."

Neuralgia of the intra-orbital branch of the fifth pair, left side. The patient was a woman of fifty-one years, who had suffered for eighteen years almost constant pain. For six months anodynes had been occasionally taken at night with advantage. Patient given half an ounce of sulphate of magnesia. "On the following day, the back and head supported by assistants, an incision made over the nerve from the orbit downward"; the seat of the nerve was determined by passing a probe into the wound. Then with the forceps a portion of the nerve was removed. As the pain persisted without much abatement and extended to the lower jaw, three teeth were extracted; and she was discharged cured in a few days.

An amputation by transfixion of the thigh, for white swelling of the knee-joint, is described as having been done in sixty-five seconds. The patient died in three days.

A carpenter, while engaged in erecting an arch in honor of Marquis Lafayette, on August 23, 1824, fell from the ladder on which he was working to the ground. He jumped, and fractured his left femur. The limb was placed in a fracture box, and an eighteen-tailed bandage applied. He was discharged cured.

From the record of a patient who submitted to the removal of a large tumor of the breast with extensive dissection: "She sustained the operation with great calmness—was much exhausted and faint."

Necrosed bone from the tibia. "Let the patient take twenty drops of tincture of opium one hour before operation. An incision from three inches below the knee, carried down over the anterior edge of the tibia to the ankle, also a cross incision at each end of the longitudinal one. This portion dissected up, leaving bare the tibia. The bone at the lower part was sawed through to the diseased part by Hey's saw. So also at upper end. Then by chisel and mallet the portions of newly-formed bone lying over the diseased bone were removed. The edges were afterwards removed by a gouge and the bone nippers, so that the diseased portion might be removed, which was then done, the lower part of it being first raised by the elevator; then the bone drawn down, as it extended a little under at upper part, and was removed. Wound was then cleansed and all parts adjusted. Compresses applied, and a roller passed around. Considerable loss of blood, faintness and vomiting during the operation; and at the termination of the operation, faintness, which lasted for some time. Was cold. Hot water and spirit was applied to the extremities, and brandy with water as freely as she could bear, with the occasional addition of six drops of ammoniated alcohol. She revived, but continued much exhausted, and became delirious. Pulse extremely rapid and feeble. Had several faint turns in the evening, with catching for breath. Hot baths and bottles were continued, with internal stimulation. She finally sank, and died at half-past nine in the evening, from the exhaustion, irritation and shock of operation, her constitution being delicate and very irritable."

An operation for the removal of a tumor of the lower jaw. Incision carried from the cheek-bone down over jaw and two inches below, in a semi-circular line. A second incision meeting the extremes of the first was made, and part of the skin, etc., included, removed. The parts covering the bony tumor were then carefully dissected up on the exterior and also on the interior parts. It was then found necessary to remove two teeth from the jaw. The surgeon then proceeded to divide by Hey's saw the middle, about one and one-half inches from the point of the chin. The bony tumor was then, by means of the elevator and with some difficulty, raised; in doing which the bone gave way in the diseased part. This portion was then removed. The remaining part was then separated from the muscles covering it, and with considerable difficulty detached at its articulation, the ligaments, etc., being exceedingly firm. The facial and maxillary arteries were secured by ligature, the wound cleared and brought together. Sponges were laid upon the parts, also a compress followed by a roller. Loss of blood inconsiderable. Had some faintness at times but bore the operation well. Tumor size of large egg.

A patient with symptoms of stone. After giving one hundred drops of laudanum, the patient was placed on the table with hands bound to feet and legs drawn up. The usual lateral operation was performed, and a stone of the size of an egg removed. Patient bore the operation well.

Cancer of penis. "Penis held fast, divided about an inch from the pubes by one stroke of the knife."

Cancer of the breast. Two semicircular incisions of five or six inches. The gland carefully dissected out. The glands of the axilla, being schirrous, were dissected out, in the course of which the axillary vein was opened. It was closed by compression.

The following brief histories appear:

January 7, 1825. "Breast was cut out with the integuments over it and the glands of the axilla."

February 4th. "Hemorrhoids cut off."

Cancer of penis. "Eighty drops of laudanum before operation. Amputation."

Up to June 26, 1826, when erysipelas was first mentioned in the records, wounds had behaved admirably, many healing by first intention, and the admissions had included many severe injuries, such as burns (largely lacerated wounds) followed by foul and suppurating discharges. The "erysipelatous affection" became so troublesome that all of the staff were requested by the trustees to propose measures fitted to eradicate the disease. They proposed the vacation of the hospital from four to six weeks. Those already sick to be isolated, and those who could bear removal to be sent to an adjoining house that could be hired for the purpose. All clothing and beds to be washed or baked. Old straw to be thrown away. The hospital wards to be exposed to the fumes of burning sulphur for three days, and one day to the strongest fumes of chlorine; then to a free current of air for at least one week, day and night. In the meantime all the sick-rooms to be whitewashed. The cellar to be thoroughly cleansed.

For the prevention of a return of this calamitous occurence, they propose that the number of beds be diminished one-third from the late establishment, and never to be increased beyond this without a formal order from the trustees upon consultation with the Medical Board; that fireplaces be constructed where it is possible; that the water-closets be more thoroughly ventilated; and that in case of any further appearance of erysipelas the patient shall be moved out of the hospital, and everything about him removed or thoroughly disinfected.

> It shall be the duty of the medical officer having such cases to report them at once to the superintendent, who shall be directed to remove such patient to some proper place with delay.
>
> John C. Warren,   James Jackson,
> Walter Channing.   George Hayward.[10]

On December 28, 1827, catgut ligatures were used for the first time. The patient was a woman with a tumor of the meatus urinarius.

In preparation for an amputation on September 20, 1832, the patient received at 10 A.M., pulv. opii, gr. ii; at 10.30, tinct. opii, gtt. xxx; at 11, tinct. opii. gtt xx; without much effect.

Dislocation of the hip. The patient was admitted October 9th. From that time to the 17th, he was given saline cathartics and a light

---

10. John Collins Warren (1778–1856) and James Jackson (1777–1867) were cofounders of the Massachusetts General Hospital. Warren was the first attending surgeon and Jackson was the first attending physician of the hospital. Both were professors of their specialties at the Harvard Medical School.

Walter Channing (1786–1876), M.D., University of Pennsylvania, 1809, was an attending physician at the Massachusetts General Hospital. He later became professor of obstetrics at Harvard and was a pioneer in the use of ether for childbirth.

George Hayward (1791–1863) received his M.D. from the University of Pennsylvania in 1812. He studied in London under several of John Hunter's pupils. He became the first clinical professor of surgery at Harvard (1835) and was the first surgeon to perform a major operation (amputation of the thigh) on an anesthetized patient (November 7, 1846).

diet. On the 18th, at 10 A.M., tartrate of antimony, one grain, and repeat every twenty minutes; omit when nauseated. At 20 minutes past 10, warm bath at 100°, increased to 110°; to remain in it one half-hour.

Patient being placed on the operating table, the cords and pulleys were attached to the dislocated limb. The fourth dose of antimony produced nausea. The vein in the left arm was opened. At this time (11.40) the extension commenced. At eight minutes before twelve o'clock faintness and great prostration. The extension was steadily continued by one person. A lengthening of the limb was perceptible. Complaint of pain in the vicinity of the head of the bone. The limb was rotated inwards across the left thigh. It now appeared longer than the second one. A broad bandage was now placed around the upper part of the thigh, passing across the shoulder of an assistant. A belt was passed around the pelvis, thus making a counter-extension to the broad bandage. The limb was again rotated inwards. No success following this direction, and the head of the bone appearing to be on the edge of the acetabulum, the limb was rotated upwards and outwards. At this time, twenty minutes before one o'clock, the patient exclaimed, "It is in!" The motion was felt by Dr. Warren while rotating, and by Dr. Hayward, whose hand was on the cervix. It was a success.

December 6, 1829. During the removal of a tumor of the lower jaw the bleeding became so profuse that it was necessary to apply the actual cautery. This checked it for a while; but as it recurred after reaching his room, it only stopped when he fainted. Five days after he had more hemorrhage, arrested by styptics.

The first case to be classed as abdominal, excepting strangulated hernias, etc., was that of a woman who entered the hospital October 28th, aged forty, with an abdominal tumor that had grown from the size of a goose-egg until it extended from the right groin to the false ribs of that side, measuring fourteen inches in that direction. It was first noticed on the same side, below and to the right of the umbilicus. Tumor movable, not tender, very firm and not fluctuating. Urine, thirty ounces, natural. No disturbance of functions. No pain. General health, appetite, and sleep good. Catamenia regular and profuse during the past ten years. Vaginal examination shows os high up above symphysis. Not tender or enlarged. Uterine fundus and body felt upon rectal examination. No tenderness or compression of gut. Enema at 10 A.M., and thirty drops of laudanum at 10.30. Operation at 11.

Directions for operation: Patient to have sixty drops of laudanum. Theatre heated carefully to 70°. Rain-water of blood-heat, and soft cloths to cover intestines. Usual instruments for an extensive operation.

Dr. Warren operated by an incision through the integuments in the linea alba, beginning three inches below the umbilicus and extending downward four inches. Subjacent muscles then carefully divided and the peritoneum opened, exposing the surface of the tumor to view. An attempt now made to reduce the size of the tumor by puncturing it with a trochar and canula. No fluid followed. It was found necessary to enlarge the incision upwards above the umbilicus. Tumor was then brought through the wound without difficulty, as it adhered only at its base. A strong cord was then tied firmly around the neck of the tumor, great care being taken to avoid including any of the intestines and to diminish the loss of blood. On cutting partly through the neck, the divided parts were found to retract, by reason of which the ligature was loosened. Another was accordingly passed around the undivided portion of the tumor, and it was then completely removed. Attempts were then made to stop the flow of blood, and several arteries were tied. After this object had been nearly or quite accomplished, the patient was found to be quite faint. Cold water was dashed upon her face, and brandy and water poured down her throat. Brisk friction of her limbs and application of blankets dipped in warm water were also made. The patient not reviving, artifical respiration was kept up for some time by inflating the lungs with a pair of bellows. The stomach-pump was then brought, and half a pint of hot brandy thrown into the stomach: but all these attempts proved fruitless, and the patient was finally given up for dead.[11]

One of the popular methods of treating sore eyes among the public at that time was to apply a *frog that had been boiled alive in a pound of butter*. A patient entered who had found this a valuable remedy; but in spite of its efficacy he was unable to open his eyes without force.

Amputation of the thigh, May 25, 1839. "Patient had one hundred drops of laudanum. He thinks that he did not feel the opium until after the operation."

Tumor of the tongue. Tumor being grasped by double hooks, it was removed by one stroke of the scalpel. Hemorrhage considerable;

---

11. This case is described by J.C. Warren in his *Surgical Observations on Tumors (Boston: Crocker & Brewster, 1837)*. His patient died from intraoperative hemorrhage. Warren wrote, "Owing to the shortness of the pedicle, the ligature partially slipped off as soon as the schirrus was taken away...." Ovariotomy was not a popular operation in Boston for some years and was not performed successfully there until 1869, by Dr. Samuel Cabot (1815–1885) of the Massachusetts General Hospital.

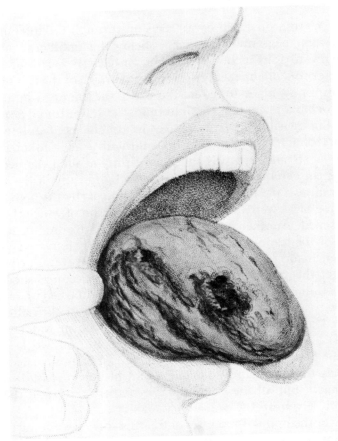

Figure 28. Tumor of the tongue. This illustration is of the patient with "tumor of the tongue" mentioned in the case report. It appears in J.C. Warren's *Surgical Observations on Tumors* (1837). (Courtesy National Library of Medicine.)

not being controlled by ligature, the actual cautery was applied. At 4 P.M., another hemorrhage compression by sponges. At 5 P.M., another hemorrhage, controlled by sponge.[12].

During an enucleation the eye was grasped by the forceps in the same way.

Removal of tongue. Tongue being protruded, it was seized with a long-bladed polypus forceps, transversely behind tumor, and firmly

---

12. This case also appears in J.C. Warren's *Surgical Observations on Tumors* with the illustration included here. In addition to a description of the surgery, Warren wrote, "The origin of the disease in this case may be traced pretty satisfactorily. The habitual application of the poisonous tobacco grad-

compressed. Tumor then being seized between the left thumb and fore-finger of the operator, a straight, sharp-pointed bistoury was passed across behind tumor through the healthy portion of the tongue, and the two lingual arteries secured by ligatures. Little blood was lost. Patient bore the operation with great fortitude.

An extensive, malignant, ulcerating growth involving the labia, nymphae, clitoris and urethra in a woman of twenty-nine years. A careful disection was made of the whole ulcerating surface. Great pain and persistent syncope accompanied the protracted dissection.

---

ually perverted the action of the parts it touched . . . we know that tobacco is a common cause of cancer in the tongue and lip." This must be one of the earliest implications of tobacco as a carcinogen. Warren states that this patient, like most suffers of cancer of the tongue and lip, was a user of chewing tobacco.

Insensibility During Surgical Operations Produced by Inhalation

HENRY JACOB BIGELOW, M.D. (1818–1890)

The following paper was the first published description of the use of ether for surgical anesthesia. It was written by Henry Jacob Bigelow, a young surgeon of Boston, who witnessed the first public demonstration of ether at the Massachusetts General Hospital. Bigelow's exact role in the events leading to the popularization of ether anesthesia is not certain. He may have been only an interested bystander as his professor, John Collins Warren, operated; or he may have been quite aware of W.T.G. Morton's previous experience with the agent in dental surgery and possibly may have witnessed such procedures. It has even been suggested that Bigelow paved the way for Morton's demonstration at the Massachusetts General Hospital on October 16, 1846.

Henry Jacob Bigelow was the son of Jacob Bigelow (1787–1879), Harvard's distinguished professor of materia medica. The younger Bigelow was born in Boston on March 11, 1818. He graduated from Harvard Medical School in 1841, determined to be a surgeon. He first served as a house pupil at the Massachusetts General Hospital and then traveled abroad to complete his surgical training. He was appointed visiting surgeon at the Massachusetts General Hospital in 1846 and then, in 1849, became the professor of surgery at Harvard. Bigelow was a brilliant surgeon and teacher who made many contributions to his specialty—particularly to the surgery of the hip and in popularizing the use of the lithotrite for the removal of bladder stones. Bigelow was

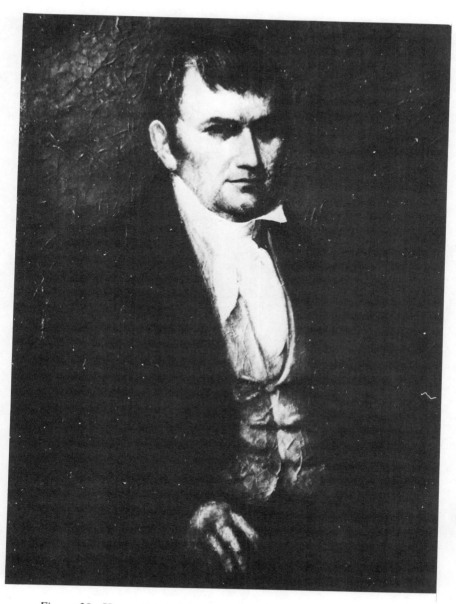

Figure 29. Henry Jacob Bigelow (1818–1890). This illustration of Bigelow, copied from a daguerreotype, was taken in Paris in 1841, five years prior to the events described in this selection. It is of interest that the photographer, Leon Foucault, made this portrait only two years after the announcement of Daguerre's discovery.

without question, the leading surgeon of Boston during his lifetime.
He died in Newton, Massachusetts, on October 30, 1890.

The following article on the use of ether for surgical anesthesia has
been shortened slightly for its inclusion here. It appeared on November
18, 1846, in the Boston Medical and Surgical Journal *(35:16).*

Insensibility During Surgical Operations Produced by Inhalation.

It has long been an important problem in medical science to devise
some method of mitigating the pain of surgical operations. An efficient agent for this purpose has at length been discovered. A patient
has been rendered completely insensible during an amputation of the
thigh, regaining consciousness after a short interval. Other severe operations have been performed without the knowledge of the patients. So
remarkable an occurrence will, it is believed, render the following details relating to the history and character of the process, not uninterest-
ing.

On the 16th of Oct., 1846, an operation was performed at the
hospital, upon a patient who had inhaled a preparation administered
by Dr. Morton,[1] a dentist of this city, with the alleged intention of producing insensibility to pain. Dr. Morton was understood to have extracted teeth under similar circumstances, without the knowledge of
the patient.[2] The present operation was performed by Dr. Warren, and
though comparatively slight, involved an incision near the lower jaw
of some inches in extent. During the operation the patient muttered,
as in a semi-conscious state, and afterwards stated that the pain was
considerable, though mitigated; in his own words, as though the skin

---

1. William Thomas Green Morton (1819–1868) was the chief protagonist
in the great ether controversy that followed the first public demonstration.
Morton was a dentist who was studying medicine at Harvard at the time that
he administered ether for this historic operation at the Massachusetts General
Hospital.

2. If we are to believe a statement made by Morton's son (a distinguished
neurologist and pioneer radiotherapist) a number of years later, Morton and
Bigelow had had considerable prior experience with ether anesthesia in surgery as well as in dentistry. Dr. William James Morton (1845–1920), the son of
W.T.G. Morton, during a discussion of anesthetic practices stated "It is not
generally known that previous to the first use of ether at the Massachusetts
General Hospital (in 1846) my father, Dr. Morton, had employed this for
thirty-seven private operations done by Henry J. Bigelow..." (*J.A.M.A.*
56:1677, 1911).

had been scratched with a hoe. There was, probably, in this instance, some defect in the process of inhalation, for on the following day the vapor was administered to another patient with complete success. A fatty tumor of considerable size was removed, by Dr. Hayward,[3] from the arm of a woman near the deltoid muscle. The operation lasted four or five minutes, during which time the patient betrayed occasional marks of uneasiness; but upon subsequently regaining her consciousness, professed not only to have felt no pain, but to have been insensible to surrounding objects, to have known nothing of the operation, being only uneasy about a child left at home. No doubt, I think, existed, in the minds of those who saw this operation, that the unconsciousness was real; nor could the imagination be accused of any share in the production of these remarkable phenomena. . . .

It remains briefly to describe the process of inhalation by the new method, and to state some of its effects. A small two-necked glass globe contains the prepared vapor, together with sponges to enlarge the evaporating surface. One aperture admits the air to the interior of the globe, whence, charged with vapor, it is drawn through the second into the lungs. The inspired air thus passes through the bottle, but the expiration is diverted by a valve in the mouth piece, and escaping into the apartment is thus prevented from vitiating the medicated vapor. A few of the operations in dentistry, in which the preparation has as yet been chiefly applied, have come under my observation. The remarks of the patients will convey an idea of their sensations.

A boy of 16, of medium stature and strength, was seated in the chair. The first few inhalations occasioned a quick cough, which afterwards subsided; at the end of eight minutes the head fell back, and the arms dropped, but owing to some resistance in opening the mouth, the tooth could not be reached before he awoke. He again inhaled for two minutes, and slept three minutes, during which time the tooth, an inferior molar, was extracted. At the moment of extraction the features assumed an expression of pain, and the hand was raised. Upon coming to himself he said he had had a "first rate dream–very quiet," he said, "and had dreamed of Napoleon—had not the slightest consciousness of pain—the time had seemed long;" and he left the chair, feeling no uneasiness of any kind, and evidently in a high state of admiration. The pupils were dilated during the state of unconsciousness, and the pulse rose from 130 to 142.

A girl of 16 immediately occupied the chair. After coughing a little, she inhaled during three minutes, and fell asleep, when a molar

3. George Hayward (1791–1863); see footnote 10, page 189.

tooth was extracted, after which she continued to slumber tranquilly during three minutes more. At the moment when force was applied she flinched and frowned, raising her hand to her mouth, but said she had been dreaming a pleasant dream and knew nothing of the operation.

A stout boy of 12, at the first inspiration coughed considerably, and required a good deal of encouragement to induce him to go on. At the end of three minutes from the first fair inhalation, the muscles were relaxed and the pupil dilated. During the attempt to force open the mouth he recovered his consciousness, and again inhaled during two minutes, and in the ensuing one minute two teeth were extracted, the patient seeming somewhat conscious, but upon actually awaking he declared "it was the best fun he ever saw," avowed his intention to come there again, and insisted upon having another tooth extracted upon the spot. A splinter which had been left, afforded an opportunity of complying with his wish, but the pain proved to be considerable. Pulse at first 110, during sleep 96, afterwards 144; pupils dilated.

The next patient was a healthy-looking middle-aged woman, who inhaled the vapor for four minutes; in the course of the next two minutes a back tooth was extracted, and the patient continued smiling in her sleep for three minutes more. Pulse 120, not affected at the moment of the operation, but smaller during sleep. Upon coming to herself, she exclaimed that "it was beautiful—she dreamed of being at home—it seemed as if she had been gone a month." These cases, which occurred successively in about an hour, at the room of Dr. Morton, are fair examples of the average results produced by the inhalation of the vapor, and will convey an idea of the feelings and expressions of many of the patients subjected to the process. Dr. Morton states that in upwards of two hundred patients, similar effects have been produced. The inhalation, after the first irritation has subsided, is easy, and produces a complete unconsciousness at the expiration of a period varying from two to five or six, sometimes eight minutes; its duration varying from two to five minutes; during which the patient is completely insensible to the ordinary tests of pain. The pupils in the cases I have observed have been generally dilated; but with allowance for excitement and other disturbing influences, the pulse is not affected, at least in frequency; the patient remains in a calm and tranquil slumber, and wakes with a pleasurable feeling. The manifestation of consciousness or resistance I at first attributed to the reflex function, but I have since had cause to modify this view.

It is natural to inquire whether no accidents have attended the employment of a method so wide in its application, and so striking in

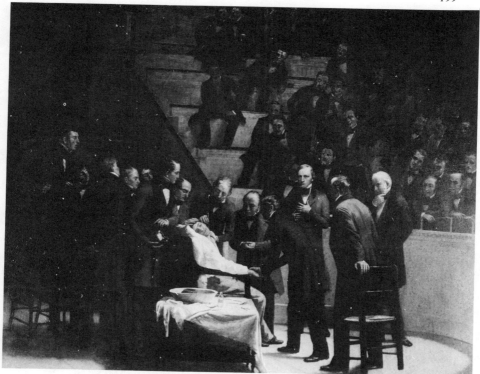

Figure 30. The first public demonstration of ether anesthesia. This painting by Robert Hinckley faithfully illustrates the operating room in the "ether dome" of the Massachusetts General Hospital. The figures have been identified and include the patient, Gilbert Abbott; his surgeon, J.C. Warren; W.T.G. Morton, holding his apparatus; and H.J. Bigelow standing with both hands clasped to his breast, the only figure not intent on the operation. (Courtesy the Boston Medical Library in the Countway Library of Medicine.)

its results. I have been unable to learn that any serious consequences have ensued. One or two robust patients have failed to be affected. I may mention as an early and unsuccessful case, its administration in a operation performed by Dr. Hayward, where an elderly woman was made to inhale the vapor for at least half an hour without effect. Though I was unable at the time to detect any imperfection in the process, I am inclined to believe that such existed. One woman became much excited, and required to be confined to the chair. As this occurred to the same patient twice, and in no other case as far as I have been able to learn, it was evidently owing to a peculiar susceptibility. Very young subjects are affected with nausea and vomiting, and for this reason Dr. M. has refused to administer it to children. Finally, in a few cases, the patient has continued to sleep tranquilly for eight or ten minutes, and once, after a protracted inhalation, for the period of an hour.

The following case, which occurred a few days since, will illustrate the probable character of future accidents. A young man was made to inhale the vapor, while an operation of limited extent, but somewhat protracted duration, was performed by Dr. Dix[4] upon the tissues near the eye. After a good deal of coughing the patient succeeded in inhaling the vapor, and fell asleep at the end of about ten minutes. During the succeeding two minutes the first incision was made, and the patient awoke, but unconscious of pain. Desiring to be again inebriated, the tube was placed in his mouth and retained there about twenty-five minutes, the patient being apparently half affected, but as he subsequently stated, unconscious. Respiration was performed partly through the tube and partly with the mouth open. Thirty-five minutes had now elapsed, when I found the pulse suddenly diminishing in force, so much so, that I suggested the propriety of desisting. The pulse continued decreasing in force, and from 120 had fallen to 96. The respiration was very slow, the hands cold, and the patient insensible. Attention was now of course directed to the return of respiration and circulation. Cold affusions, as directed for poisoning with alcohol, were applied to the head, the ears were syringed, and ammonia presented to the nostrils and administered internally. For fifteen minutes the symptoms remained stationary, when it was proposed to use active exercise, as in a case of narcotism from opium. Being lifted to his feet, the patient soon made an effort to move his limbs, and the pulse became more full, but again decreased in the sitting posture, and it was only after being compelled to walk during half an hour that the patient was able to lift his head. Complete consciousness returned only at the expiration of an hour. In this case the blood was flowing from the head, and rendered additional loss of blood unnecessary. Indeed the probable hemorrhage was previously relied on as salutary in its tendency.[5]

Two recent cases serve to confirm, and one I think to decide, the great utility of this process. On Saturday, the 7th of Nov., at the Mass. General Hospital, the right leg of a young girl was amputated above the knee, by Dr. Hayward, for disease of this joint.[6] Being made to inhale

---

4. John Homer Dix (1812–1884). M.D., Jefferson Medical College, 1836. An ophthalmic surgeon of Boston.

5. This was probably the first case in which the patient was taken down to stage III, or true surgical anesthesia.

6. This apparently was the first major operation performed on an etherized patient. The knee joint was damaged by tuberculous arthritis.

the preparation, after protesting her inability to do so from the pungency of the vapor, she became insensible in about five minutes. The last circumstance she was able to recall was the adjustment of the mouth piece of the apparatus, after which she was unconscious until she heard some remark at the time of securing the vessels—one of the last steps of the operation. Of the incision she knew nothing, and was unable to say, upon my asking her, whether or not the limb had been removed. She refused to answer several questions during the operation, and was evidently completely insensible to pain or other external influences. This operation was followed by another, consisting of the removal of a part of the lower jaw, by Dr. Warren. The patient was insensible to the pain of the first incision, though she recovered her consciousness in the course of a few minutes.

The character of the lethargic state, which follows this inhalation, is peculiar. The patient loses his individuality and awakes after a certain period, either entirely unconscious of what has taken place, or retaining only a faint recollection of it. Severe pain is sometimes remembered as being of a dull character; sometimes the operation is supposed by the patient to be performed upon somebody else. Certain patients, whose teeth have been extracted, remember the application of the extracting instruments; yet none have been conscious of any real pain.

As before remarked, the phenomena of the lethargic state are not such as to lead the observer to infer this insensibility. Almost all patients under the dentist's hands scowl or frown; some raise the hand. The patient whose leg was amputated, uttered a cry when the sciatic nerve was divided. Many patients open the mouth, or rise themselves in the chair, upon being directed to do so. Others manifest the activity of certain intellectual faculties. An Irishman objected to the pain, that he had been promised an exemption from it. A young man taking his seat in the chair and inhaling a short time, rejected the globe, and taking from his pockets a pencil and card wrote and added figures. Dr. M. supposing him to be affected, asked if he would now submit to the operation, to which the young man willingly assented. A tooth was accordingly extracted, and the patient soon after recovered his senses. In none of these cases had the patients any knowledge of what had been done during their sleep.

I am, as yet, unable to generalize certain other symptoms to which I have directed attention. The pulse has been, as far as my observation extends, unaltered in frequency, though somewhat diminished in volume, but the excitement preceding an operation, has, in almost every instance, so accelerated the pulse that it has continued rapid for a length of time. The pupils are in a majority of cases dilated; yet they are in certain cases unaltered, as in the above case of amputation.

The duration of the insensibility is another important element in the process. When the apparatus is withdrawn at the moment of unconsciousness, it continues, upon the average, two or three minutes, and the patient then recovers completely or incompletely, without subsequent ill effects. In this sudden cessation of the symptoms, this vapor in the air tubes differs in its effects from the narcotics or stimulants in the stomach, and, as far as the evidence of a few experiments of Dr. Morton goes, from the ethereal solution of opium when breathed. Lassitude, headache and other symptoms lasted for several hours, when this agent was employed.

But if the respiration of the vapor be prolonged much beyond the first period, the symptoms are more permanent in their character. In one of the first cases, that of a young boy, the inhalation was continued during the greater part of ten minutes, and the subsequent narcotism and drowsiness lasted more than an hour. In a case alluded to before, the narcotism was complete during more than twenty minutes, the insensibility approached to a coma. . . .

The process is obviously adapted to operations which are brief in their duration, whatever be their severity. Of these, the two most striking are, perhaps, amputations and the extraction of teeth. In protracted dissections, the pain of the first incision alone is of sufficient importance to induce its use; and it may hereafter prove safe to administer it for a length of time, and to produce a narcotism of an hour's duration. It is not unlikely to be applicable in cases requiring a suspension of muscular action; such as the reduction of dislocations or of strangulated hernia; and finally it may be employed in the alleviation of functional pain, of muscular spasm, as in cramp and colic, and as a sedative or narcotic.

The application of the process to the performance of surgical operations is, it will be conceded, new. If it can be shown to have been occasionally resorted to before, it was only an ignorance of its universal application and immense practical utility that prevented such isolated facts from being generalized.

It is natural to inquire with whom this invention originated. Without entering into details, I learn that the patent bears the name of Dr. Charles T. Jackson,[7] a distinguished chemist, and of Dr. Morton, a skilful dentist, of this city, as inventors–and has been issued to the latter gentleman as proprietor.

----

7. Charles Thomas Jackson (1805–1880) was a graduate of Harvard Medical School (1829) and was both a physician and a chemist. His merits in the controversy for the credit of introducing ether are difficult to assess, al-

It has been considered desirable by the interested parties that the character of the agent employed by them, should not be at this time announced; but it may be stated that it has been made known to those gentlemen who have had occasion to avail themselves of it.

I will add, in conclusion, a few remarks upon the actual position of this invention as regards the public.

No one will deny that he who benefits the world should receive from it an equivalent. The only question is, of what nature shall the equivalent be? Shall it be voluntarily ceded by the world, or levied upon it? For various reasons, discoveries in high science have been usually rewarded indirectly by fame, honor, position, and occasionally, in other countries, by funds appropriated for the purpose. Discoveries in medical science, whose domain approaches so nearly that of philanthropy, have been generally ranked with them; and many will assent with reluctance to the propriety of restricting by letters patent the use of an agent capable of mitigating human suffering. There are various reasons, however, which apologize for the arrangement which I understand to have been made with regard to the application of the new agent.

1st. It is capable of abuse, and can readily be applied to nefarious ends.

2nd. Its action is not yet thoroughly understood, and its use should be restricted to responsible persons.

3d. One of its greatest fields is the mechanical art of dentistry, many of whose processes are by convention, secret, or protected by patent rights. It is especially with reference to this art, that the patent has been secured. We understand, already, that the proprietor has ceded its use to the Mass. General Hospital, and that his intentions are extremely liberal with regard to the medical profession generally, and that so soon as necessary arrangements can be made for publicity of the process, great facilities will be offered to those who are disposed to avail themselves of what now promises to be one of the important discoveries of the age.

---

though he probably did little more than suggest to Morton that he substitute pure sulfuric ether for the impure product with which he was experimenting. It is of interest that Jackson also claimed to have suggested the telegraph to S.F.B. Morse.

Inhalation of Ethereal Vapor for the Prevention of Pain in Surgical Operations

JOHN COLLINS WARREN, M.D. (1778–1856)

The following paper is Dr. John Collins Warren's account of the operation that he performed on 20-year-old Gilbert Abbott. This was not the first time that ether had been used for surgery, but it might as well have been, for it was only following this demonstration that the merciful benefits of inhalation anesthesia were recognized and put to use.

John Collins Warren, the son of John Warren (1753–1815), was born in Boston, August 1, 1778. He studied medicine with his father and then went to Europe to complete his education. He learned surgery as a dresser under Astley Cooper and later took his M.D. degree at Edinburgh in 1801. He traveled to Paris and studied under the great surgeons of that city, returning to the United States during the following year. John Collins Warren practiced with his father and eventually succeeded him as professor of surgery at Harvard in 1815. He became one of America's great surgeons. He was instrumental in founding the Massachusetts General Hospital and the New England Journal of Medicine and Surgery—*both institutions flourish today (although the latter has dropped "Surgery" from its title). Warren wrote the first American text on tumors and frequently operated for cancer with a boldness that made him well aware of the need for lessening pain during surgery.*

John Collins Warren was 68 years old in 1846. He had been a capable and effective surgeon and teacher whose name would have lived for

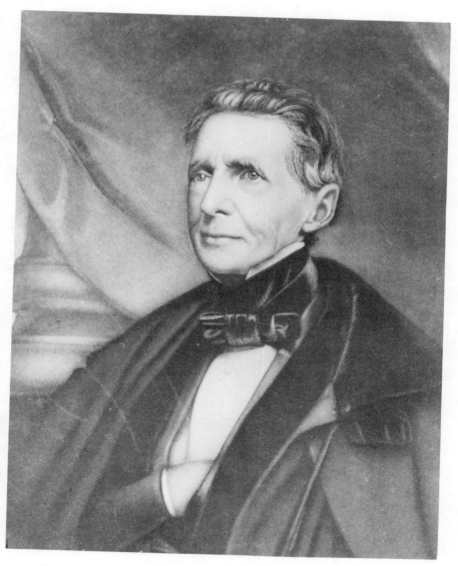

Figure 31. John Collins Warren (1778–1856). (Courtesy National Library of Medicine.)

his other contributions. It seems particularly fitting, however, that this aging professor should cap his career with the operation described in the following paper. Warren's willingness to allow the public demonstration of ether, coupled with his prominence as a surgeon, made its immediate acceptance a certainty. He lived for another decade and died in Boston on May 4, 1856.

The following account by John Collins Warren appeared in the Boston Medical and Surgical Journal *(36:375) on December 9, 1846.*

Inhalation of Ethereal Vapor for the Prevention of Pain in Surgical Operations

Application has been made to me by R.H. Eddy, Esq.,[1] in a letter dated Nov. 30th, in behalf Dr. W.T.G. Morton, to furnish an account of the operations witnessed and performed by me, wherein his new discovery for preventing pain was employed. Dr. M. has also proposed to me to give him the names of such hospitals as I know of in this country, in order that he may present them with the use of his discovery. These applications, and the hope of being useful to my professional brethren, especially those concerned in the hospitals which may have the benefit of Dr. M.'s proposal, have induced me to draw up the following statement, and to request that it may be public through your Journal.

The discovery of a mode of preventing pain in surgical operations has been an object of strong desire among surgeons from an early period. In my surgical lectures I have almost annually alluded to it, and stated the means which I have usually adopted for the attainment of this object. I have also freely declared, that notwithstanding the use of very large doses of narcotic substances, this desideratum had never been satisfactorily obtained. The successful use of any article of the materia medica for this purpose, would therefore be hailed by me as an important alleviation to human suffering. I have in consequence admitted the trial of plans calculated to accomplish this object, whenever they were free from danger.[2]

---

1. R.H. Eddy, Esq., was the patent agent representing W.T.G. Morton.

2. J.C. Warren in 1844 had allowed Horace Wells (1815–1848), a dentist, to demonstrate nitrous oxide before a class at the Harvard Medical School. Unfortunately he was unable to achieve complete anesthesia, his patient cried out, and Wells was jeered by the skeptical students. Wells, of course, was vindicated, but only after his suicide in 1848. His pupil, Morton, was fortunate enough to find an agent potent enough to be effective.

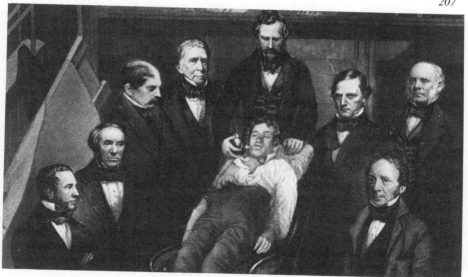

Figure 32. The first public demonstration of ether anesthesia. This depiction of the historic operation on Gilbert Abbot appeared in N.P. Rice's *Trials of a Public Benefactor* (New York: Rodney & Russell; 1859), a book that defended Morton in the great ether controversy about priority. Bigelow is on the far left, J.C. Warren stands just to the left of Morton.

About five weeks since, Dr. Morton, dentist of this city, informed me that he had invented an apparatus for the inhalation of a vapor, the effect of which was to produce a state of total insensibility to pain and that he had employed it successfully in a sufficient number of cases in his practice to justify him in a belief of its efficacy. He wished for an opportunity to test its power in surgical operations, and I agreed to give him such an opportunity as soon as practicable.

Being at that time in attendance as Surgeon of the Massachusetts General Hospital, a patient presented himself in that valuable institution a few days after my conversation with Dr. Morton, who required an operation for a tumor of the neck, and agreeably to my promise I requested the attendance of Dr. M.

On October 17th, the patient being prepared for the operation, the apparatus was applied to his mouth by Dr. Morton for about three minutes, at the end of which time he sank into a state of insensibility. I immediately made an incision about three inches long through the skin of the neck, and began a dissection among important nerves and blood-vessels without any expression of pain on the part of the patient. Soon after he began to speak incoherently, and appeared to be in an agitated state during the remainder of the operation. Being asked immediately afterwards whether he had suffered much, he said that he had felt as if his neck had been scratched; but subsequently, when inquired of by me, his statement was, that he did not experience pain at the time, although aware that the operation was proceeding.[3]

The effect of the gaseous inhalation in neutralizing the sentient faculty was made perfectly distinct to my mind by this experiment, although the patient during a part of its prosecution exhibited appearances indicative of suffering. Dr. Morton had apprised me, that the influence of his application would last but a few minutes after its intermission; and as the operation was necessarily protracted, I was not disappointed that its success was only partial.

On the following day, October 18th, an operation was done by Dr. Hayward,[4] on a tumor of the arm, in a female patient at the Hospital. The respiration of the gas was in this case continued during the whole of the operation. There was no exhibition of pain, excepting some occasional groans during its last stage, which she subsequently stated to have arisen from a disagreeable dream. Noticing the pulse in this patient before and after the operation, I found it to have risen from 80 to 120.

Two or three days after these occurrences, on meeting with Dr. Charles T. Jackson,[5] distinguished for his philosophical spirit of inquiry, as well as for his geological and chemical science, this gentleman informed me that he first suggested to Dr. Morton the inspiration of ether, as a means of preventing the pain of operations on the teeth. He did not claim the invention of the apparatus, nor its practical application; for these we are indebted to Dr. Morton.

The success of this process in the prevention of pain for a certain period being quite established, I at once conceived it to be my duty to introduce the apparatus into the practice of the Hospital, but was immediately arrested by learning that the proprietor intended to obtain an exclusive patent for its use. It now became a question, whether, in accordance with that elevated principle long since introduced into the medical profession, which forbids its members to conceal any useful

---

3. The operation on Gilbert Abbott was not the first time that ether had been used for surgical anesthesia. Its prior use by Crawford Williamson Long (1815–1878) of Georgia is well known. Long had attended ether frolics while a medical student in the University of Pennsylvania (1839). He first used ether as an anesthetic in 1842, but, for reasons that will be forever unknown, did not publish his experience until 1849. For all practical purposes the advent of ether as an anesthetic dates from its use at the Massachusetts General Hospital. Its immediate acceptance was a result of its endorsement by surgeons of the stature of Warren, Hayward and Bigelow.
4. George Hayward (1791–1863); see note, page 189.
5. Charles Thomas Jackson (1805–1880); see note, page 202.

discovery, we could continue to encourage an application we were not allowed to use ourselves, and of the components of which we were ignorant. On discussing this matter with Dr. Hayward, my colleague in the Hospital, we came to the conclusion, that we were not justified in encouraging the further use of this new invention, until we were better satisfied on these points. Dr. Hayward thereupon had a conversation with Dr. Morton, in consequence of which Dr. M. addressed to me a letter. In this he declared his willingness to make known to us the article employed, and to supply assistance to administer the inhalation whenever called upon. These stipulations he has complied with.

This being done, we thought ourselves justified in inviting Dr. Morton to continue his experiments at the Hospital, and elsewhere; and he directly after, Nov. 7th, attended at a painful and protracted operation performed by me, of the excision of a portion of the lower jaw, in which the patient's sufferings were greatly mitigated. On the same day an amputation of the thigh of a young woman was performed at the Hospital by Dr. Hayward. In this case the respiration of the ethereal vapor appeared to be entirely successful in preventing the pain of the operation; the patient stating, afterwards, that she did not know that anything had been done to her.

On Nov. 12th, an operation for the removal of a tumor from the arm of a young woman was performed by Dr. J. Mason Warren.[6] The vapor was administered for three minutes, when the patient became unconscious; the operator then proceeded, the inspiration being continued. Standing myself on one side of the patient, while the operator was on the other, so entirely tranquil was she, that I was not aware the operation had begun, until it was nearly completed.

On Nov. 21st an operation was performed by Dr. J. Mason Warren on a gentleman for the removal of a tumor, which covered nearly the half of the front of the right thigh. The patient lying upon a bed, the vapor was administered by Dr. Morton in the presence of Drs. Charles T. Jackson, Reynolds, J.V.C. Smith, Flagg, Gould, Shurtleff, Lawrence, Parsons, Briggs,[7] and others. After he had breathed the vapor for three minutes his head fell, and he ceased to respire it, but presently awakening, the inhalation was renewed till he

---

6. Jonathan Mason Warren (1811–1867); see note 5, page 181.

7. This operation was performed at the Bromfield House—a Boston hotel—apparently on a private patient. The tumor was a large lipoma of the thigh. The operation seems to have been arranged as a demonstration so that a number of prominent medical men could observe etherization. Of those whom Warren lists, the following have been identified:

Charles Thomas Jackson (1805–1880); see note, page 202.

Edward Reynolds (1793–1881) had been a pupil of J.C. Warren. He was

again appeared insensible. The operation was then commenced. At the first stroke of the knife he clapped his hand on the wound, but I immediately seized and held it during the remainder of the operation, though not without some difficulty in consequence of his struggles. The operation was completed in two or three minutes, and the patient remained quietly on his back with his eyes closed. On examination the pupils were found to be dilated; the pulse was not materially affected. After he had lain about two minutes, I roused him by the inquiry, "how do you do to-day?" to which he replied, "very well, I thank you." I then asked what he had been doing. He said he believed he had been dreaming; he dreamed that he was at home, and making some examination into his business. "Do you feel any pain?" "No." "How is that tumor of yours?" The patient raised himself in bed, looked at his thigh for a moment, and said, "it is gone, and I'm glad of it." I then inquired if he had felt any pain during the operation, to which he replied in the negative. He soon recovered his natural state, experienced no inconvenience from the inhalation, was remarkably free from pain, and in three days went home into the country.

---

a general and ophthalmic surgeon and a founder of the Massachusetts Eye and Ear Infirmary, a sister institution to the Massachuetts General Hospital.

Jerome Van Crowningshield Smith (1800–1879) graduated from the Berkshire Medical Institution in 1825. He was a prominent medical journalist and author of a number of books on various subjects. He was the editor of the *Boston Medical and Surgical Journal* (today's *New England Journal of Medicine*) in which Bigelow's and Warren's articles were published. He was also the port physician of Boston.

Josiah Foster Flagg (1789–1853) was a pupil of J.C. Warren and a graduate of Harvard Medical School (1815). A versatile man, he was not only a physician but also a dentist and an engraver. He had illustrated several of Warren's books on anatomical subjects.

Augustus Addison Gould (1805–1866), M.D., Harvard, 1830. Gould was also an author and zoologist. He was Morton's neighbor and befriended him during the ether controversy. Gould was a visiting physician, on the staff of the Massachusetts General Hospital.

Nathaniel Bradstreet Shurtleff (1810–1874) graduated from Harvard Medical School in 1834. He was also a historian and prominent in many organizations. He later became an overseer of Harvard College and a mayor of Boston.

Usher Parsons (1788–1868) of Providence, Rhode Island. Parsons was an early apprentice of J.C. Warren. He was well known for his brave and competent behavior under fire while serving as a naval surgeon under Commodore Perry on Lake Erie in 1813. He had a distinguished career in the navy after the war and then became a prominent surgeon in Providence. Parsons served on the faculty of several medical schools and wrote a number of papers on surgical subjects.

In all these cases there was a decided mitigation of pain; in most of them the patients on the day after the operation, and at other times, stated, that they had not been conscious of pain. All those who attended were, I think, satisfied of the efficacy of the application in preventing, or, at least, greatly diminishing the suffering usual in such cases. The phenomena presented in these operations afford grounds for many interesting reflections, but it being my principal intention at this time to give a simple statement of facts, I shall not pursue the subject further, but close with two or three remarks.

1st. The breathing of the ethereal vapor[8] appears to operate directly on the cerebral affection.

2d. Muscular power was for the time suspended in some cases, in others its loss was partial, and in one instance was scarcely sensible. The great relaxation of muscular action produced by a full dose of the application, leads to the hope that it may be employed with advantage in cases of spasmodic affection, both by the surgeon and by the physician.

3d. The action of the heart is remarkably accelerated in some cases, but not in all.

4th. The respiration is sometimes stertorous, like that of apoplexy.

All these changes soon pass off without leaving any distinct traces behind them, and the ordinary state of the functions returns. This has been the course of things in the cases I have witnessed, but I think it quite probable, that so powerful an agent may sometimes produce other and even alarming effects. I therefore would recommend, that it should never be employed except under the inspection of a judicious and competent person.

Let me conclude by congratulating my professional brethren on the acquisition of a mode of mitigating human suffering, which may become a valuable agent in the hands of careful and well-instructed practitioners, even if it should not prove of such general application as the imagination of sanguine persons would lead them to anticipate.

Boston, Dec. 3, 1846.

---

8. Warren speaks here of "ethereal vapor," for by now Morton had made known its composition. Warren may have recognized its odor, for he had used sulfuric ether himself as early as 1805 to give relief in advanced pulmonary disease. Dr. Warren wrote in his journal on October 16 (the date of his operation on Gilbert Abbott, instead of 17 as he states in this paper), "Did an interesting operation at the Hospital this morning, while the patient was under the influence of Dr. Morton's preparation to prevent pain. The substance employed was sulphuric ether."

Operation for Vesico-Vaginal Fistula

JAMES MARION SIMS, M.D. (1813–1883)

There were, to be sure, women's doctors before Marion Sims. Their therapy was chiefly limited, however, to the prescribing of medicine, douches, and tampons, and to the fitting of pessaries. Sims was one of the first surgeons to adapt the techniques of surgery to diseases of the female generative tract: in so doing he helped found a specialty. He and his disciples dedicated themselves to developing operations that were curative for women's ailments that hitherto had been, for the most part, incurable.

James Marion Sims was born in Lancaster County, South Carolina, on January 25, 1813. He received his medical education at the Charleston Medical School (today's Medical College of South Carolina), which he attended for a year, and then at Jefferson Medical College in Philadelphia, receiving his M.D. degree there in 1835. Sims was greatly influenced by George McClellan (1796–1847), Jefferson's founder and professor of surgery, a dynamic man and daring surgeon. After graduating, Sims practiced for a time in Montgomery, Alabama. He subsequently moved to New York and then, during the Civil War, traveled and practiced in Europe. During the later years of his life, Sims was known, in this country and in Europe, as one of the world's leading surgeons, both for his skill in treating diseases of the female generative tract and as a pioneer in advancing surgery of the abdominal cavity. He was quick to realize the value of aseptic techniques and

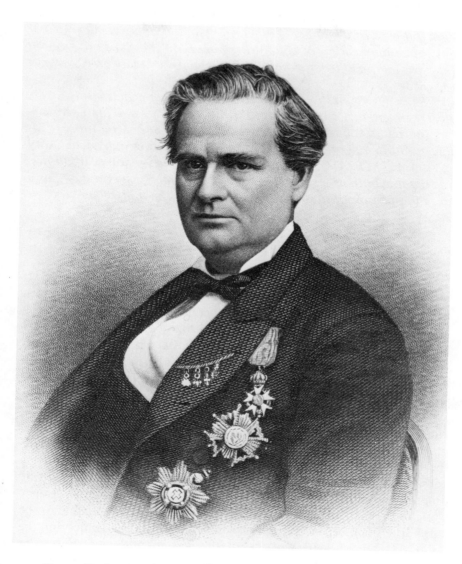

Figure 33. James Marion Sims (1813–1883).

popularized their use. Sims is best known today for his treatment of vesico-vaginal fistula. He performed his first successful operation for this condition in Montgomery, Alabama, in 1849. His first case was soon followed by a number of others; his patients thus were liberated of this foul complication of childbirth. James Marion Sims practiced in New York during the latter part of his life and died there on November 13, 1883.

Sims described his operative technique in an article entitled "On the Treatment of Vesico-Vaginal Fistula" that appeared in the American Journal of the Medical Sciences *in (23:59) 1852. A far more readable account, however, is to be found in his autobiography,* The Story of My Life *(N.Y.: D. Appleton, 1884). This is the version that follows; it is notable both as a success story of a determined surgeon and as a revealing picture of life in the deep South in the mid 1800s.*

The First Operation for Vesico-Vaginal Fistula

Early in the month of June (1845) Dr. Henry[1] asked me to go out to Mr. Wescott's, only a mile from the town, to a case of labor which had lasted three days and the child not yet born. He said, "I am thinking that you had better take your instruments along with you, for you may want to use them." We found a young colored woman, about seventeen years of age, well developed, who had been in labor then seventy-two hours. The child's head was so impacted in the pelvis that the labor-pains had almost entirely ceased. It was evident that matters could not long remain in this condition without the system becoming exhausted, and without the pressure producing a sloughing of the soft parts of the mother. So I agreed with Dr. Henry that the sooner she was delivered the better, and without any great effort the child was brought away with forceps. She rallied from the confinement and seemed to be getting on pretty well, until about five days after her delivery, when Dr. Henry came to see me, and said that there was an extensive sloughing of the soft parts, the mother having lost control of both the bladder and the rectum. Of course, aside from death, this was about the worst accident that could have happened to the poor young girl. I went to see her, and found an enormous slough, spreading from the posterior wall of the

---

1. Most of the practitioners that Sims mentions in this selection have not been identified but "Dr. Henry" was probably Hugh William Henry, who practiced in Montgomery. His son, John Hazard Henry (1829–1905), was a pupil in Sims's office in 1847.

vagina, and another thrown off from the anterior wall. The case was hopelessly incurable.

I went home and investigated the literature of the subject thoroughly and fully. Then, seeing the master of the servant the next day, I said: "Mr. Wescott, Anarcha has an affection that unfits her for the duties required of a servant. She will not die, but will never get well, and all you have to do is to take good care of her so long as she lives." Mr. Wesscott was a kind-hearted man, a good master, and, accepting the situation, made up his mind that Anarcha should have an easy time in this world as long as she lived.

I had practiced medicine ten years, and had never before seen a case of vesico-vaginal fistula. I looked upon it as a surgical curiosity, although a very unfortunate one. Strange to say, in one month from that time Dr. Harris, from Lowndes County, came to see me, and he said: "Well, doctor, one of my servant girls, Betsey, a young woman seventeen or eighteen years old, married last year, had a baby about a month ago. Since than she has not been able to hold a single drop of water."

I replied, "I am very sorry, doctor, but nothing can be done for her. There is a similar case here in town."

He said, "I thought myself it was incurable. But I am going to tell my overseer to send her up to you tomorrow and let you examine her case." So the next day Betsey came, and I examined her. The base of the bladder was destroyed, and her case was certainly a very miserable one. I kept her a day or two in Montgomery and then sent her home, writing a note to the doctor, giving him my opinon of the case and its incurability. I supposed that I should never see another case of vesico-vaginal fistula.

About a month after this, however, Mr. Tom Zimmerman, of Macon County, called on me. I was his family physician when I lived in Cubahatchee, but I had not seen him since I left there, four or five years before. He began immediately by saying that his negro girl, Lucy, about eighteen years old, had given birth to a child two months ago, and that since that time she had been unable to hold any water.

I said, "Tom, I know all about this case, and there is no doctor in this town or country who can afford any relief. I have just been reading up the subject; I have consulted all the authorities I can find in every doctor's library in this city. She has a fistula in the bladder—a hole in it. It may be no larger than a pipe-stem, or it may be as large as two or three inches in diameter; but, whether big or little, the urine runs all the time; it makes no odds what position she is in, whether asleep or awake, walking or standing, sitting or lying down. The case is absolutely incurable. I don't want to see her or the case. You need not send her to town. I have just seen two cases, one in this town, and another that was sent to me from Lowndes County, and I have sent the last one back because there is no hope for it."

"Is there no chance for your being mistaken about the case, without having seen it?"

I said, "No, there is no chance for me to be mistaken. It is absolutely incurable."

"Are you not disposed to investigate it," he said, "and see if there is not some chance?"

I said, "No, I don't want to see it."

"But you would have done so before you moved from the piney woods and came to the city. Moving to a city sets a man up wonderfully. You are putting on airs. When you were my family doctor, and used to see my family or my niggers, you never objected to an investigation of their cases, and you didn't say what you would do and what not. I am going to send Lucy in. What day do you want her to come down?"

I said, "I don't want to see her. I can do her no good."

"Well," said he, "I am going to send her down to you at your office, by Monday's train, whether you want to see her or not." And so, sure enough, Monday came, and Lucy was at my office. I had a little hospital of eight beds, built in the corner of my yard, for taking care of my negro patients and for negro surgical cases; and so when Lucy came I gave her a bed. As soon as I could get to her I examined the case very minutely. I told her that I was unable to do anything for her, and I said, "To-morrow afternoon I shall have to send you home." She was very much disappointed, for her condition was loathsome, and she was in hopes that she could be cured. I told her that she must go home on the next afternoon.

It was my usual habit to start off at nine o'clock to visit my patients, and I seldom had less than from eighteen to twenty visits to make in a morning. Just as I was starting off, and was about to get into my buggy, a little nigger came running to the office and said, "Massa doctor, Mrs. Merrill done been throwed from her pony, and is mighty badly hurt, and you must go down there right off to see her, just as soon as you can get there." So, as this was a surgical case, and not knowing whether it was a fractured limb or a broken skull, I looked upon it as a case of urgency, and instead of making my usual morning round. I started upon "the hill," three fourths of a mile, to see old Mrs. Merrill. She was not an old woman, but she was the wife of a dissipated old man, who was supposed to be of not much account, as he was gambling and leading an otherwise disreputable life. Mrs. Merrill, however, was a respectable woman who obtained a living by washing and taking in sewing, and was much appreciated and respected among her neighbors. She was about forty-six years of age, stout and fat, and weighed nearly two hundred pounds. She had been riding along on a pony, and when within about fifty yards of her own house a hog lying by the roadside, in the corner of the fence, jumped out and made a noise that frightened the pony, and it sprang from under the rider. She fell with all her weight on the pelvis. She had no broken bones. She was in bed, complaining of great pain in her back, and a sense of tenesmus in both the bladder and rectum, the bearing down making her condition miserable.

If there was anything I hated, it was investigating the organs of the female pelvis. But this poor woman was in such a condition that I was obliged to find out what was the matter with her. It was by a digital examination, and I had sense enough to discover that there was retroversion of the uterus. It was half turned upside down, and I took it for granted that this sudden dislocation, or disturbance of the pelvic organs, was the result of the fall on the pelvis. The question was, what I should do to relieve her. I remembered, when a medical student in Charleston Medical College, that old Dr. Prioleau[2] used to say: "Gentlemen, if any of you are ever called to a case of sudden version of the uterus backward, you must place the patient on the knees and elbows—in a genu-pectoral position—and then introduce one finger into the rectum and another into the vagina, and push up, and pull down; and, if you don't get the uterus in position by this means, you will hardly effect it by any other." This piece of information at the time it was given went into one ear and out at the other. I never expected to have any use for it. Strangely enough, all that Professor Prioleau said came back to me at once when the case was presented. So I placed the patient as directed, with a large sheet thrown over her. I could not make up my mind to introduce my finger into the rectum, because only a few days before that I had had occasion to examine the rectum of a nervous gentleman who had a fissure, and he made so much complaint of the examination that I thought that this poor woman was suffering enough without my doing so disagreeable a thing. So, as she raised herself and rested on her knees, just on the edge of the bed, and by putting one finger into the vagina I could easily touch the uterus by my pushing, but I could not place it in position, for my finger was too short; if it had been half

---

2. "Old Dr. Prioleau" was Thomas Grimball Prioleau (1786–1876), a graduate of the University of Pennsylvania in 1808. He was a founder of the Medical College of South Carolina and held the chair of obstetrics in that school for 43 years.

an inch longer, I could have put the womb into place. So I introduced the middle and index fingers, and immediately touched the uterus. I commenced making strong efforts to push it back, and thus I turned my hand with the palm upward, and then downward, and pushing with all my might, when all at once, I could not feel the womb, or the walls of the vagina. I could touch nothing at all, and wondered what it all meant. It was as if I had put my two fingers into a hat, and worked them around, without touching the substance of it. While I was wondering what it all meant Mrs. Merrill said, "Why, doctor, I am relieved." My mission was ended, but what had brought the relief I could not understand. I removed my hand, and said to her, "You may lie down now." She was in a profuse perspiration from pain and unnatural position, and in part from the effort. She rather fell on her side. Suddenly there was an explosion, just as though there had been an escape of air from the bowel. She was exceedingly mortified and began to apologize, and said, "I am so ashamed." I said: "That is not from the bowel, but from the vagina, and it has explained now what I did not understand before. I understand now what has relieved you, but I would not have understood it but for that escapement of air from the vagina. When I placed my fingers there, the mouth of the vagina was so dilated that the air rushed in and extended the vagina to its fullest capacity, by the natural pressure of fifty-five pounds to the square inch, and this, conjoined with the position, was the means of restoring the retroverted organ to its normal place."

Then, said I to myself, if I can place the patient in that position, and distend the vagina by the pressure of air, so as to produce such a wonderful result as this, why can I not take the incurable case of vesico-vaginal fistula, which seems now to be so incomprehensible, and put the girl in this position and see exactly what are the relations of the surrounding tissues? Fired with this idea, I forgot that I had twenty patients waiting to see me all over the hills of this beautiful city. I jumped into my buggy and drove hurriedly home. Passing by the store of Hall, Mores & Roberts, I stopped and bought a pewter spoon. I went to my office where I had two medical students, and said, "Come, boys, go to the hospital with me."

"You have got through your work early this morning," they said.

"I have done none of it," I replied; "come to the hospital with me." Arriving there, I said, "Betsey, I told you that I would send you home this afternoon, but before you go I want to make one more examination of your case." She willingly consented. I got a table about three feet long, and put a coverlet upon it, and mounted her on the table, on her knees, with her head resting on the palms of her hands. I placed the two students one on each side of the pelvis, and they laid hold of the nates, and pulled them open. Before I could get the bent spoon-handle into the vagina, the air rushed in with a puffing noise, dilating the vagina to its fullest extent. Introducing the bent handle of the spoon I saw everything, as no man had ever seen before. The fistula was as plain as the nose on a man's face. The edges were clear and well-defined, and distinct, and the opening could be measured as accurately as if it had been

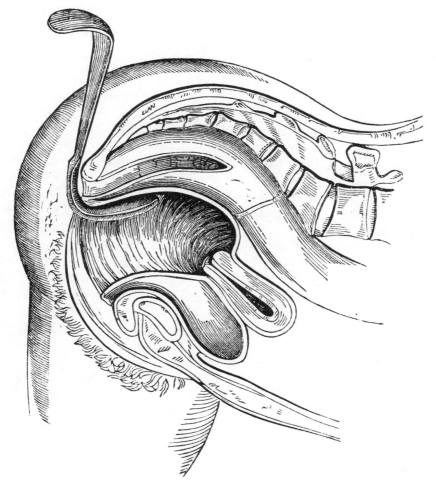

Figure 34. "Sims's retractor" and "Sims's position." Today Sims's position refers to a left decubitis position. Sims originally used the upright knee-chest position, however. (Courtesy National Library of Medicine.)

cut out of a piece of plain paper. The walls of the vagina could be seen closing in every direction; the neck of the uterus was distinct and well-defined, and even the secretions from the neck could be seen as a tear glistening in the eye, clear even and distinct, and as plain as could be. I said at once, "Why can not these things be cured? It seems to me that there is nothing to do but to pare the edges of the fistula and bring it together nicely, introduce a catheter in the neck of the bladder and drain the urine off continually, and the case will be cured." Fired with enthusiam by this wonderful discovery, it raised me into a plane of thought that unfitted me almost for the duties of the day. Still, with gladdened heart, and buoyant spirits, and rejoicing in my soul, I went off to make my daily rounds. I felt sure that I was on the eve of one of the greatest discoveries of the day. The more I thought of it, the more I was convinced of it.

I immediately went to work to invent instruments necessary for performing the operation on the principles that were self-evident on the first inspection of the first case. The speculum, or retractor, was perfectly clear from the very beginning. I did not send Lucy home, and I wrote to her master that I would retain her there, and he must come and see me again. I saw Mr. Wescott, and I told him that I was on the eve of a great discovery, and that I would like to have him send Anarcha back to my hospital. I also wrote to Dr. Harris saying that I had changed my mind in regard to Betsey, and for him to send her back again. I ransacked the country for cases, told the doctors what had happened and what I had done, and it ended in my finding six or seven cases of vesico-vaginal fistula that had been hidden away for years in the country because they had been pronounced incurable. I went to put another story on my hospital, and this gave me sixteen beds; four beds for servants, and twelve for the patients. Then I made this proposition to the owners of the negros: If you will give me Anarcha and Betsey for experiment. I agree to perform no experiment or operation on either of them to endanger their lives, and will not charge a cent for keeping them, but you must pay their taxes and clothe them. I will keep them at my own expense. Remember, I was very enthusiastic, and expected to cure them, every one, in six months. I never dreamed of failure, and could see how accurately and how nicely the operation could be performed.

It took me about three months to have my instruments made, to gather the patients in, and to have everything ready to commence the season of philosophical experiment. The first patient I operated on was Lucy. She was the last one I had, and the case was a very bad one. The whole base of the bladder was gone and destroyed, and a piece had fallen out, leaving an opening between the vagina and the bladder, at least two inches in diameter or more. That was before the days of anaesthetics, and the poor girl, on her knees, bore the operation with great heroism and bravery. I had about a dozen doctors there to witness the series of experiments that I expected to perform. All the doctors had seen my notes often and examined them, and agreed that I was on the eve of a great discovery, and every one of them was interested in seeing me operate. The operations were tedious and difficult. The instruments were on the right principle, though they were not as perfect as they were subsequently, and improvements had to be made slowly. I succeeded in closing the fistula in about an hour's time, which was considered to be very good work. I placed my patient in bed, and it does seem to me now, since things were so simple and clear, that I was exceedingly stupid at the beginning.

But I must have something to turn the urine from the bladder, and I thought that if I could make a catheter stay in the bladder I could succeed. But I knew that the books said that the doctors had tried to do it for ages past and had never succeeded. The great Wurtzer, of Germany, attempted to cure fistula, many years ago, and, failing to retain the catheter in the bladder, he adopted the plan of fastening the patient face downward, for a week at a time, to prevent the urine from dripping through the vagina. I said, "I will put a little piece of sponge into the neck of the bladder, running a silk string through it. This will act as a capillary tube; the urine will be turned, and the fistula cured." It was a very stupid thing for me to do, as the sequel will show. At the end of five days my patient was very ill. She had fever, frequent pulse, and real blood-poisoning, but we did not know what to call it at that day and time. However, I saw that everything must be removed; so I cut loose my sutures, which had been held by a peculiar mechanical contrivance which it is not necessary here to detail. Then I attempted to remove the little piece of sponge from the neck of the bladder. It was about two inches long. One inch occupied the urethra, half an inch projected into the bladder, and half an inch into the meatus. As soon as it was applied, the urine came dripping through, just as fast as it was secreted in the bladder, and so it continued during all the time it was worn. It performed its duties most wonderfully; but when I came to remove it I found what I ought to have known, that the sponge could not rest there simply as a sponge, but was perfectly infiltrated with sabulous matter, and was really stone. The whole urethra and the neck of the bladder were in a high state of inflammation, which came from the foreign substance. It had to come away, and there was nothing to do but to pull it away by main force. Lucy's agony was extreme. She was much prostrated, and I thought she was going to die; but by irrigating the parts of the bladder she recovered with great rapidity, and in the course of a week or ten days was as well as ever.

After she had recovered entirely from the effects of this unfortunate experiment, I put her on a table, to examine and see what was the result of the operation. The appearance of the parts was changed entirely. The enormous fistula had disappeared, and two little openings in the line of union, across the vagina, were all that remained. One was the size of a knitting-needle, and the other was the size of a goose-quill. That encouraged me very much in the operation, for I said, "If one operation can produce results such as this, under such unfavorable circumstances, why may it not be perfectly successful when I have something to draw the urine that will not produce inflammation of the soft parts?"

This operation was performed in December, 1845. It inaugurated a series of experiments that were continued for a long time. It took Lucy two or three months to recover entirely from the effects of the operation. As soon as I had arranged a substitute for the sponge, I operated on Betsey. The fistula was favorable, and would be considered a favorable one at the present day. Of course, I considered it very unfavorable. The fistula occupied the base of the bladder, and was very large, being quite two inches in diameter. I repeated the operation, in the same way and manner as performed on Lucy, with the exception of placing in the bladder a self-retaining catheter, instead of the sponge. I started out very hopefully, and, of course, I waited anxiously for the result of the operation. Seven days rolled around; she had none of the chills or fever, either violent or sudden, or the disturbance attending the previous operation. At the end of seven days the sutures were removed. To my great astonishment and disappointment, the operation

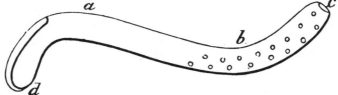

Figure 35. Sims's inlying catheter, to allow the bladder to remain empty after the repair of a vesicovaginal fistula. This and the following figures are taken from Sims's original article in the *American Journal of the Medical Sciences.* (Courtesy National Library of Medicine.)

was a failure. Still, the opening had been changed entirely in character, and, instead of being two inches in diameter, it was united across entirely, with the exception of three little openings, one in the middle, and one at each end of the line of union. The line of union was transverse.

I thought I could make some improvements in the operation, and Anarcha was the next case. Anarcha was the first case that I had ever seen, having assisted Dr. Henry in her delivery. She had not only an enormous fistula in the base of the bladder, but there was an extensive destruction of the posterior wall of the vagina, opening into the rectum, by which gas—intestinal gas—escaped involuntarily, and was pass- The urine was running day and night, saturating the bedding and clothing, and producing an inflammation of the external parts wherever it came in contact with the person, almost similar to confluent smallpox, with constant pain and burning. The odor from this saturation permeated everything, and every corner of the room; and, of course, her life was one of suffering and disgust. Death would have been preferable. But patients of this kind never die; they must live and suffer. Anarcha had added to the fistula an opening which extended into the rectum, by which gas–intestinal gas–escaped involuntarily, and was passing off continually, so that her person was not only loathsome and disgusting to herself, but to every one who came near her.

I made some modifications in the suture apparatus, such as I thought important, and in the catheter, and then operated on the fistula of the bladder. But, like the others, she was only partially cured. The large fistula was contracted, leaving only two or three smaller ones in the line of union, as in the other two instances. The size of the fistula makes no difference in the involuntary loss of urine. It will escape as readily and as rapidly through an opening the size of a goose-quill as it will when the whole base of the bladder is destroyed. The patient is not cured so long as there is the involuntary loss of a single drop of urine. It would be tiresome for me to repeat in detail all the stages of improvement in the operation that were necessary before it was made perfect. These I have detailed in a surgical history of the facts, and to professional readers are still well known. Besides these three cases, I got three or four more to experiment on, and there was never a time that I could not, at any day, have had a subject for operation. But my operations all failed, so far as a positive cure was concerned. This went on, not for one year, but for two and three, and even four years. I kept all these negroes at my own expense all the time. As a matter of course this was an enormous tax for a young doctor in country practice. When I began the experiments, the other doctors in the city were all willing to help me, and all seemed anxious to witness the operations. But, at last, two or three years of constant failure and fruitless effort rather made my friends tired, and it was with difficulty that I could get any doctor to help me. But, notwithstanding the repeated failures, I had succeeded in inspiring my patients with confidence that they would be cured eventually. They would not have felt that confidence if I had not felt confident too; and at last I performed operations only with the assistance of the patients themselves.

So I went on working without any progress, or at least permanent result, til my brother-in-law, Dr. Rush Jones, came to me one day, and he said:

"I have come to have a serious talk with you. When you began these experiments, we all thought that you were going to succeed at once, and that you were on the eve of a brilliant discovery that would be of great importance to suffering humanity. We have watched you, and sympathized with you; but your friends here have seen that of late you are doing too much work, and that you are breaking down. And, besides, I must tell you frankly that with your young and growing family it is unjust to them to continue in this way, and carry on this series of experiments. You have no idea what it costs you to support a half-dozen niggers, now more than three years, and my advice to you is to resign the whole subject and give it up. It is better for you, and better for your family."

I was very much surprised at what he said. But I said: "My dear brother, if I live I am bound to succeed; and I am as sure that I shall carry this thing through to success as I am that I now live, or as sure as I can be of anything. I have done too much already, and I am too near the accomplishment of the work to give it up now. My patients are all perfectly satisfied with what I am doing for them. I can not depend on the doctors, and so I have trained them to assist me in the operations. I am going on with this series of experiments to the end. It matters not what it costs, if it costs me my life. For, if I should fail, I believe somebody would be raised up to take the work where I lay it down and carry it on to successful issue."

The experiments were continued at least a year after this conversation with Dr. Jones. I went on improving the methods of operating, eliminating first one thing and then another, till I had got it down to a very simple practice. Then I said: "I am not going to perform another operation until I discover some method of tying the suture higher up in the body where I can not reach." This puzzled me sorely. I had been three weeks without performing a single operation on either of the half-dozen patients that I had there. They were clamorous, and at last the idea occurred to me about three o'clock one morning. I had been lying awake for an hour, wondering how to tie the suture, when all at once an idea occurred to me to run a shot, a perforated shot, on the suture, and, when it was drawn tight, to compress it with a pair of forceps, which would make the knot perfectly secure. I was so elated with the idea, and so enthusiastic as I lay in bed, that I could not help waking up my kind and sympathetic wife and telling her of the simple and beautiful method I had discovered of tying the suture. I lay there till morning, tying the suture and performing all sorts of beautiful operations, in imagination, on the poor people in my little hospital; and I determined, as soon as I had made my round of morning calls, to operate with this perfected suture. Just as I had got ready to perform my operation I was summoned to go twenty miles into the country, and I did not get back until late in the night. I looked upon it as a very unfortunate thing, and one of the keenest disappointments of my life, because it kept me from seeing all the beautiful results of my method. However, the next day, in due time, the operation was

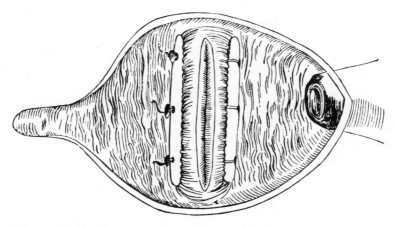

Figure 36. Sims's method of suturing the vesicovaginal defect, showing the silver wire suture, the small strips of lead through which the sutures were passed, and the lead shots used to fasten the wire. Sims called this his "clamp suture." (Courtesy National Library of Medicine.)

performed on Lucy. When it was done, I said, "Could anything be more beautiful? Now I know that she will be cured very soon, and then all the rest might be cured." It was with great impatience that I waited a whole week to see what the result of the operation would be. When I came to examine it, it was a complete failure.

I then said to myself. "There must be a cause for this. I have improved the operations till the mechanism seems to be as perfect as possible, and yet they fail. I wonder if it is in the kind of suture that is used? Can I get some substitute for the silk thread? Mettauer,[3] of Virginia, had used lead, and I had used a leaden suture and failed. What can I do?" Just in this time of tribulation about the subject, I was walking from my house to the office, and picked up a little bit of brass wire in the yard. It was very fine, and such as was formerly used as springs in suspenders before the days of India-rubber. I took it around to Mr. Swan, who was then my jeweler, and asked him if he could make me a little silver wire about the size of the piece of brass wire. He said Yes, and he made it. He made it of all pure silver. Anarcha was the subject of this experiment. The operation was performed on the fistula in the base of the bladder, that would admit of the end of my little finger; she had been cured of one fistula in the base of the bladder. The edges of the wound were nicely denuded, and neatly brought together with four of these fine silver wires. They were passed through little strips of lead, one on one side of the fistula, and the other on the other. The suture was tightened, and then secured or fastened by the perforated shot run on the wire, and pressed with forceps. This was the thirtieth operation performed on Anarcha. She was put to bed, a catheter was introduced, and the next day the urine came from the bladder as clear and as limpid as spring water, and so continued during all the time she wore the catheter. In all the preceding operations, where the silk was used for a suture at the base of the bladder, cystitis always resulted. The urethra was swollen continually, and the urine loaded with a thick, ropy mucus. With the use of the silver suture there was a complete change in these conditions.

I was always anxious to see the result of all experiments; but this was attended with such marked symptoms of improvement, in every way, that I was more anxious now than ever. When the week rolled around—it seemed to me that the time would never come for the removal of the sutures—Anarcha was removed from the bed and carried to the operation-table. With a palpitating heart and an anxious mind I turned her on her side, introduced the speculum, and there

---

3. James Peter Mettauer (1785–1875) of Prince Edward County, Virginia, was a pupil of P. S. Physick (q.v.) and graduated from the University of Pennsylvania in 1809. Mettauer was a superbly skillful surgeon who had one of the largest practices in the United States in his day. He operated until the time of his death at 90. Mettauer is said to have had between forty-five and sixty patients under his care at all times. He performed over eight hundred operations for cataract, and over four hundred lithotomies—a truly astronomical number.

lay the suture apparatus just exactly as I had placed it. There was no inflammation, there was no tumefaction, nothing unnatural, and a very perfect union of the little fistula.

This was in the month of May, I think, though possibly it was June (1849). In the course of two weeks more, Lucy and Betsey were both cured by the same means, without any sort of disturbance or discomfort. Then I realized the fact that, at last, my efforts had been blessed with success, and that I had made, perhaps, one of the most important discoveries of the age for the relief of suffering humanity.[4]

---

4. Sims may not have been aware of previous successful operations for vesico-vaginal fistula when he first became interested in this condition, but a number had been performed that antedated his own. Later, when he wrote up his cases for the *American Journal of the Medical Sciences*, he mentioned several prior successful cases that had come to his attention. These (and several others not mentioned by Sims) included the cases of Mettauer, who was probably the first surgeon to repair successfully a vesico-vaginal fistula (1838). Mettauer eventually was able to compile a series of six cures. Hayward of Boston had three successes in twenty operations on nine patients (1851); his first cure was in 1839. Mussey of New Hampshire also had a successful case antedating Sims', as did Pancoast of Philadelphia (1847). In Europe the operation had been performed a number of times by Jobert de Lamballe of Paris with several successes (1852). Maisonneuve of Paris also had a successful case (1848).

Sims's contribution was not one of priority. Rather, he devised a successful and reproducible operation.

Notes on Arrow Wounds

JOSEPH HOWLAND BILL, Jr. (1835?–1885)

Joseph Howland Bill, Jr. was an assistant surgeon in the United States Army serving on the Arizona-New Mexico frontier when he wrote the following monograph, which appeared in the American Journal of Medical Sciences *(154: 365–87, 1862). The original is typical of American medical writing of that time—poorly organized and verbose. Nevertheless, it does contain a great deal of information and must be considered the definitive work on American Indian arrow wounds. Bill's article clearly depicts the brutal nature of frontier warfare as fought among southwestern Indian tribes and the troops and settlers who were appropriating Indian lands during the years immediately preceding the Civil War. It also indicates what an effective and lethal weapon the "Nabajoe" and warriors of other tribes had in their bows and arrows.*

Bill, in writing this article, saw what the future held for the native Americans, who were so effectively harrassing the troops that he served. Warfare with the bow and arrow would soon be relegated to history as the western Indians were suppressed. The young surgeon appreciated that there was nothing in the medical literature that described the specialized military surgery that he was then practicing on our western frontier. His article would have been read with interest when it appeared; today it is of historical importance and it deserves

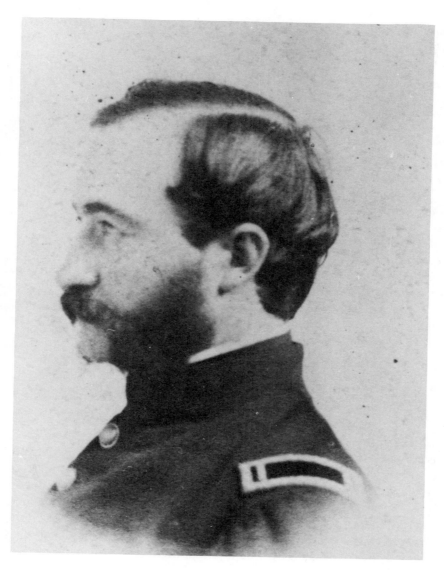

Figure 37. Joseph Howland Bill, Jr. (1835?–1885). (Courtesy National Library of Medicine.)

to be reprinted. This paper, as it appeared in the The American Journal of Medical Sciences, *was in essence a monograph; it has been shortened considerably for its inclusion here (readers who are interested in this may wish to consult the original article). Bill eventually devised an instrument for extracting arrows, described in* The Medical Record *(11:245, 1876); the entire article has been reproduced as Figure 38.*

There apparently is no proper biographical account of J. H. Bill; the following has been pieced together from a number of sources. He was a Philadelphian who graduated from Jefferson Medical College in 1858. He was appointed 1st Lieutenant and assistant surgeon in the army in 1860 and was immediately assigned to Fort Defiance, New Mexico, where he was stationed when he wrote his essay on arrow wounds. He remained on the frontier only for about a year, and we next find "Assistant Surgeon J. H. Bill, U.S.A." mentioned on a number of occasions in the Medical and Surgical History of the War of the Rebellion; *his reports as an operating surgeon during a number of battles are frequently quoted. He served with distinction and was cited for "faithful and meritorious service" during the war. He had achieved the rank of Brevet Lieutenant Colonel by the war's end, and in 1866 he became a Major (a higher rank than today) and a surgeon in the peacetime army. He apparently served in the army until his death in 1885.*

Notes on Arrow Wounds

The arrow is a weapon of the greatest antiquity. It is one with which, in this country, at least, we are all familiar; nevertheless, there is nowhere now extant an account of wounds produced by it sufficiently accurate or definite to guide a surgeon in their treatment, or to give to the medical antiquary a record of their history and appearance. Before long these wounds will become of infrequent occurrence, for our Indian tribes are fast being exterminated. We propose, in the first place, as a matter of historical interest, to state in this article what we know of arrow wounds. The subject still presents much of practical interest to the surgeon, and must continue so to do, in a greater of less degree, for the future. It will be some time before all our Indian tribes are "civilized off the face of all creation," and many a soldier and settler has yet to pay the death penalty for courage or hardihood. Arrow wounds are, therefore, and for some time likely to be, of practical interest.

So much as an apology for the appearance of this article.

The arrow is the favorite weapon of all our Indian tribes, and it is such because in skilful and desperate hands the wound which it inflicts is attended with a fatality greater than that produced by any other weapon—particularly when surgical assistance cannot be obtained. The weapon is constructed not only to disable an antagonist, but also to kill sooner or later its victim.

In order fully to appreciate the subject of arrow wounds, it will be necessary to understand the mechanism and construction of the arrow itself. Let us briefly explain this.

The arrow is composed of two parts, a shaft and a head. The shaft varies in length from two to three feet. Usually it is made from a *limb* of the dogwood tree. A limb of a quarter-inch diameter is taken, soaked in water, the bark peeled off, and then cut into suitable lengths. The straightening process is now commenced. The ends of the piece to be straightened are squared off, and two small and flat strips of wood placed transversely, as regards the long axis of the piece, and firmly lashed one to each end of the latter, in the manner of a cross. One of these sticks is held between the teeth, whilst the other is grasped by the hand. This end is now twisted to and fro by rotating the slip grasped by the hand, after the manner of a trephine. The fibres of the stick to be straightened after a while assume a spiral twist at the same time the stick itself is found to be straight. It often will require three days to straighten a single shaft. A notch is now filed at one end for the bowstring, and a slit made in the other to receive the straight quadrangular stem which comes off from the base of the head. The head is made of soft hoop iron filed into the form of an isosceles triangle, and furnished with a stem to attach it to the shaft. This stem is an inch long by one-eighth of an inch broad, and is of one piece with the rest of the head. An arrow-head varies in length from half an inch to two inches, and half an inch to three–quarters of an inch in breadth at its base. No two arrows are alike. The stem at the base of the arrow-head is pushed into the slit made for it in the shaft, and held there by wrapping narrow ribbons of tendon spirally around the split sides of the latter, thus clamping these together, and the stem itself closely in their embrace. If it were not for these ribbons the head would be held losely. It is then this ribbon of tendon that gives solidity to the arrow, and makes of a head and a shaft a perfect and a most dangerous weapon. The tendon removed and the weapon falls to pieces.

Such being the mechanism of the arrow, we can readily understand the danger peculiar to arrow wounds in general, a danger often seen in pistol-ball wounds of the chest. Let us suppose a case to illustrate and explain our meaning. An arrow is shot at a man at a distance of fifty yards. It penetrates his abdomen, and without wounding an intestine or a great vessel, lodges in the body of one of the verterbrae. The arrow is grasped by the shaft by some officious friend, and after a little tugging is pulled out. We said the arrow is pulled. This was a mistake; it is the shaft only of the arrow that is pulled out. The angular and jagged head has been left buried in the bone to kill—for so it surely will—the victim. The explanation of such mishaps is this: the ribbon of tendon which compressed together the split sides of the end of the arrow, and so clamped the head and the shaft together, had become wetted with the fluids effused in the course of the wound. It ceased longer to bind together the split sides of the shaft; this and the head were, consequently, very feebly united and readily detached. Experience has abundantly shown, and none know the fact better than the Indians themselves, that any arrow wound of chest or abdomen, in which the arrow-head is detached from the shaft and lodged is mortal. From this we conclude that the danger *peculiar* to all arrow wounds is, *that the shaft becoming detached from the head of an implanted arrow, leaves this so deeply imbedded in a bone that it cannot be withdrawn, and that, remaining, it kills.* It is not possible with forceps to extract an arrow-head so lodged (if lodged deeply), throwing aside the difficulty of discovering and the danger of searching for it. The blades of forceps long enough for this purpose (supposing the foreign body deeply lodged in the chest) would bend too readily with the force required for the removal of the missile. The greatest force is sometimes required for the extraction of arrow heads so lodged. We have seen an arrow shot at a distance of one hundred yards, so deeply embedded in an oak plank that it required great force, applied by strong tooth forceps to remove it. In the case of a man shot in the shaft of the humerus by an arrow, it was only after using both knees, applied to the ends of the bone as a counter-extending force, and a stout pair of tooth-forceps, that we succeeded in removing the foreign body. Arrow wounds are often complicated by profuse hemorrhage, and for the same reason that in bayonet wounds abscesses form, through inability of matter to find a ready outlet; in arrow wounds haematomata result. In fact, when arrow wounds suppurate, they generally do so through disorganization of these collections of blood.

What parts of the body are oftenest wounded by the arrow, and what is the relative fatality? The following table of cases, falling principally under our own observation, will show:

Table 1

	Number of Cases Saved	Number of Cases Died	Total
Head			
Brain wounded	1	2	3
Brain not wounded	2	0	2
Spinal marrow	0	1	1
Neck	2	0	2
Chest			
Lung wounded	2	4	6
Lung not wounded	9	0	9
Heart	0	2	2
Abdomen			
Intestine wounded	0	15	15
Intestine not wounded	3	3	6
Upper extremity	27	1	28
Lower extremity	5	1	6
Total	51	29	80

An expert bowman can easily discharge six arrows per minute, and a man wounded with one is almost sure to receive several arrows. In the above table, when a man was wounded in more places than one, the most serious wound, or that which immediately caused his death, is recorded. We have not seen more than one or two men wounded by a single arrow only. In three of our soldiers shot by Nabajoes, we counted forty-two arrow wounds; this is an extreme case, as the manufacture of the arrow costs the Indian too much labour and time to expend one unnecessarily. The cause of death in the twenty nine fatal cases [has been] thus summed up [in Table 2].

Keeping in view the real cause of dread in arrow wounds, to wit, the lodging and fixation of the iron head in a bone, let us now proceed to consider the subject from a more limited view, and investigate the arrow wounds of each separate part of the body.

First then for the simplest case; an arrow wound involving no parts essential to life. Let us suppose a case.

Table 2

Cause of Death	Number of Cases
Immediate hemorrhage	7
Peritonitis	13
Compression of brain	2
Wound of heart	2
Empyema	1
Tetanus	1
Pneumonia	1
Wound of spinal cord	1
Other injuries	1
Total	29

A man is shot by an arrow which passes through integuments and muscle, and grazing the bone, makes its exit on the other side of a limb. We will find at the spot where the arrow entered, a very small and narrow slit, surrounded by a circular patch of bruised integument of a dusky red colour. On the other side of the limb another slit, somewhat larger than that above described, is seen, but not surrounded by the red areola. This is the exit wound. What is the treatment? Apply cold or evaporating lotions, place the limb at perfect rest, let the patient diet himself and the chances are favourable of such a wound healing by first intention.

If an arrow, instead of passing through a limb, strikes a bone, it will lodge, and that too, so deeply, that nothing but forcible traction and judicious movement will extract it. The wound should be enlarged with a bistoury, as the shaft of an arrow is always so tightly grasped by the tissues through which it passes, that a forceps cannot be introduced for its extraction. An incision an inch to two inches in length will suffice, but it must divide to this extent all the tissues, through which the arrow has passed. After this has been made, pass down a finger, and explore the parts; ascertain the position, seat, and depth of the arrow-head in the bone. Then guide down upon the finger a pair of straight tooth forceps, and make these embrace the arrow–head; remove the finger gently, til the arrow shifts from side to side, so as to loosen its seat in the bone. A gentle rocking motion of the handles of the forceps, such as a dentist uses to extract a tooth, will, if enough of the arrow-head projects out of the bone, suffice to disengage it. If it is deeply buried, nothing but sheer brute force will accomplish its extraction. The following is a case in point:

Private Bishop was shot in the head of the humerus with an arrow, and the shaft having been plucked out, the iron head was left deeply imbedded in the bone. I introduced forceps, seized it by its base, but could obtain scarcely any "purchase". I at last succeeded in grasping it tightly, and bracing my knees against the patient's thorax, I applied all the traction I could muster. Suddenly the arrow-head flew out of its seat, and I would have fallen of the floor, had not the steward caught me. The wound healed well. It was treated by evaporating lotions, and a rigorously antiphlogistic diet for the patient. Motion in the joint was not lost, though somewhat impaired.

If a surgeon is called to a case in which an arrow-head is left lodged in a bone, and in which, from any cause, immediate extraction is impossible, what should be the treatment? In such a case, the treatment must be expectant. Place the limb on a splint, make the orifice of the wound the most depending portion thereof, and finally introduce a sponge-tent, or what is better, perhaps, a drainage-tube of Chassaignac.[1] From a fair trial of this instrument in several cases of gunshot wound, we can cordially recommend it both in gun shot wounds, and in all wounds where deep suppuration is expected. In addition to a tent or drainage-tube, bandages and compresses will be found necessary, particularly towards the conclusion of the case. They should never be applied so tightly as to produce uneasiness, but should always keep up just that amount of pressure which will serve to prevent the burrowing of matter, and check motion of the muscles. Perhaps, after pursuing this course for while, the arrow-head may be detected, and if detected, extracted with facility. In any event, frequent search should be made for it. Generally, we will at length succeed in removing the foreign body; but all things else failing, as time, strength, and patience may, we must operate.

It is not possible to lay down any fixed rules for such an operation. The incisions should be large and free-boldness rather than prudence governing our actions. We might as well cut the patient's limb up until we do find the arrow-head, for if it is left, amputation will be necessary, and worse than this can hardly ensue from the "cutting up" we have advised. We would, if we undertook such an operation, make up our

---

1. Edouard Pierre Marie Chassaignac (1804–1879). Surgeon of Paris who was the first to use and advocate effective surgical drainage, using india-rubber tubes for the purpose. He wrote a two-volume work on the subject, *On Suppuration and Surgical Drainage* (Paris: 1859).

mind to find the arrow-head, even if it were necessary to tear up every fasciculus of every muscle of the injured member. It is just in such cases as this that the motto, "Operative surgery is the art of cutting and tying what you cut," finds its best exemplification. As such a wound will be attended with hemorrhage, rendering all its steps more difficult, it will be proper to compress the main artery of the limb by the hand of an assistant. Having thus briefly considered the subject of arrow wounds of parts not essential to life, let us recapitulate:

1st. An arrow passing through a limb makes a clean half punctured, half incised wound, which will generally heal by first intention, if proper treatment be instituted.

2d. An arrow lodging in bone requires some force, much tact, strong forceps, and an ample incision for its removal.

3d. This removal should always be effected as soon as possible after the receipt of the injury, *and the greatest care taken in doing so not to detach the shaft from the head of the arrow.*

4th. Always use the finger to explore the lodgment of an arrow-head, and to determine whether it is bent or straight.

5th. If we fail to detect or to extract an arrow-head lodged in bone, we wait a few days, trusting to suppuration, tents, position, etc. and then search again and again for it.

6th. If we fail in removing the foreign body by these means, we operate, making large incisions and compressing the artery of the limb.

Let us now proceed to consider arrow wounds of the head. An arrow will usually glance off, making a scalp wound a wound here requiring no particular notice, as it presents nothing peculiar. If however, an arrow should strike the skull at a short range and perpendicularly to its surface, it will probably penetrate. In doing this the arrow-head makes in the outer table by compressing the particles of bone surrounding it, a narrow puncture the width of the thickness of the arrow-head. In addition to this a crack usually commences from both ends of this puncture, and extends itself in an opposite direction from its fellow, over a distance proportional to the momentum which the arrow possessed. In its passage through the outer table, the arrow-head loses its momentum, and strikes the inner table with a greatly reduced velocity, a velocity not sufficient to allow the arrow-head to penetrate it and pass into the substance of the brain; but enough to cause a scale of the inner table to be fractured off; and whilst still sticking to the point of the arrow-head, to be slightly driven upon (seldom into) the brain itself. Under these circumstances, the usual symptoms of compression will arise, as in any other case. The man fails insensible to the ground. Hence it happens that the surgeon is seldom called to treat such cases.

The man being so wounded and insensible falls an easy prey to the vindictive savage who shot him, and such a chance is never neglected. If, however, we do have such a case to treat, we remove the arrow-head and elevate the depressed bone. Both of these indications will usually be filled by making gentle traction on the arrow-head; for as the arrow-head is withdrawn, it draws with it the scale of depressed bone, which is sticking to its point, until this last is elevated into its proper place. If, on removing the foreign body in the manner indicated, we find the symptoms of compression still present, we infer that we have failed to elevate the depressed bone. But in any such event we must trephine. We trephine not so much with the purpose of elevating the depressed bone as with the object of removing the cause of the compression, whatever this may be. The after treatment of such a case must be most strictly anti-inflammatory, the first signs of cerebral disturbance being met with bleeding and one smart purge. Croton oil has answered best in our hands. After the elevation of the fragment, close the wound with collodion, shave the head, apply cold unremittingly, and if inflammation does ensue, as indicated by cerebral derangements, treat it as above indicted. The bleeding, however must be *ad deliquium*. If in any case suppuration should commence, and abscess form , then also we must resort to the trephine. Such a case will almost surely end fatally.

Miguel "Nigro", the post-guide at Fort Union, was shot with an arrow by a Utah Indian. I found the arrow-head sticking in the left parietal bone, the shaft having been detached. I made traction on it, and drew it out of the wound. The symptoms of compression present at once vanished, the man turned over and sneezed, and rose up on his feet. I had made arrangements to trephine the skull if necessary, but I had probably restored to its proper level that portion of the inner table which was depressed, so that measure was unnecessary. The cause of the compression was gone, and I had nothing to trephine for. The next day the man complained of headache. His face was flushed, eyes suffused, pulse hard, and irregular. I ordered croton oil, shaved his head, and applied cold. Presently, when delirium came on, I bled him until he fainted. This bleeding was repeated the night of the same day. The next day he was greatly better; the croton had operated well. The man was left to recover, which he did in three weeks.

Arrow wounds of the trunk, from their greater importance and more frequent occurrence, comprise the greater part of our subject. The Indians know well the fatality of such wounds, and aim always at the umbilicus; hence one cause of the frequency of these wounds.

An arrow sometimes goes through the chest and passes out. It would always do so if it were not that it can scarcely miss hitting a bone.

Hence it happens that a lung is not nearly so often wounded by an arrow as an intestine. Of fifteen cases of arrow wound of the chest falling under our notice, in New Mexico, in seven cases only was the lung wounded, and in one of these, the heart was wounded also; and in four of these (rejecting the case complicated with heart wound) the patients died. In two, the death was by hemorrhage; in one, by empyema; in one by pneumonia, complicated with peritonitis.

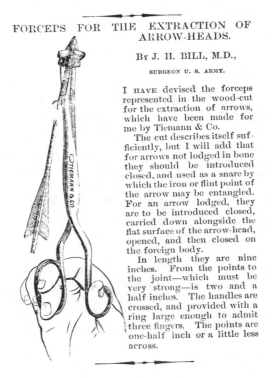

FORCEPS FOR THE EXTRACTION OF ARROW-HEADS.

By J. H. BILL, M.D.,
SURGEON U. S. ARMY.

I HAVE devised the forceps represented in the wood-cut for the extraction of arrows, which have been made for me by Tiemann & Co.

The cut describes itself sufficiently, but I will add that for arrows not lodged in bone they should be introduced closed, and used as a snare by which the iron or flint point of the arrow may be entangled. For an arrow lodged, they are to be introduced closed, carried down alongside the flat surface of the arrow-head, opened, and then closed on the foreign body.

In length they are nine inches. From the points to the joint—which must be very strong—is two and a half inches. The handles are crossed, and provided with a ring large enough to admit three fingers. The points are one-half inch or a little less across.

Figure 38. Bill's forceps for the extraction of arrowheads. Bill eventually devised an instrument that could be used to extract arrows with their heads intact. His contribution is reproduced here in its entirety as it appeared in the *Medical Record* in 1876.

An arrow wound of the lung is from first to last more dangerous than a gunshot wound of the same parts. There are three reasons for this. First the hemorrhage occuring at the time of the injury, or a few hours after, is much more profuse than in an ordinary gunshot wound. Secondly, an arrow wounding the lung, is almost sure to lodge, whilst a ball generally passes. If an arrow-head becoming detached from its shaft is *permanently* lodged in a vertebra, or a rib, empyema will result.

The third danger peculiar to arrow wounds of lung is the supervention of emphysema twelve or fifteen hours after the receipt of the injury. It is rather an inconvenience than a danger.

[Five very lengthy case reports follow that serve to illustrate arrow wounds of the lungs. Two of Bill's patients died of immediate hemorrhage, and two died of sepsis. One patient who was shot five times in the lungs also sustained a wound of the liver. He developed a troublesome biliary fistula but eventually recovered. In this case, fortunately, none of the arrowheads were retained. Bill described in great detail several methods that could be used to extract arrowheads from the chest. These consisted of introducing various instruments that served to place one or more wire loops below the flare of the arrowhead. Traction on the wire then enabled the head and shaft to be extracted together.]

Arrow wounds of the heart are generally fatal, although not always instantaneously so. In one case falling under my notice the man perished instantly. I found the ventricles of the heart and the descending aorta pierced by an arrow and spiked to a rib. In another case the man lived five minutes. The case was interesting in a medico-legal view, as it was devolved upon us to determine whether the man had been shot with a pistol ball from the weapon of a comrade, or with an arrow, so much did the wound resemble that made by a navy-sized Colt's revolver. I found the arrow-head lodged in a vertebra. It had pierced the top of the auricle.

Arrow wounds of the abdomen are generally fatal. An arrow can scarcely pass through the abdomen and fail to open a vessel or wound an intestine. We have seen twenty-one cases of arrow wound of the abdomen. All save one, of those cases in which the abdominal cavity was implicated, terminated fatally. In three the integuments only were wounded, and in one the arrow had lodged in the crest of the ilium without wounding an intestine.

Of the seventeen fatal cases, thirteen perished from peritonitis and four from hemorrhage. All save two were wounded in the intestine, although two of those so wounded died from hemorrhage. Nine of the cases of peritonitis had been exposed to a broiling sun, without water, for two days. Five were dead, and none lived to reach the Post. The remaining four cases of peritonitis occurred in the persons of United States soldiers engaged against Nabajoes. In all, fecal matter was found discharged into the peritoneal cavity, the intestine being wounded.

The Mexicans, on entering into an Indian fight, wrap many folds of a blanket around the abdomen. Thus it happens that an arrow, after penetrating these folds, has not momentum enough left to do more than wound the integument, and fails to reach the abdominal cavity.

From all that has been stated it must appear that the prognosis in all cases of arrow wounds of the abdomen is very unfavorable. Much, however will depend upon the seat and extent of the injury, and upon the facilities for treatment and transportation. The treatment should take into consideration the extraction of the missile, the checking of hemorrhage, the removal of any discharged excrementitious matters, the suturing of the wounded intestine, and the preventing or suppressing of peritonitis. If the arrow-head is lodged, or feces [are] extruded through the wounded intestine, we consider that no surgeon should be satisfied without operating. It is difficult, however, to arrive at this information with certainty.

If called to another case of arrow-wound of the abdominal cavity we would feel almost justified in enlarging the wound, laying open the abdomen, searching gently for wounded intestine, and removing the arrow-head if lodged firmly in bone, with strong short forceps. In any event, if this is not done the patient will die. For suturing the intestine we should look upon *very* fine gold wire with great favour; on gold wire because this metal is possessed of greater ductility than any other. If we are certain that an arrow-head has lodged in a bone of the pelvis, the course above indicated must be pursued, for in addition to the facility which an enlarging of the wound gives for extracting the arrowhead, there is thus afforded also an opportunity of suturing intestine requiring it, of removing foreign matters, and perhaps of checking hemorrhage. If it is decided upon to adopt an expectant plan, and, in fact, after any operation for removal of arrow-heads, opium must be given in full doses very frequently, until narcotism ensues, and starvation and absolute rest must be enforced. The patient must not be allowed to rise from the recumbent position for at least two weeks, and milk and light custard must be his only diet. We know of at least one instance in which an officer lost his life by insisting on leaving his bed before the tenth day. In every case, however, of arrow-wound of the abdomen, it is necessary to remember that the arrow-head must be extracted or the patient will die. It is the great distinctive rule between arrow and gunshot wounds of all other parts of the body as well as of the abdomen, *always extract the foreign body, if it be an arrow.*

Such then, arrow wounds as we have seen them—a class of wounds as troublesome to the surgeon as dangerous to the patient. But in no class of wounds does surgical skill avail the patient so much or reward the surgeon so well for his trouble. Only never let him despair of his patient until he has operated in vain. An expectant treatment in such cases is really no treatment at all.

Fort Craig, New Mexico, January 1, 1862

Extract from a Narrative of His Services in the War of the Rebellion

JOHN SHAW BILLINGS, M.D. (1838–1913)

In marked contradistinction to the Revolutionary War, a flood of accounts became available from many pens describing surgery during the Civil War. Few give a picture as vivid as John Shaw Billing's dispassionate, formal report on his activities during the battle of Chancellorsville in 1863. Billings was one of America's foremost men of medicine. He "achieved excellence and gained distinction in no less than six different fields," according to his biographer, F.H. Garrison. Garrison's list did not include surgery, but it should have, for this was Billings's first field of distinction following his graduation from medical school in 1860.

John Shaw Billings was born in Switzerland County, Indiana, on April 12, 1838. He was a precocious child and was given an excellent education. In 1858 he entered the Medical College of Ohio in Cincinnati and two years later, after his graduation, joined the Union Army. He soon became a skilled military surgeon. Billings remained with the Army Surgeon-General's office after the war. During his 30 years, in the army, and afterwards as a civilian, he made many contributions to such diverse fields as hospital and library design, sanitation, medical statistics, administration, and especially as a librarian and as a bibliographer. Billings died in New York City on March 11, 1913.

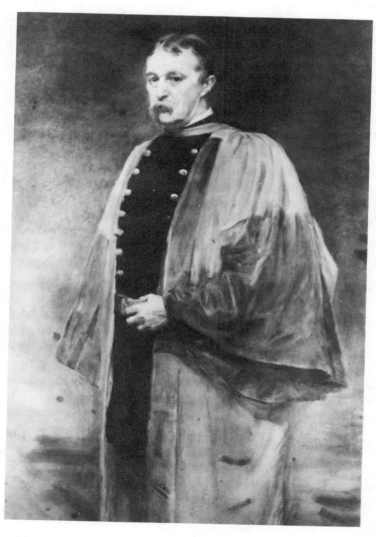

Figure 39. John Shaw Billings (1838–1913). (Courtesy New York Academy of Medicine.)

*The following account of the battle of Chancellorsville appeared
on page 135 of the appendix to the first medical volume of the* Medical and Surgical History of the War of the Rebellion, *published by the
Government Printing Office, Washington, D.C., in 1875.*

Extract from a Narrative of His Services in the Medical Staff

I reported for duty to Surgeon J. Letterman,[1] medical director of
the army of the Potomac, on the 31st of March, 1863, and was immediately assigned to duty with the 11th U.S. Infantry, 2d brigade, 2d division, Fifth Corps. On the 27th of April, the division commenced the
march across the Rappahannock.[2] In anticipation of the forthcoming
battle, the detail of officers for the division hospital was made out by
Assistant Surgeon Wagner,[3] then chief medical officer of the division
and I was designated as one of the operators, my assistants being
Assistant Surgeon Bacon,[4] U.S.A., and Acting Assistant Surgeon
Hichborn.[5] But two ambulances were allowed to the division, and no

---

1. Jonathan Letterman (1824–1872) graduated from Jefferson Medical
College in 1849 and entered the army the same year. He contributed greatly
to the efficient organization of the medical department during the Civil War.
Letterman is best known for the development of ambulance evacuation facilities—one of the few noteworthy advances in military medicine to come out of
that war.
2. The Union troops at Chancellorsville were under the command of
General Joe Hooker. As Billings mentions, Hooker deployed his forces on the
further side of the Rappahannock River, and so had the river at his back during the battle—not best tactical position. The Union forces had a numerical
advantage, but two big disadvantages: their commander's indecision, and the
ability of the opposing generals, Robert E. Lee and Stonewall Jackson.
Hooker was worried about how he would retreat if this became necessary: and
weighed down by this negative consideration, he was unable to attack with
sufficient enthusiam to exploit his larger force.
   The Confederacy sustained a severe loss at Chancellorsville, however,
for Stonewall Jackson fell here after sustaining a gunshot fracture of his right
humerus. Ironically, the bullet was fired by confused Confederate troops.
Amputation was performed but he succumbed to infection ten days later.
3. Clinton Wagner (1837–1914) was a graduate of the Medical School
of the University of Maryland (1858). He achieved prominence as a Civil War
surgeon and subsequently became a nose and throat surgeon in New York
City.
4. Francis Bacon (1831–1912) was a graduate of Yale Medical School
(1851). He served as a surgeon throughout the entire war and later became
professor of surgery at Yale.

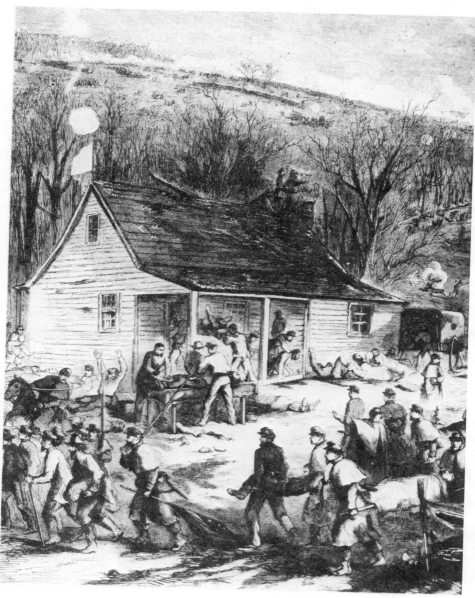

Figure 40. Civil War aid station. This illustration (a detail from a larger one) appeared in *Harpers Weekly*. The artist, Thomas Nast, might well have been illustrating Billings's account of his experiences at Chancellorsville.

---

5. I have not been able to identify Hichborn further. He was killed in this battle.

stretchers or stretcher bearers, nor did any medical supply or Auten-rieth wagons[6] accompany us across the river. After a rapid march over muddy roads, the division reached the brick house of Doctor Chan-cellor[7] on the evening of the 30th of April, and encamped in the woods about half a mile beyond, on the road leading from that place to Bank's Ford. After marching about one mile, the enemy opened fire with rifled shell from a section of artillery so posted as to sweep the road. The column immediately debouched to the left, forming a line of battle at right angles to the road, and advanced at a double quick. Soon after leaving the road, I received orders to repair to a small frame house on a little knoll near by, which was to be used as a temporary hospital. On reaching it, I found several men with slight shell wounds. I had hardly dismounted, when the fire seemed to be concentrated on the spot; shells fell on all sides, one passing through the house; and, in five min-utes, I was the only person left about the place. I then rode back about three hundred yards to another small frame house by the roadside, where I found my assistants, and was soon after joined by the other members of the staff of the hospital. By this time Surgeon John Moore, U.S.A.,[8] medical director of the Fifth Corps, had come up with the ambulances and stretchers, and an Autenrieth wagon, having, by great personal exertion, succeeded in getting them, that morning, across the river. The infantry being now engaged, the wounded began to come in very rapidly, and I proceeded to the relief of the more urgent cases, performing several amputations, among others, two at the shoulder joint, also, one exsection of the same joint and one of the elbow. In about two hours, we were informed that our troops were falling back, and were ordered to remove the wounded to the brick house of Dr. Chancellor, then occupied as headquarters by General Hooker. We succeeded in removing all of the wounded, and within ten minutes after we left the house, the rebel lines came up to it.

---

6. The Autenrieth medicine wagon appeared fairly late in the war. It was a four-wheeled, horse-drawn wagon with a complete supply of medicine, drugs, and instruments.

7. This house and the land were named Chancellorsville and gave the battle its name. It was owned by James Edgar Chancellor, M.D. (1826–1896), and by his family before him. Dr. Chancellor graduated from Jefferson Medi-cal College in 1848 and joined the Confederate Army as a surgeon at the out-break of the war. After the war he served on the faculty of the medical school of the University of Virginia.

8. John Moore (1826–1907) was a graduate of the medical school of New York University (1850). He entered the army in 1853, served during the Civil War, and remained with the Army Medical Department after the war. In 1886 he became surgeon-general.

On reaching the brick house, everything was found in confusion. All the large rooms in the house were locked and filled with furniture; the wounded were lying about in the veranda, in the halls, and wherever space could be found; while a crowd of teamsters, orderlies, contrabands and stragglers filled the kitchen and outbuildings. I immediately broke open the doors; had the furniture carried out, and the wounded taken into the parlors; cleared out the kitchen, and ordered a cook to prepare soup; after which, I resumed the care of the wounded. At this place, the most extensive shell wounds that I have ever seen came under my notice. In two instances, the abdominal walls were entirely carried away; and, from a third patient, I removed the entire head of a three-inch shell which had passed into the abdominal cavity, and was slightly impacted in the bodies of the lumbar vertebrae. This man suffered but little pain, was sensible of his desperate condition, but was very importunate to have the fragment removed, as he said it felt heavy and gave him the colic. After its removal, he expressed himself as much relieved. He lived forty-eight hours. In a fourth case, a large fragment of a three-inch shell had passed through the pelvis from one trochanter to the other. In another, the arm had been torn entirely off, and three inches of the brachial artery was hanging out of the wound and pulsating to within an inch of its extremity. I also observed four cases of wounds of the abdominal walls, with protrusion of unwounded intestines and omentum. In two of them, it was very difficult to return the protruded mass, which was as large as the fist, the muscles of the abdominal walls being strongly and spasmodically contracted. At first, I supposed that the difficulty was due to constriction at the base of the tumor, and enlarged the opening slightly with a probe-pointed bistoury, but the protrusion increased, and all attempts to replace the slippery mass were futile, as it glided out at one angle when pushed in at the other, until I caused one attendant to lift the patient by his head, and another by his heels, the nates just touching the ground, thus relaxing the abdominal walls, while, with silver spatulas, I lifted the abdominal walls away from and over the tumor. I then closed the wound by means of sutures and collodion. Our labors continued all night, as fresh cases were constantly coming in. Every wounded man in the house had soup and coffee served to him. But little operating was done, as few cases required it. I performed exsections of the shoulder and elbow joints, and three or four amputations here.

On the 2d of May, we were ordered to remove our wounded and rejoin our division, then lying about a mile and a half to the rear. Doctor Hichborn was left at the Chancellor house to receive and care for such men as might be brought in from the field. He was killed the next day in attempting to escape from the house. On reaching the division.

I found it just preparing to march to the right of our line, to strengthen or replace the flying columns of the Eleventh Corps. It was then about four in the afternoon, but it was dusk before the column got fairly in motion. A confused medley of wagons, artillery and stragglers blocked up the road; while, to add to the confusion, the First Corps, under General Reynolds, was coming up at right angles to the line of march. The woods were full of stragglers, who were lighting fires in every direction, while a body of cavalry was attempting to drive them in and to extinguish the fires.[9] At daybreak, I was ordered to establish a hospital in a hollow in the woods, on the road to Bank's Ford, about six hundred yards to the rear of our line of battle. Doctor Doolittle,[10] of the 5th N.Y. Volunteers, who had been detailed as surgeon-in-chief of the hospital, having gone away, I was ordered to assume the duties of that post as well as those of operator. An old saw-mill near by furnished boards enough to make a shelter for about forty men, and this was extended by means of evergreens and pieces of shelter tents, as far as was found necessary. Two hundred and fifty rations were obtained from the commissary of the corps, and in the afternoon, the brigade medical supply wagons were brought up. While at this point, we received and treated about eighty wounded men, very few of whom, however, belonged to our corps. I excised the shoulder joint in two cases at this place. I operated, also, in three cases in which a ball had entered the cranium through the frontal bone, and penetrated the substance of the brain. In the first case, I merely removed the fragments and spiculae of bone which had been forced into the cerebral substance, the ball not being found by any examination which I deemed prudent to attempt. In the second case, I removed the ball, the fragments of bone and the letter of the man's cap, which had been forced into the anterior lobe of the brain. I may add that I saw this man, four weeks afterward, in the corps hospital. At that time, the wound had nearly healed, and no unfavorable symptoms of any kind had occurred. In the third case, a Confederate, I removed the ball and fragments of bone from the centre of the anterior lobe, and forty-eight hours after, when I left, the man was leaning against a tree, smoking a pipe and observing my proceedings with great interest. In none of these cases was there any disturbance of the mental faculties, after the first two hours, during the time that they

---

9. All this confusion was the result of Lee and Jackson's successful plan to sweep the Union Army's right flank, held by the Eleventh Corps. Billings's division, as well as other units, was shifted to the right amid the usual confusion of battle.

10. "Dr. Doolittle" has not been identified.

remained under my observation. On the 5th of May, by the order of Surgeon J. Moore, U.S.A., I removed all the supplies from the brigade wagons, except about fifty blankets and a few bottles of whiskey, and sent them off with all the wounded belonging to our corps. I then had the wounded belonging to other corps transfered to their respective hospitals, leaving no patients except fifteen wounded rebels. All the other medical supplies of the division and about two hundred rations were left in charge of Assistant Surgeon Bacon, U.S.A. One hospital steward, one cook and one nurse were also detailed to remain. At five o'clock of the morning of the 6th of May, we joined the division, which was then on its way towards the river, acting as rear guard, and crossed about nine o'clock. Before leaving, I suggested to Doctor Bacon the propriety of burying, or otherwise concealing, a box of whiskey and some chloroform and morphine. This was done, and I have since been informed by Doctor Bacon that it proved a very useful precaution, as the greater part of the stores not so concealed were appropriated for the rebel wounded as soon as they came up. On the evening of the 6th of May, in a pouring rain, the division reached its old camp near Potomac creek.

A March in
the Ranks Hard-Prest

WALT WHITMAN (1819–1892)

Walt Whitman wrote in later life, "The War of Attempted Se-
cession has, of course, been the distinguishing event of my time. I commenced at the close of 1862, and continued steadily through '63, '64,
and '65, to visit the sick and wounded of the army, both on the field and
in the hospitals in and around Washington City." Whitman worked in
Washington for these years, supporting himself as a secretary and as a
part-time correspondent for several newspapers, including the New
York Times; during that time he estimated that he made 600 hospital
visits. Part of his Civil War writings, including the following brief selection, were incorporated into Leaves of Grass. His prose notes appeared in Specimen Days, and still others have been published since his
death (Walt Whitman's Civil War, ed. Walter Lowenfels; [N. Y. Alfred
A. Knopf, 1961]). None contain descriptions of actual surgery, although the following brief selection, from "Drum-Taps" (in Leaves of
Grass), comes closest.

Whitman's Civil War writings are like the photographs that came
out of the war. There are many pictures of hospitals and the wounded;
there are almost none of actual surgery (and the few that there are appear to have been carefully posed). Whitman probably wrote "A
March in the Ranks Hard-Prest" during a trip to the battlefield at

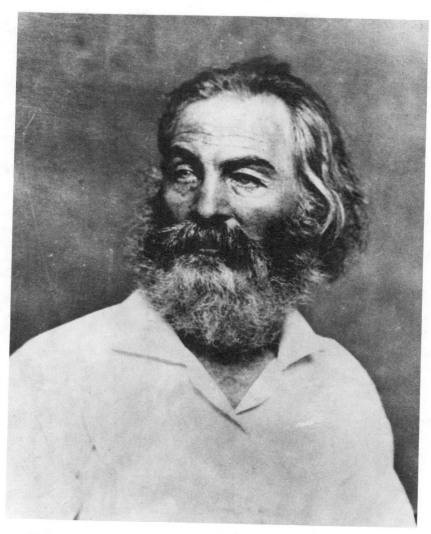

Figure 41. Walt Whitman in 1862. (Courtesy the National Archives.)

Chancellorsville, where he had gone to care for his younger brother, George, who had been wounded. Walt may have seen more than he cared to of the battle, judging from a grim and explicit description of battlefield carnage that he penned at the time—the strongest in Specimen Days. *The description that follows is presumably a scene that Whitman came across at Chancellorsville. His impression—the hospital in a church, the wounded and dying men, the surgeons working by torchlight—provides us with a far less dispassionate glimpse of Civil War field surgery than was penned by J. S. Billings writing about the same battle.*

A March in the Ranks Hard-Prest

A march in the ranks hard-prest, and the road unknown.
A route through a heavy wood with muffled steps in the darkness,
Our army foil'd with loss severe, and the sullen remnant retreating.
Till after midnight glimmer upon us the lights of a dim-lighted
      building,
We come to an open space in the woods, and halt by the dim-
      lighted building,
'Tis a large old church at the crossing roads, now an impromptu
      hospital,
Entering but for a minute I see a sight beyond all the pictures
      and poems ever made,
Shadows of deepest, deepest black, just lit by moving candles and
      lamps,
And by one great pitchy torch stationary with wild red flame and
      clouds of smoke,
By these, crowds, groups of forms vaguely I see on the floor, some
      in the pews laid down,
At my feet more distinctly a soldier, a mere lad, in danger of
      bleeding to death, (he is shot in the abdomen,)
I stanch the blood temporarily, (the youngster's face is white as
      a lily,)
Then before I depart I sweep my eyes o'er the scene fain to
      absorb it all,
Faces, varieties, postures beyond description, most in obscurity,
      some of them dead,
Surgeons operating, attendants holding lights, the smell of
      ether, the odor of blood,

The crowd, O the crowd of the bloody forms, the yard outside also
    fill'd,
Some on the bare ground, some on planks or stretchers, some in
    the death spasm sweating,
An occasional scream or cry, the doctor's shouted orders or
    calls,
The glisten of the little steel instruments catching the glint of
    the torches
These I resume as I chant, I see again the forms, I smell the
    odor,
Then hear outside the orders given, *Fall in, my men, fall in:*
But first I bend to the dying lad, his eyes open, a half-smile
    gives he me,
Then the eyes close, calmly close, and I speed forth to the darkness,
Resuming, marching, ever in darkness marching, on in the ranks,
The unknown road still marching.

A New Use of
Carbolized Catgut Ligatures

HENRY ORLANDO MARCY, M.D. (1837–1924)

Henry O. Marcy was born in Otis, Massachusetts, on June 23, 1837, He graduated from Harvard Medical School in 1863 and then served as an army surgeon during the last years of the Civil War. Marcy traveled abroad and in 1870 became Joseph Lister's (1827–1912) first American pupil, studying surgery in Edinburgh under this man whose doctrines changed all of surgical practice. Marcy returned to America well indoctrinated with the techniques of antiseptic surgery, and he was one of the first surgeons in America to follow the rituals of Listerism as it was then taught. Marcy and a few others spread the gospel of antisepsis, but its principles were accepted only slowly by American surgeons. In 1876 Joseph Lister came to this country on an "evangelistic journey." He traveled over much of the United States, sightseeing, teaching, and occasionally operating. This trip did much to advance the use of antiseptic methods in America.

Marcy continued to be an enthusiastic advocate of Listerism for the remainder of his professional life. He died in Boston on January 1, 1924.

The paper that follows records Henry O. Marcy's results using the antiseptic method in the surgical treatment of two inguinal hernias. These two cases were worth reporting: not only did the wounds heal without infection—a most unusual event—but the hernias were cured

254

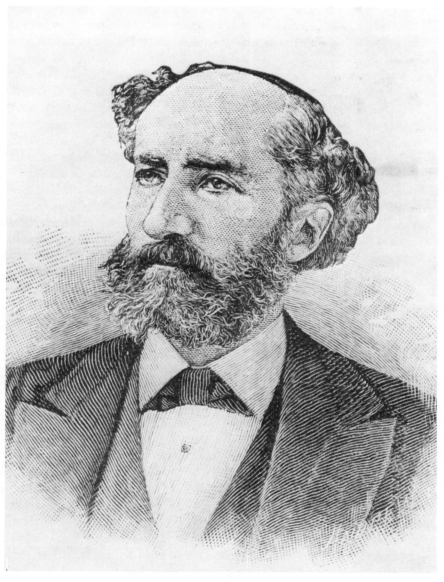

Figure 42. Henry Orlando Marcy (1837–1924). (Courtesy National Library of Medicine.)

as well! This early contribution to antiseptic surgery appeared in the Boston Medical and Surgical Journal *(85: 315) on November 16, 1871.*

A New Use of Carbolized Catgut Ligatures

Among the benefits conferred by carbolic acid on the medical profession, the antiseptic carbolized catgut ligature of Lister promises to take a prominent position.

This ligature is prepared by soaking the ordinary catgut of the shops, made from the intestines of the sheep, in five parts of fixed oil (olive or linseed), and one part of carbolic acid rendered liquid by adding five per cent of water. Catgut, before being thus prepared, is rendered soft and slippery by being immersed in water, is by no means strong, and is entirely unfitted for the purpose of ligatures; but after a few weeks' suspension in this fluid, it is translucent, firm, hard, but pliable, makes a strong knot, and upon immersion in water or the fluids of the body, it undergoes no immediate change, and for days together the knots retain a firm hold.

Prof. Lister, after experimenting with carbolized silk ligatures, found that, although the wound healed easily, leaving the ligature enclosed, usually the softened fibres of the silk acted as an irritant, and were discharged later by the processes of suppuration. He had frequently noticed under antiseptic dressings that clots of blood and large pieces of dead skin and other tissues had disappeared without suppuration, and therefore inferred that small pieces of animal texture, if applied antiseptically, would be similarly disposed of. Acting upon this thought, he has given us the before-mentioned, prepared catgut ligature.

Lister has shown that this ligature, in a wound kept antiseptic, is converted into a form of germinal matter, and is either transformed into, or replaced by connective tissue cells, thus making a living band to enclose, construct and support the surrounded part.

The importance of these results, as applied to the ligature of vessels, especially those of large size in close proximity to important branches, can be seen at a glance. Accepting these results as satisfactory, it has occured to me that the use of these ligatures may have a wider application than for the obliteration of vessels, and in illustration of this, I would cite the two following cases of direct inguinal hernia which have recently fallen under my observation.[1]

---

1. It is difficult to attempt to assign priority for the introduction of Lister's antiseptic techniques in this country. Carbolic acid dressings were tried

On the 19th of last February, I was called in consultation, by Dr. A. P. Clarke,[2] of Cambridge, to see Mrs. M., a washer-woman, æt. 60, who had for years suffered from hernia. Five days previous she had been suddenly seized with severe pain and vomiting, with chill, and had been confined to her bed since that time. Long-continued and careful taxis had failed to reduce the hernia, and for twenty-four hours the vomiting had been stercoraceous, and the patient seemed in extremis. The hernial tumor was the size of an egg, protruding from the external inguinal ring. A careful dissection exposed the sac, composed of the fascia lata and conjoined tendon which was closely adherent to the surrounding parts. The constriction was in the ring, bounded below by Poupart's ligament and above by the transversalis fascia and conjoined tendon. The stricture was divided in the usual way, with the hernial knife carefully introduced upon the finger. This was with some difficulty accomplished, owing to the constriction of the ring. The sac, unopened, was then pushed up with its contents into the abdominal cavity, and two stitches of medium-sized catgut ligature were taken directly through the walls of the ring. The wound was dressed antiseptically, and from Dr. Clarke's notes, taken at the time—which he has kindly furnished me—I find the patient complained of no pain, and steadily progressed without serious accident, and was discharged, convalescent, March 12th.

The wound was not entirely closed by first intention, but a careful daily examination showed no trace of our ligatures, and an abundant deposition of new tissue could be felt in the line of the opening about the walls of the ring. This has proved a radical cure of the hernia,[3] and a

---

in the United States almost as soon as Lister's original papers were received in 1867. Carbolic acid was used in the Boston City Hospital as early as October of that year (*Boston Medical and Surgical Journal* 77:271, 1867; cited by Churchill).

Several American surgeons after Marcy visited and observed Lister during the early years of antisepsis. They all brought back the details of his methods, and a few practiced them with varying degrees of enthusiasm. Marcy was one of the first to write about his results. He continued to be an enthusiastic disciple of Lister's and campaigned vigorously for the use of antiseptic methods in surgery.

2. Augustus Peck Clarke (1833–1912) graduated with an M.D. from Harvard in 1862, served throughout the Civil War, and then studied in Europe. He became known especially as an obstetrician and gynecologist in Cambridge, Massachusetts.

3. For "radical," read "complete." Marcy was a pioneer in developing surgical techniques for the permanent cure of hernia. His method of repair was similar to that of Bassini and of Halsted, both of whom he antedated by several years. Marcy's technique gradually evolved from the simple method

firm, hardened deposit may still be felt marking the closure. The ligatures were first suggested to my mind because the patient suffered severely from an asthmatic cough, and it was at least desirable to secure a temporary strengthening of the weakened ring.

Mrs. L., aged about 45, approaching the climacteric period, had been very much reduced by excessive menorrhagia, and upon March 10th, my attention was called to an old, direct, inguinal hernia of the left side, usually supported by a truss, which had come down the night previous and defied the patient's efforts to replace.

After two attempts to reduce the hernia, under ether, had failed, assisted by Dr. W. W. Wellington,[4] of this city, I operated as in the first instance, dividing the constricting ring and replacing the sac and its contents unopened. Three carbolized ligatures were applied through the walls of the ring, and the wound carefully dressed with carbolized lac plaster. As in the first place, there was complete absence of pain—the wound united without suppuration—there was an abundant deposit of new material about the ring, and when last examined, in June, the cicatrix was linear, but a firm, hard deposit of new tissue could be felt marking the site of the sutures. It is, perhaps, needless to add, the cure is radical, and in neither case has the patient used a truss since the operation. On the 7th of April, my attention was called to the wound by the patient, who felt then a slight uneasiness, and I discovered a small swelling in the cicatrix, about the size of a bean. This, upon being opened, discharged a drop or two of pale, serous-looking fluid, which microscopic examination proved free from pus cells, but containing abundance of epithelium and a few shreds of connective tissue cells. It might be a question of doubt, but the latter appeared to be minute portions of one of the ligatures.

As far as my observation has extended, this is a new use of the carbolized catgut ligature, and suggests a still wider field of application. No method of operation for radical cure of hernia appears more feasible, is probably attended with less danger, and at the same time affords a means of closing and strengthening the weakened ring, which is so desirable, and yet, with all the ingenious devices of surgery, is so difficult to obtain.

---

of repair described in his paper. By 1887 he advocated high ligation of the sac, with suture of the overlying tissues firmly about the cord (*J.A.M.A.* 8:589, 1887)—essentially the operation described independently by both Bassini and Halsted in 1889. All these men continued to modify and perfect their repairs.

4. William Williamson Wellington (1814–1896), M.D., Harvard, 1838, was a physician and obstetrician of Cambridge, Massachusetts.

The Report of the Case of President Garfield

D. W. BLISS (1825–1889)

President James Abram Garfield (1831–1881) was shot on July 2d, 1881. He died two-and-a-half months later, on September 19, 1881. His lingering illness and his death occasioned a great outpouring of surgical opinion, debate, and criticism all pertaining to the care the president had received. At that time, surgery in America was in transition; the events and discussion surrounding the presidential assassination forced the medical profession to take a hard look at surgery as it was then being practiced in the United States. The story is told here in two parts: the first is by the president's surgeon, D. W. Bliss; the second, which follows, is a critical summing-up of the presidents's care and also a condemnation of American surgery by one of Europe's leading surgeons, Friedrich Esmarch.

James Garfield was a man well suited for the presidency. He had been in turn a teacher, a successful lawyer, and a notable military leader, achieving **the rank of major-general** *in the Union Army within two years of the outbreak of the Civil War. In 1863 he resigned his commission to serve the first of nine consecutive terms in Congress as a politically effective representative from his native Ohio. Garfield was then elected to the Senate (in 1880) but was never seated; a short time later he became the compromise Republican presidential candidate (he was nominated on the 35th ballot) and won the election. The first few months of his presidency were stormy, marred by squabbles over pa-*

tronage. On the day that he was shot, President Garfield was leaving Washington to give the commencement address at Williams College, his alma mater. His assassin was a disgruntled and mentally disturbed lawyer, Charles Julius Guiteau (1841–1882), who had worked for the Republican victory and then had been denied a political appointment under the spoils system.

Guiteau had unsuccessfully stalked the president before, but this time he was waiting in the right place as the presidential party walked through the Baltimore and Potomac Railroad depot (the departure time, unwisely, had been published in the newspapers). Guiteau approached Garfield from behind and shot twice with his handgun, an English .44 caliber centerfire Bulldog revolver. One shot missed; the second dropped the President. Within minutes a physician from the District of Columbia Health Department reached the scene; he was the first of many to probe the wound with his (presumably unwashed) finger. A carriage was then sent for Dr. D. W. Bliss. Bliss, who was to care for the wounded president until his death, arrived within the hour and found the president lying on a mattress near the scene of the shooting. D. W. Bliss (his initials stood for "Doctor Williard"; his biographer does not further identify the physician for whom he was named) had embarked on a nightmare; he would be hurt more by the assassination than anyone outside of the president's immediate circle of family and friends.

Bliss was a prominent Washington surgeon and a logical person to call to provide care for the president. He had graduated from Cleveland Medical College in 1846 and then practiced in the Midwest for some years before going to war in 1861 with a regiment of Michigan volunteers. Bliss apparently served capably and was thought of as a competent surgeon. Later in the war, he was posted to Washington, first to supervise construction of the Armory Square Hospital and then to serve as its surgeon-in-chief (he is mentioned as a surgeon there by Walt Whitman, who referred to Bliss as "one of the best surgeons in the army . . ."[Specimen Days, entry for May 1, 1865]). At the war's end he remained in the capital. Bliss's accounting of the president's illness and death is the best of many and presumably the most accurate. It has been condensed to about half the length of his original paper, which appeared in The Medical Record (20:393–402, 1881).

The Report of the Case of President Garfield

The great interest which has been manifested by the medical public in the surgical history of the case of President Garfield, and my close direct connection with it as surgeon in charge, from the time I was summoned, until his death, imposes upon me the obligation of giving, even at this early date, a general summary of the salient points connected with diagnoses, treatment, and pathology.

Immediately after the shooting of President Garfield, on the morning of July 2d, I was summoned by the Secretary of War[1] to take charge of this case. I was conducted to an upper room in the building where I found the President lying upon a mattress, in a semiprone position, on the left side. He presented the appearance of perfect collapse, the lines of expression were lost, there was extreme pallor, sighing respiration (about eight or ten per minute); pulse exceedingly small, feeble, and frequent, and ranging about 120. The ingesta lying upon the mattress indicated that he had recently vomited and large beads of perspiration stood upon his face, forehead, hands, and forearms. The President's coat had previously been removed; the remainder of his clothing was intact, except that over the region of the wound which was so arranged as to expose the point of entrance of the ball.

The President complained of a sense of weight and numbness, and subsequently of a tingling sensation and pain in the lower extremities. With a view of exploring the wound to ascertain the course of the ball the organs involved in its passage, I introduced a Nelaton probe[2], which took a direction downward and forward, on a line which would represent a point of exit four inches to the right, and nearly directly opposite to the umbilicus. The point of entrance of the ball, which was oval and sharply cut, was on the right side, four inches from the median line of the spine, and on a line with the eleventh rib. A slight discharge of blood was oozing from this orifice, and had soiled the clothing. I passed the probe in the direction previously indicated, through the tenth intercostal space, for a distance of three and one-half inches from the surface of the body, to what appeared to be a cavity, and I was unable to detect any foreign substance beyond the rib to indicate the presence of fragments of bone or the missile. In attempting to withdraw the probe it became engaged between the fractured fragments and the end of the rib, and could not be liberated until pressure was made upon the sternal end of the rib so as to slightly elevate its fractured

---

1. Robert Todd Lincoln (1843–1926), the son of the president, was Garfield's secretary of war. The secretary of state, James Gillespie Blaine (1830–1893), was also with Garfield when he was shot. An impromptu cabinet meeting was probably held after the event, and it was decided that Dr. Bliss was the most suitable surgeon to be called to care for the president.

2. The Nelaton probe was ceramic tipped so that it would be marked if it came in contact with a lead bullet. Auguste Nelaton (1807–1873) first used it successfully in 1862 to locate the bullet in the wounded Italian patriot Guiseppe Garibaldi (1807–1882).

extremity. I then passed the little finger of my left hand to its full extent into the wound, which developed the character and extent of the fracture of the rib, and was only able to reach a point on a line with the inner surface of the rib, where it came in contact with what appeared to be lacerated tissue or comparatively firm coagula, probably the latter. After withdrawing my finger I made an exploration with a long, flexible silver probe, which I suitably curved before entering, and gently passed it downward and forward, and downward and backward in several directions, with a view of indicating the course of the ball, if it had been deflected by contact with the rib, and meeting with resistance from soft parts I desisted and excluded the probability of deflection, being inclined to the opinion that the ball had entered the liver, which, if true, would not warrant further exploration in that direction.

The President repeatedly requested that he be taken to the White House, and after further consultation and a full understanding of the manner and detail of his transfer, his speedy removal was agreed upon. Temporary dressings were applied to the wound, when the President was lifted on to the mattress, carefully placed upon a stretcher, conveyed down-stairs, and placed in an ambulance in waiting.

On his arrival thither a careful examination was made of his condition, The pulse continued feeble, frequent, and extremely compressible; the respiration was slow and sighing; extremities and surface cold, with occasional vomiting and profuse perspiration over the entire body; voice husky, with constant complaint of severe pains in the inferior extremities. He was placed upon his right side, so as to make the wound dependent, to facilitate drainage, and keep the viscera in contact with the injured parietes, with a view of preventing further hemorrhage and looking to the possible adhesion of the injured parts to the peritoneum. After consultation it was deemed improper to remove the clothing, as such a proceeding would thus increase the dangers. Water was given in small quantities often repeated. This was necessitated by the extreme thirst from which the patient suffered.

[The president arrived at the White House before 10:00 A.M. on July 2d, the morning of the attack. By this time a number of other physicians had been called; there were now a total of ten doctors in attendance. He was given morphine injections twice during the day for control of pain. Nausea and vomiting continued until the following morning.]

At 5:30 P.M., in accordance with a previous understanding with the physicians, the clothing was removed by being cut from the body in such a manner as to prevent any motion or agitation, and to permit the more successful application of dry heat by warm flannels to the entire body, which had been imperfectly accomplished before. Upon examination, a well defined field of dulness over the region of the wound, thought to be due to hemorrhage in the substance of the liver, along the supposed track of the ball, extended seven and one-half inches antero-posteriorly and five and one-half inches laterally.

The urine was retained until 6 o'clock P.M., when a flexible, velvet-eyed catheter was introduced, and about six ounces of normal urine drawn. At 10:00 P.M. the pulse was 158, temperature 96.5, respiration 35, which was the most critical period attending the collapse. The carbolized absorbent cotton which had previously sealed the wound having become displaced, was reapplied.

At the evening consultation, July 2d (7:00 P.M.) the gentlemen invited by me to visit the bedside were Surgeon-General Wales,[3] Surgeon J. J. Woodward,[4] and Dr. Reyburn.[5] On that occasion the opinion was expressed that the field of dulness heretofore referred to, the boundaries of which were well defined, was thought to be due to hemorrhage in the substance of the liver, from the passage of the ball into or through it. [Bliss later mentions that Surgeon-General Wales also probed the wound with his finger during this consultation.] The opinion obtained, and was so expressed to the council, that internal hemorrhage was then taking place, and that the extreme prostration and feebleness of the respiration were due to that cause, and that the President would not survive the night.

There was some oozing of dark venous blood during the entire night, sufficient to saturate the carbolized cotton and stain the bed. On the following morning the hemorrhage had entirely ceased, and the dressings became adherent to the skin. At this time Dr. D. Hayes Agnew[6] of Philadelphia, and Dr. Frank H. Hamilton[7] of New York were summoned to visit the patient in consultation. A careful review of

---

3. Philip Skinner Wales (1837–1906), M.D., University of Pennsylvania, 1861. He served in the U.S. Navy during the Civil War and remained in it for his entire professional life. He served as surgeon-general of the navy from 1879–1884.

4. Joseph Janvier Woodward (1833–1884), M.D., University of Pennsylvania, 1853, practiced in Philadelphia and then joined the Union Army in 1861, making this his career. He was a leading microscopist, became a prolific writer, and served as the editor of the three medical volumes of the *Medical and Surgical History of the War of the Rebellion* (1875).

5. Robert Reyburn (1833–1909), M.D., Philadelphia College of Medicine, 1856; M.A., Harvard, 1861. Commissioned a surgeon in the U.S. Army, he subsequently practiced in Washington. He was on the faculties of both Georgetown and Howard universities.

6. David Hayes Agnew (1818–1892), professor of surgery at the University of Pennsylvania; see footnote 6, page 281.

7. Frank Hastings Hamilton (1813–1886), M.D., University of Pennsyl-

the case from the time I first saw the President was given to these gentlemen. They individually examined the wound with great care. These examinations consisted in the introduction, in different directions, of probes and flexible bougies, in order, if possible, to determine the course of the ball.

[The consultants conferred and weighed all the evidence; the position of the assassin, the direction that the ball seemed to have taken as indicated by the various probings, the pain and hyperaesthesia of the scrotum and feet, the broken rib that did not permit adequate probing, and the President's profound shock.]

With all the facts before them it was impossible to determine the position of the ball. The propriety of making extensive incisions and dissections so as to explore the fractured ribs and remove as much as might be necessary to reveal the true course of ball, was duly considered. But the opinion was maintained that the favorable progress of the President thus far did not warrant any interference.

The case progressed, with slight fluctuations, up to July 23d, when a rigor occurred at 7 p.m., followed by a pulse of 124, respiration 26, and temperature 104 F. Two days previous to this a pus-sac was observed in the integument, extending down below the twelfth rib toward the erector spinae muscle, and underneath the latissimus dorsi, and was carefully evacuated by gentle pressure into the original opening on the occasion of each dressing. We did not feel satisfied that this superficial and limited collection of pus, which was so readily evacuated, was the principal cause of the aggravation of the symptoms present. However, a free incision was made into the pus-sac, which afforded a more direct and dependent channel to the fractured rib, from which a small fragment of bone was removed.

Pressure made backward and upward upon the abdominal wall, between the umbilicus and anterior spine, gave exit to a flow of peculiarly white and firm pus. I remarked at the time to the council that the appearance of this pus gave assurance that it had never been exposed to the air, and must have come from a deep-seated source.

[After this incision and drainage on July 23, the president did not improve as much as his physicians had hoped that he would. Alexander Graham Bell (1847–1922) twice came to the president's bedside, on July 26 and again on August 1, and attempted unsuccess-

---

vania, 1835, was on the surgical faculty of at least five medical schools during his lifetime, the last being Bellevue. He was a senior surgeon at the end of a distinguished career when he was called to assist in the care of President Garfield; see also footnote 5, page 281.

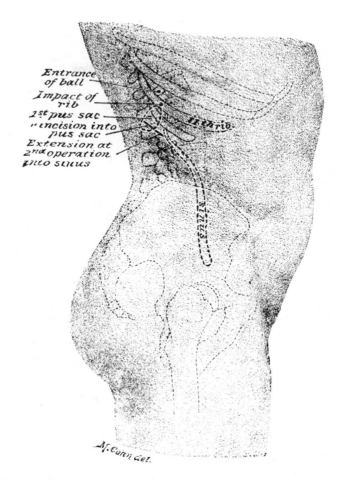

Entrance of ball
Impact of rib
1st pus sac
" incision into pus sac
Extension at 2nd operation into sinus

11th rib

sinus

N. Conn del.

Figure 43. President Garfield's wound: operative findings. Illustration showing the operative findings in President Garfield's case, from D. W. Bliss's account.

fully to locate the bullet with an induction device that he had constructed for this purpose.[8] On August 8, under ether anesthesia, another incision was made into the president's flank. This uncovered a long sinus tract that extended from the first incision, deep under the muscles of the right flank, and into the pelvis (Figure 43). Garfield

8. "Bell, A.G., upon the electrical experiments to determine the location of the bullet in the body of the late President Garfield; and upon a successful form of induction balance for the detection of painless masses in the human body." *American Journal of Science* 25:22–61, 1883.

showed little improvement, however, and his fever, prostration, and vomiting continued. On August 18 a further complication developed:]

On August 18th a slight tumefaction of the right parotid gland was noticeable, unaccompanied by pain or tenderness on pressure, until the suppurative period was established, when mental disturbance, vomiting, restlessness, and jactitation[9] supervened; nor was there any increase of temperature, local or systemic, to indicate the probability of its metastatic origin. The parotitis presented many of the characteristics of an ordinary carbuncle, and was unaccompanied by any other abscesses in the adjoining tissue. During the progress of the parotitis facial paralysis occurred, and continued, with slight improvement, until the time of his death. When the climax of suppuration was reached, a free discharge of laudable pus followed, with a rapid abatement of the more urgent symptoms, and after the separation of the slough (which was limited in extent) reparation was rapid and complete throughout the entire suppurating surface, as well as in the several incisions which had been previously made to liberate the pus. These lesions had entirely healed at the time of death, except an opening behind the right ear.

[The president's condition continued slowly but inexorably to deteriorate as manifestations of chronic sepsis continued to surface. By August 23 he had lost over 80 pounds. The tract in his right flank discharged a slough, he developed furunculosis and then sacral bedsores; he continued to vomit and "acute bronchial catarrh" developed associated with "hypostatic congestion" of the lungs, more extensive on the right side. His doctors discussed the possibility of moving him to the New Jersey seashore,[10] but the right parotid abscess had not been adequately drained and his condition worsened. He was given "stimulants" in the form of beef-tea and peptone broths in the hope that the "President might be sustained until suppuration was established in the parotid, and the constitutional disturbances incident thereto had subsided...."]

---

9. jactitation: restlessness, particularly while delirious.

10. Caring for the president in the heat of a Washington summer was difficult. An air conditioning unit—possibly the first ever—was built. It made use of an ice-cooled chamber with electrically driven fans. According to articles in various medical journals ("How President Garfield's room is cooled," *Medical Record* 20:620–24, 1881; also *Boston Medical and Surgical Journal* 105:470–71, 1881) it was capable of cooling ambient air at 99 F. down to 54 F. and was able to deliver 22,000 cubic feet per hour. In spite of this innovation, the move to new Jersey must have been welcomed.

Our efforts were rewarded on August 26th by a free discharge of pus from the external auditory canal; also in the mouth. It was believed that the pus which discharged in the mouth dissected its way along the course of Steno's duct. There being rigidity of the masseter muscle, the jaw was fixed so as to preclude the possibility of opening the mouth sufficiently for a satisfactory examination. A tenacious mucus was secreted from that side in large quantities, and occasioned great annoyance. The patient during this period was occasionally wandering in his mind especially after rousing from sleep. When his attention was fixed by an attendant, his mental condition seemed to be comparatively perfect.

[On September 6 the president was transferred to Long Branch on the New Jersey seashore. There was some improvement in his condition after this move, enough so that he reduced the number of physicians in attendance.]

September 17th, at 11 a.m., a severe rigor occurred of half an hours duration, followed by a sharp rise in temperature. At 12 m. the pulse was 120, temperature 102 F., and respiration 24. This chill was accompanied by severe pain over the anterior mediastinum, and the President said to me that it was similar to what he understood as angina pectoris. It is evident that this pain, which occurred on several occasions at intervals of six to twelve hours prior to his death, was occasioned by first a rupture of the aneurismal sac, and the progressive dissection, at irregular intervals, of the blood into the surrounding tissue, until finally it burst into the peritoneum.

[Severe chills, fever, and pain continued as the president worsened over the next two days. Dr. Bliss told the family, "There is a gravity in this case that portends serious trouble."]

At 10:10 p.m. I was summoned hastily to the bedside, and found the President in an unconscious and dying condition, pulseless at the wrist, with extreme pallor, the eyes opened and turned upward, and respiration eight per minute and gasping. Placing my finger upon the carotid, I could not recognize pulsation; applying my ear over the heart, I detected an indistinct flutter, which continued until 10:35, when he expired. The brave and heroic sufferer, the nation's patient, for whom all had labored so cheerfully and unceasingly, had passed away.

[Bliss's article rambles on rather defensively for another page; he had been under great and continuous pressure from the medical profession and from the press—most of it unjustified and unfair—for the treatment that the president had received during his illness. The criticism was mainly centered on the failure to locate the bullet—a

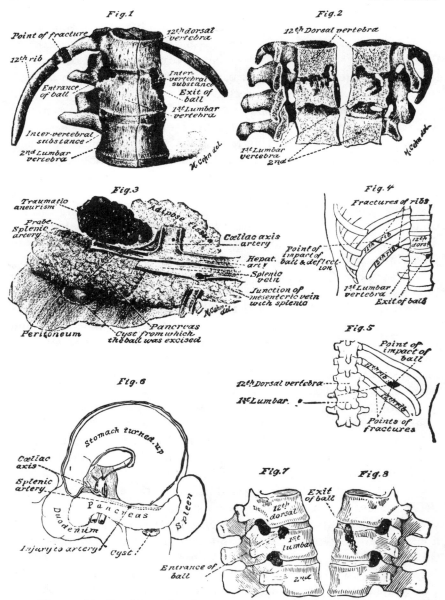

Figure 44. President Garfield's wound: autopsy findings. Autopsy findings showing the course of the ball, from D. W. Bliss's account.

failure that was considered, at that time, tantamount to malpractice. As the autopsy showed later, this would have been impossible by any means then available. The following illustrations (Figure 44), taken from the detailed autopsy report that accompanied Bliss's article, are self explanatory. The twelfth thoracic, the first and second lumbar vertebrae, and their cartilages were all found to be involved by infection. The immediate cause of death had been rupture of the traumatic (and presumably septic) aneurysm of the splenic artery.

Garfield's death must have been a blessed relief for Bliss, who at 56 was not a young man. He had been in constant attendance, day and night, on a desperately ill and important man. We can imagine the pressure under which he worked, seemingly efficiently, serving his patient as well as he knew how, for two and a half months. Bliss submitted a bill of $25,000, a great deal of money for that day, but reasonable in view of the services rendered. Congress awarded him $6,500. Bliss refused this, claiming—with justification—that his health had been damaged and his practice ruined. A bill was pending in Congress to pay him for his services at the time of his death in 1889.

I keep wondering whether, in later years, Bliss thought about all those fingers in President Garfield's wound.]

The Treatment of
the Wound of
President Garfield

JOHANN FRIEDRICH AUGUST VON ESMARCH (1823–1908)

The following selection is unusual in that, unlike all the other selections in this anthology, it was not written by an American surgeon. Nevertheless, it is important to American surgery, for it indicates how wide the gap was between surgical practice in the United States and in the Germanic countries of Europe in the year 1881. Friedrich von Esmarch's contribution also must be considered as the final word in the most widely debated surgical case of the last century.

The drama of the assassination, the illustrious patient, the lingering course, all gave impetus to endless argument concerning President Garfield's care. Every newspaper carried a daily press bulletin from Washington as well as speculation and discussion about the president's condition and the effect of his prolonged illness on the nation. Every medical journal had articles on the president's treatment; editorials and innumerable letters commented on the case. Every well-known surgeon had an opinion, suggestion, or criticism; each spoke out during the president's illness and after his death.

Surgeons in Europe watched the drama unfold with interest. Many, including Johann Friedrich August von Esmarch (1823–1908), were experienced and capable military surgeons. Esmarch had been a pupil of Langenbeck and later became professor of surgery at Kiel (1857–1899). He had also served in three Prussian military campaigns between 1838 and 1871, writing extensively on many aspects of military

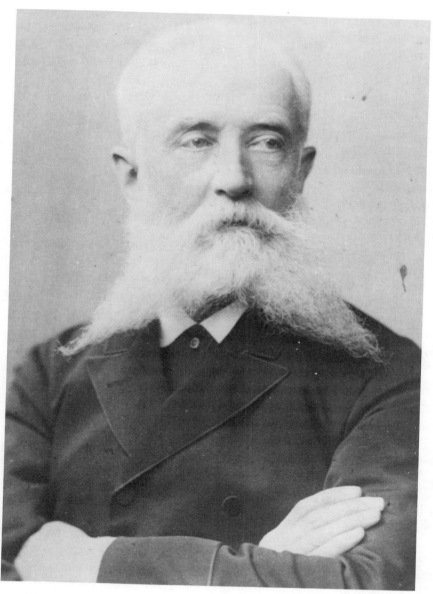

Figure 45. Johann Friedrich August von Esmarch (1823–1908). (Courtesy New York Academy of Medicine.)

surgery: resection of joints after gunshot wounds, establishment of field hospitals and aid stations, battlefield first aid (he introduced first aid dressings), and hemostasis (the Esmarch bandage is in use today). Esmarch had adopted antiseptic surgery some years before, and one wonders what his feelings were (disbelief? sorrow? indignation?) as he followed the president's course in the American medical press.

Esmarch did not prepare the following critique for publication, but for a talk before the Physiological Society of Kiel, given on February 2, 1882. It appeared later, on September 7, 1882, in the Boston Medical and Surgical Journal *(107:234–37). Esmarch's talk had been translated by "Stansbury Sutton, M.D., of Pittsburgh, Pa." Rhodes Stansbury Sutton, M.D. (1841–1906), was a practitioner of Pittsburgh, Pennsylvania. It is unclear how he happened to translate the article.*

It is impossible to guess how much effect Esmarch's criticisms may have had. Certainly they were justified. He was not alone in condemning the care given to the president, but his was the most authoritative voice to do so; his criticisms were valid, others were not. Esmarch's communication could not make believers of all American surgeons, but it must have given at least some of them food for thought; that may have been the greatest good to come from the death of the president.

The Treatment of the Wound of President Garfield

In the Boston Medical and Surgical Journal of November 24, 1881, I find a letter from the senior surgeon of the Pennsylvania Hospital, Dr. William Hunt,[1] in which he speaks of the symptoms of President Garfield's wound, defends the attending physicians against the charge that they had not done enough, and finishes with an attack on the antiseptic method in the following language:—

"Much has been said about antiseptic treatment in the case. It was practiced, I believe, to a very great extent. Its *practice* is grand, except the spray; I heartily agree with the German surgeon who said 'fort mit dem spray'.[2] Could there be a better commentary on the

---

1. William Hunt (1825–1896), M.D., University of Pennsylvania, 1849. Surgeon, teacher, and surgical writer on the staff of the Pennsylvania and other hospitals in Philadelphia.

2. Bergmann (see footnote 7 below) and others said, "Away with the

unproved theory of antiseptic surgery than the President's case? Against its theory, or at least the effects of it on many minds, namely, that all sources of contamination which produce septic poisoning come from without, I earnestly protest. I have too much respect for Mr. Lister[3] to think that he believes what the extremists among his disciples teach.

"The influence of such teaching on the rising generation of physicians and surgeons is bad, in this, that it leads to narrow views and interferes with clear diagnosis. It leads outwardly too much, for contamination comes from within, I believe, more frequently than from without. Was not the decaying vertebra in the President's case enough to account for the septicaemia?

"To get all the rats out and then stop the hole with poison and stuffing is a good thing, but to poison and plug the hole and leave the rats in, is a very bad thing. They only undermine and make other holes. A narrow antiseptic [surgeon?] looks around the room instead of at the patient, whereas he should look at both and give due weight to all septic possibilities."[4]

These utterances of an esteemed American surgeon induce me to communicate my opinion of the treatment of President Garfield's wound, inasmuch as I see in different American and English medical periodicals, of which I get a sight, that the wound of the President and its treatment has been publicly discussed by the most celebrated surgeons of America, and very different opinions have been expressed. The *North American Review* for December, 1881, contains four articles, which emanate from well known authors.[5] In the first article,

---

spray"; the carbolic acid spray was dangerous and unnecessary and should be replaced by the aseptic techniques that he and others were introducing into surgery.

3. Joseph Lister (1827–1912) was indeed respected (quite aside from his doctrines) in the United States and especially in Philadelphia. He had been an invited speaker to the International Medical Congress, held in that city in 1876 as part of the centennial celebration, and had impressed everyone who heard and met him.

4. Hunt's quotation is typical of the complete nonsense being written in the United States at that time about antiseptic technique. As is evident by his remarks, he had little or no understanding of the germ theory, on which Lister's teachings were based.

5. Esmarch plainly was well acquainted with all of the facts, and all of the debate concerning President Garfield's wound and its subsequent treatment. The *North American Review* solicited and published the opinions of the four prominent doctors that Esmarch listed:

Dr. Hammond, author of the *Handbook of Military Hygiene*, finds fault with the attending physicians, because they have not tried to remove the ball. He further says, "The original injury was not a fatal one, but the President has not had all the advantages that modern surgery offers." Marion Sims, on the contrary, asserts that the wound of the President was absolutely mortal; that the injury of the vertebra was of necessity a cause of septicaemia; that it was impossible that the President could have died without it, and that it was impossible that he could live with it. John Ashhurst and Hodgen then again defend the treatment of the attending physicians and the former intimates that there has not been sufficient care taken to nourish the patient. On the whole, I am compelled to agree with Dr. Hammond's last sentence [i.e., "the President has not had all the advantages that modern surgery offers"], but from quite a different stand-point.

In order to argue my opinion of the case, I will premise an abridgment of the history of the illness which Dr. Bliss has published in the *Medical Record* of October 8, 1881, and to this I will append at appropriate places, short critical remarks.

[Esmarch then quotes almost all of Bliss's account as given in the preceding selection; Esmarch's synopsis is accurate, but it suffers from double translation, first by Esmarch into German, then by Sutton back into English. I have omitted this part of Esmarch's paper because of the previous inclusion of Bliss's original account; Esmarch's conclusions follow:]

From the history of the case, including the post mortem, I draw the following conclusions:

1. President Garfield did not receive an absolutely mortal wound.

Neither liver nor peritonaeum were injured. There was no peritonitis. No important organ was injured, excepting the bony spinal column. The vertebral canal was not opened, the spinal marrow was found uninjured. The injury to the vertebra was not of itself mortal:

William Alexander Hammond (1828–1900), M.D., University of the City of New York, 1848. He was appointed surgeon-general of the army in 1862 because of exceptional administrative ability. This precocious appointment, coupled with necessary reforms, made many enemies. Hammond was unfairly court-martialed but later exonerated. He subsequently became an outstanding neurologist, medical writer, and educator.

Marion Sims (1813–1900); see introduction to "Operation for Vesico-vaginal Fistula, page 212.

John Ashhurst (1839–1900); see footnote 3, page 281.

John Thompson Hodgen (1826–1882), teacher and surgeon of St. Louis, had a distinguished army career during the Civil War. He was Missouri's leading surgeon and became known nationally for many surgical innovations, particularly for the care of fractures (Hodgen's splint).

it might have healed very well had it not been for the suppuration. There are in military surgery enough examples of the healing of such wounds.

2. The bullet was not the cause of the suppuration; it probably carried no septic material into the wound, for it was encapsulated, and the adjoining part of its track was healed.

3. The cause of the suppuration, the septic material, must have been put in from outside, and different actions in the treatment are to be accused of that.

First. The immediate examination of the wound with the bullet probe and finger, which were probably not disinfected (without antiseptic precautions).

Second. The repeated examination on the third day (probably in the same way) by several physicians.

Third. The entirely insufficient antiseptic method in the treatment of the wound (bandage technics deficient).

Fourth. The squeezing of the wound on July 21st.

Fifth. The then daily probing and spouting [sic: the surgeons had used dilute potassium permanganate solution to irrigate the president's wounds] of the wound with an insufficiently antiseptic fluid. (A method of disinfection out of use.)

Sixth. The omission of a free incision of the pus cavity (August 8th).

A metastatic inflammation[6] of the parotid gland did not appear before the 18th of August; it did not amount to real pyaemia. The President did not die of pyaemia, but of haemorrhage after his strength was exhausted by the septic fever, the bronchial catarrh, and the hypostatic pneumonia. The blood came from an opening in the splenic artery, which was perhaps made by the bullet or a bone splinter; but probably extended afterwards, slowly by reason of the suppurative process, from a point bruised by the bullet or a bone splinter.

It is probable that before the fatal haemorrhage occurred a spurious aneurism had formed, which opened under the suppurative process. If suppuration had not occurred, the injury to the artery might not have been followed by evil consequences. It seems that our exhortations to place first in the treatment of shot wounds the principle "do not do any damage," and the fine observations of Pirogoff, Klebs, Reyher, Bergmann,[7] and others on the manner of curing the worst

---

6. It was felt that Garfield's severe parotitis represented metastatic infection. It probably did not, for parotitis is common in chronically ill patients, the result of the salivary stasis that follows dehydration and lack of the secretory stimulation provided by a normal diet.

7. The four names that Esmarch mentions all made significant contri-

bullet wounds, without suppuration, have not made any influence on our colleagues beyond the ocean. It is true that the public still think the bullet most dangerous: the soldier is happy when you put into his hand the bullet which you have cut out. But the surgeon should know that the bullet itself does not do any damage in most of the cases: the damage which proceeds from it is caused by it in its course; the damage which is added to it mostly proceeds from the examiners fingers.

It seems that the attendant physicians were under the pressure of the public opinion that they were doing far too little. But according to my opinion they have not done too little but far too much.

If they had entirely omitted the search after the bullet, and immediately after the injury dressed the wound in a real antiseptic way, the President might perhaps be still alive, like our Emperor, from whom Von Langenbeck[8] did not cut out a single one of all his many small shots.

---

butions to the surgery of gunshot wounds—contributions that (as Esmarch noted) were unknown to American surgeons:

Nikolai Ivanovich Pirogoff (1810–1881) was the most notable figure in Russian surgery. He studied in Berlin and in 1840 became professor of surgery at St. Petersburg. Pirogoff worked chiefly in the preantiseptic era and believed that surgical interference with gunshot wounds resulted in pyemia.

Edwin Klebs (1834–1913), pathologist and bacteriologist (Klebsiella), did pioneer work in relating specific organisms to infection. Klebs studied the bacteriology of gunshot wounds during the Franco-Prussian War (1872) and showed that the wound itself is sterile; pyemia followed bacterial contamination. He taught at various medical schools in Germany and then joined the faculty of Rush Medical College in Chicago in 1896.

Carl Reyher (1846–1890) was a brilliant young Russian surgeon who studied with Bergmann and then served in the Prussian army during the Franco-Prussian War and wrote on sepsis in battle wounds. Later he left Bergmann, joined the Russian Army, and served in the Russo-Turkish War. In 1881 Reyher attended the International Medical Congress in London and gave a landmark paper entitled "Primary Debridement for Gunshot Wounds," in which he showed that wound mortality could be lowered significantly if debridement were carried out using antiseptic wound treatment. (See the Wangensteens' *Rise of Surgery* [Minneapolis, Minn.: University of Minnesota Press, 1978], pp. 57–60.)

Ernst von Bergmann (1836–1907), born in Riga (Latvia), educated at Dorpat (1860). He served in the Franco-Prussian War and returned to Dorpat as professor of surgery and then went on to Berlin, where he succeeded von Langenbeck (see footnote 8 below). Bergmann was an early disciple of Lister; by 1886 he had given up antiseptic surgery completely in favor of aseptic techniques. He introduced heat sterilization and contributed as much as any surgeon to the introduction of the whole aseptic ritual.

8. Bernhard Rudolph Conrad von Langenbeck (1810–1887), professor of surgery at Berlin, was the most illustrious German surgeon of the mid-nineteenth century. Famed both as a superb clinician (said to have devised 21 new operative procedures) and as a teacher of many of Europe's great surgeons (Esmarch, Bergmann, Billroth, to name only a few), Langenbeck taught his students to apply science to surgery. He had a particular interest in military surgery. Langenbeck cared for William I, the German Emperor, when he was wounded in assassination attempts in May and again in June, 1878.

Surgical Operations in the Antiseptic Era

RUDOLPH MATAS, M.D. (1860–1957)

Anesthesia gained immediate acceptance after its first public demonstration in 1846; but 21 years were required for the adoption of Joseph Lister's principles following their enunciation in 1867. Lister's methods were epitomized by complicated, frequently revised rituals. These tended to confuse the surgeons of that day, and the underlying principles of the germ theory were generally ignored. The following selection, written by Rudolph Matas, was published in 1942, but the events that it describes occurred 60 years earlier. It is one of the best available descriptions of surgical practice during the transitional period between the septic and aseptic eras.

Rudolph Matas was born in Bonnet Carre, Louisiana, on September 12, 1860. He graduated from the medical school of Tulane University in 1880. He soon built up a surgical practice in New Orleans and in 1895 became the professor of surgery at Tulane. Matas made many contributions to his specialty. He was a pioneer in the use of local anesthesia for regional and subarachnoid block. He was especially well known as a vascular surgeon and introduced the operation of endoaneurysmorrhaphy (the ligation of the vessels entering an aneurysm, from within the aneurysmal sac) in 1902. Rudolph Matas was one of America's best known and most respected surgeons. He died in New Orleans in his ninety-eighth year on September 23, 1957.

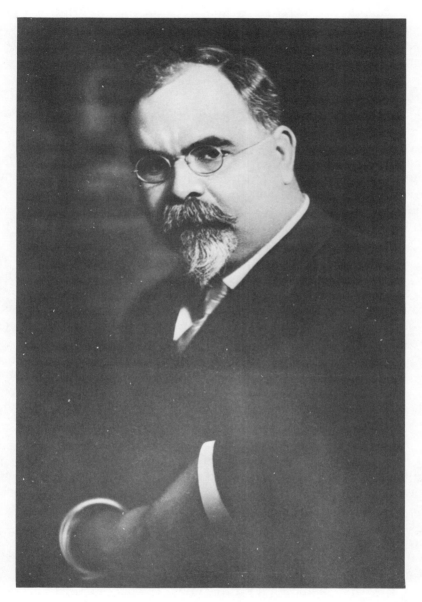

Figure 46. Rudolph Matas (1860–1957). (Courtesy National Library of Medicine.)

The following selection by Rudolph Matas has been abridged for its inclusion here. It appeared originally in the American Journal of Surgery *(51:40, 1942) under the title "Surgical Operations Fifty Years Ago."*

Surgical Operations in the Antiseptic Era

Since I am expected to give some account of personal impressions and experiences, I trust I may be excused for speaking in the first person. I might as well begin with the earliest recollections of my medical career which began as a matriculate of the Medical School of the University of Louisiana (now Tulane) in the fall of 1877, and as an intern of the Charity Hospital of New Orleans from 1878 to 1880, when I was graduated as an M.D.

In this transition between the old septic and the new antiseptic period there were many modes of treating wounds, almost as many as there were senior surgeons on the staff. These variations were most notable in the treatment of compound fractures, lacerated and incised wounds and especially amputations, which were the most frequent major performances at a time when the field of surgery was much restricted in its indications and limitations.

Notwithstanding the seeming indifference or reluctance to adopt the typical Listerian dressing, there were certain prominent features of the antiseptic ritual which found general acceptance, even when the doctrine itself was subject to doubt and criticism. These were:

1. The use of carbolic acid as the preferred antiseptic.

2. The revival of drainage with Chassaignac's[1] rubber tube in wounds and in closed amputations, leaving the stumps open and unclosed.

3. The gradual adoption of the buried, short cut, carbolated ligatures, preferably Lister's catgut or silk. But even this marvelous improvement in technic was slow in coming, for, in 1878 and 1879, I saw a number of amputation stumps from which long ligatures dangled, waiting to ripen in pus to drop off.

4. At an amputation it was the most frequent practice to irrigate the wound with a 5 per cent carbolic solution, then insert the rubber drains and suture the flaps, leaving large intervals between the sutures, after which adhesive strips were applied to support the whole stump, while compressing with gentle pressure to avoid dead spaces.

---

1. Edouard Pierre Marie Chassaignac (1804–1879); see footnote 1, page 235.

5. The stump and limb were wrapped in cotton batting (later sterilized absorbent cotton was used) and bandaged with the wide heavy cotton or linen rollers of that period.

While this mode of treatment gradually became part of the routine management, the procedure was something of a compromise with the early Listerian ritual in which many of the minor features were missing. It was virtually the same dressing which Lister himself had modified from Syme,[2] his father-in-law, in Edinburgh, long before Lister had arrived at the conclusion that infection was the assault of a bacterial invasion.

As relics of the pre-antiseptic period, various methods of dressing and treating stumps were still in evidence before 1880. These varied considerably, according to the school in which the surgeons had been trained. The surgeons who were graduates of American schools were largely inspired by the American texts of Ashhurst,[3] Gross,[4] Hamilton[5] and Agnew,[6] with a fundamental leaning toward British traditions (Astley Cooper, Erichsen, Bell, Paget, etc.[7]). Those of French origin still held allegiance to the great Parisian masters, Dupuytren, Velpeau, Lisfranc, Broca, Nelaton; while the few Germans swore by Von Graefe, Langenbeck, Volkmann and Billroth.

---

2. James Syme (1799–1870), professor of surgery at Edinburgh. He was Lister's teacher and father-in-law. Lister succeeded him at Edinburgh in 1869.

3. John Ashhurst (1839–1900), graduate of the medical school of the University of Pennsylvania (1860), and later professor of surgery in this school. His *Principles and Practice of Surgery* appeared in 1871 and went through six editions.

4. Samuel David Gross (1805–1884) graduated from Jefferson Medical college in 1828. His *System of Surgery* appeared in 1859 and went through four editions: it was the best American surgical text to be published during the last century. Gross was professor of surgery, first in Louisville and then at Jefferson. He wrote extensively. His subjects included surgical pathology, urology, intestinal surgery, surgery of the airways, and medical history. S. D. Gross must be considered one of the truly great American surgeons of the last century. See also page 165.

5. Frank Hastings Hamilton (1813–1886) was a graduate of the University of Pennsylvania (1835). His *Treatise on the Principles and Practice of Surgery* appeared in 1872 and went through three editions. He was on the faculty of several medical schools.

6. David Hayes Agnew (1818–1892) was also a graduate of the University of Pennsylvania (1838). He was an industrious surgeon with a large practice in Philadelphia. His text, *The Principles and Practice of Surgery*, appeared in 1878.

7. This and succeeding lists of British, French, and German surgeons are too long to identify individually. They are made up of the greatest names in European surgery during this era; some are identified in subsequent selections.

As a result of this international medley, a number of methods were devised to protect the amputations from infection or to combat it when it occurred. These procedures if catalogued would embrace over twenty to twenty-five designated titles, and can be generally classed under two heads:

A. Methods which aimed at a free contact of the open stump with the air, with or without approximation of the flaps, kept wet or dry according to the circumstances. The open or dry methods were advocated in Britain by Teale, of Leeds, Humphrey, of Oxford, Stimpson, of Edinburgh (1860), and with some modifications by Volkmann, Thiersch, Nussbaum and Billroth (1855 to 1876) before their conversion to Listerism.

1. A typical dressing of the *open dry type* was that practiced systematically by Dr. James R. Wood,[8] of New York, which is graphically described by Dr. Frederic S. Dennis,[9] his devoted intern (1876):

> After the limb has been amputated, the flaps are not even coaptated but left entirely open. A pillow of oakum is placed under the stump, which is allowed to rest upon this support until the wound is nearly healed. A small piece of gauze is placed over the contour of the stump and a cradle over the limb, so as to avoid contact with the clothing. This is all the dressing that is employed; no sutures are used except in lateral skin flap methods, no adhesive plaster, no oil silk, no bandage. No dry charpie[10] is stuffed into the wound, no fenestrated compresses are placed between the flaps; in other words, the stump is left entirely alone, naked, just as the surgeon made it in his amputation. . . . As the wound drains freely, it is irrigated at frequent intervals with carbolic solution, after which Balsam of Peru (which makes a fine stimulating application) is poured over the granulating surface. When suppuration has subsided the flaps are gradually approximated by strips of adhesive plaster.

2. In the *wet division* of the open methods, the most prominent was the "cold water dressing" of Robert Liston,[11] used in bad septic cases as late as 1885 and later. This consisted in holding the stump on a

---

8. James Rushmore Wood (1813–1882) was a noted surgeon of New York and a founder of Bellevue Hospital.

9. Frederic Shepard Dennis (1850–1934) was a surgeon of the Bellevue Hospital and the author of a surgical text (*System of Surgery*, 1895), which was especially noteworthy for the introduction by John Shaw Billings on the history of surgery—one of the best ever written.

10. Charpie was the lint of scraped linen. It was widely used as a dressing material.

11. Robert Liston (1794–1847), noted English surgeon and professor of surgery at University College, London.

rubber covered pillow, keeping it constantly wet by a drip of cold water (plain or medicated), falling on a thin gauze cloth from an overhanging receptacle, the water draining by a gutter to a bucket on the floor.

3. In this group also was the *"simple open wet dressing"* of Prof. John Ashhurst, of Philadelphia (1870 to 1885), in which the sutured stump was drained with rubber tubing and kept wet by loose surface dressings soaked in laudanum, substituting this by alcohol at the end of forty-eight hours.

4. An extension of the *open wet method* was that advocated by Langenbeck, in Germany, Lefort and Verneuil, in France, and Hamilton, in New York, which consisted in keeping the patient himself immersed, with his open undressed stump, in a tub with flowing plain or medicated water. This was carried out on the same principle as the Hebra continued tub baths utilized to this day in the Austrian and Germany dermatological clinics.

B. Methods which aimed at the total *exclusion of air* from the stump, under the impression or belief that the infection, whatever it was, was transmitted through the air, in manifest contradiction to the principles held by advocates of Class A.

1. Perhaps the most typical of these was the method to be described later, the *"pansement ouate"* [cotton dressing] of Alphonse Guerin,[12] with which I was most familiar, as I had seen it applied at the Charity Hospital.

2. Other methods which were remarkable because of the devices used to exclude air from the stump were: the "pneumatic occlusion" of Jules Guerin (1865); the "incubation method" of Jules Guyot; the "pneumatic aspiration" method of Maisonneuve, which aimed at the constant aspiration of air and secretions; the dry closed covered dressing, with drainage, practiced by Syme and Lister before Pasteur's discoveries (1850 to 1860).

3. Among others were the "Bordeaux method," a compromise between the Guerin and Lister methods (1864); the "earth pack" dressing of Addinell Hewson,[13] of Philadelphia (1872); the coagulating "perchloride of iron dressing" of the open stump of Bourgade, of Clermont Ferrand, France, which created with the perchloride a "tough leathery

---

12. Alphonse Guerin (1816–1894) was a prominent surgeon of Paris during the second half of the nineteenth century. In 1847, prior to the work of Pasteur and Lister, he postulated a theory of "miasmatic" contamination of wounds.

13. Addinell Hewson (1828–1889), M.D., Jefferson, 1850, was a surgeon of Philadelphia who was best known for the "earth dressing" mentioned here.

cuirass of necrotic tissue which completely isolated the subjacent tissues from the influence of the contaminating air and other surrounding agents. This mass was detached slowly after the sixth or tenth day, and in becoming detached, left a surface covered with healthy granulations. The wound was then dressed with aromatic wine and the flaps brought together to induce union by second intention."

This multitude of dressings and their variants, of which the titles just referred to are only samples, and in which the advocate of each mode deplored the great mortality of amputations in the hands of other surgeons and confidently put forward his own method as superior, which, by his own experience, he had proved best—showed by the complexity of methods and their contradictory principles and ideas— how, in ignorance of the essential causative factor of infection, the surgeons of the pre-antiseptic period, in despair at the fearful and prohibitive mortality of their operations, sought frantically anywhere and everywhere, for some mode of relief.

Of these international and pre-Listerian methods, I was most impressed by the strips or interrupted sutures until complete union and cicatrization had taken place, the stump being again immobilized in a copious cotton dressing, which was cheaper and more available in Louisiana than in any other part of the world. The most notable feature of this cure was that, despite its stench and offensiveness after the dressing had been on for over two or three weeks, the patient recovered without any of the usual local and systemic complications of rival methods.[14] The reasons for the success of this method according to the author were: (1) that it kept away atmospheric contamination during the process of healing; (2) it allowed free drainage; (3) it kept the wound

---

14. This method of dressing was essentially the one advocated by the Frenchman Guerin and alluded to earlier by Matas. Guerin's "cotton bale dressing" was widely used during the Franco-Prussian War of 1870 and was quite successful until supplanted by aseptic techniques. Guerin's dressing represented the rediscovery of the surgical truth that septic wounds will often heal if put completely to rest. Napoleon's surgeon, the great Dominique-Jean Larrey (1766–1842), used this technique quite successfully. In America, Benjamin Winslow Dudley (q.v.), a pupil of Larrey, used the roller bandage to provide rest and support for healing wounds. Most recently this principle has been refurbished and described by Joseph Trueta (1897–1977) during the Spanish Civil War and subsequently used in World War II. Trueta's method consisted of debriding and then packing war wounds with sterile petrolatum gauze. He subsequently immobilized the wounded extremity in a plaster-of-Paris cast. As Matas points out, it is often amazing how well healing occurs beneath the stinking layer of saprophytic bacteria.

free from irritating washes and disturbing manipulations; and (4) it kept the amputated limb at rest while healing was going on.

When Lister came to the United States in 1876, to preside at the International Medical Congress held in connection with the Centennial Exposition at Philadelphia, which was ten years after his first pronouncement of the antiseptic doctrine, he was no doubt disappointed at the indifferent impression that his teachings had produced in the United States. This was even more remarkable in view of the much closer relations of the United States to England than any other country and that the Germans, whose clinics were much frequented by admiring Americans, had adopted Listerism with great enthusiasm.

The reasons why American surgeons had been so slow in subscribing to the Listerian doctrine were well stated by Professor Robert F. Weir,[15] who, writing in 1877 (*N. Y. Med. J.*, December, 1877–January, 1878) stated: "It is only lately that in America attention has been given practically to the teachings of Lister in respect to the treatment of wounds. In fact, aside from an article by Schuppert in the New Orleans Med. & Surg. J., little or nothing has appeared in our medical journals relative to the result of the so-called antiseptic method." The reasons given by Weir to account for the tardiness of American surgeons to try this mode of treatment were: that the treatment, as enunciated by Mr. Lister (1) "has been repeatedly changed in its details: (2) that it was too complicated and demanded the supervision of the surgeon himself, or, in a hospital of a carefully trained staff of assistants; (3) that many who had tried it had been unsuccessful in the cases where the essay had been made; (4) but the most weighty objection which was asserted or entertained was the positiveness of the enunciation of the germ-theory in explanation of the process of decomposition in the secretions of a wound." While this was true, there was still another reason which Dr. Weir did not mention and that was the indifference and the hostility of some of the leading British surgeons themselves who sought to minimize the importance of the Listerian movement at home (Nunnelly, Savory, Paget, Wood, Humphrey, Spence, Callender, Bantock, and above all, Tait[16]). But this opposition was offset later by the loyalty of

---

15. Robert Fulton Weir (1838–1927), M.D., College of Physicians and Surgeons of New York, 1859, was a surgeon of New York City. He served on the faculty of several medical schools there.

16. Robert Lawson Tait (1845–1899), "the bull of Birmingham," deserves special mention among this list of eminent British surgeons. Tait, a hefty but capable surgeon, was the most vocal of Lister's detractors. He ridiculed both the germ theory and Lister's methods. Tait's results in abdominal surgery,

Lister's pupils and associates and by the enthusiasm of the Germans, French and all the leading surgeons of the continental European countries, who ultimately recognized the merit of his labors and accorded him the homage due to one of the world's greatest benefactors.

In New Orleans (1877 to 1880) as previously stated, the faculty and the staff of the Hospital, in common with all the leading surgeons of the United States, were undecided, skeptic or frankly hostile to the method, the only exception being a German surgeon, Dr. Moritz Schuppert,[17] graduate of the University of Marburg (1849) where he was born in 1817, who championed the cause in New Orleans. He had settled in New Orleans in the early fifties, soon rising to distinction as a very able operator and prolific writer, despite the short time he had to acquire a knowledge of the language. He was soon a member of the Hospital Staff, a professor in the Charity Hospital Medical School and prominent at Medical meetings. Always a diligent student and omnivorous reader, he kept in touch with German literature, and it was from this source that he gathered the enthusiasm of his old friends and teachers in acclaiming the new era that had dawned in surgery with the advent of Lister and the antiseptic doctrine. In a lecture published in the New Orleans Med & Surg. J. for January, 1878, Schuppert stated: "The astonishing reports which had reached me from the interior of Germany at the end of 1874, that the antiseptic treatment of wounds recommended by Lister promised to cause a revolution in surgical practice, did not permit me to rest, and the Spring of 1875 found me already on the road to visit those places where such stunning facts were reported. After my return to this city in the fall of 1875, I gave a resume of what I had absorbed in some of the most renowned hospitals of the European continent in a few lectures delivered in the amphitheatre of the Charity Hospital and reported in this Journal."

In this extensive monograph, Schuppert gives a most minute description of the antiseptic treatment, the progress it had made, especially in Germany under the leadership of Volkmann, whom he admired intensely and followed most closely; and he closes finally with a complete summary of his own experience based on his personal operations in New Orleans at the Charity Hospital in strict pursuance of the Listerian method during the period of 1875 to 1878.

---

especially ovariotomy, were excellent for that era. He made use of no antiseptics but boiled his instruments and used soap and water copiously—thus, essentially, using aseptic techniques.

17. Moritz Schuppert (1817–1887) became one of New Orleans' leading surgeons. He quite deserves the credit that Matas gives him as an early proponent of Listerism in the United States.

His summary embraces 120 miscellaneous operations including twenty-three amputations (major and minor), seventeen resections of bones and joints, two compound comminuted fractures of leg and thigh, five ligations of arteries in continuity, thirty-four cuts and stabs including larynx and pharynx, stab of chest, two gunshot wounds of abdomen (one death), three penetrating stabs of abdomen with no deaths, altogether 120 operations, besides forty-four chronic ulcers of the leg, treated antiseptically, with a total mortality of only 4 per cent.

He describes in minute detail the antiseptic treatment in the complicated and methodical ritual-like form of the early Listerian dressings, but modified and simplified by Volkmann and later by himself after his return to New Orleans. These details I learned personally under very impressive circumstances when it was my fortune to be called, as intern, to carry out the full program of antiseptic preparation for the extirpation of an enormous ovarian cyst in a patient admitted in the summer of 1878. The chief of my service, Dr. Wm. Carson, called on Dr. Schuppert to direct and assist him in the prospective ovariotomy which was to be the first performed in the Hospital under strict antiseptic precautions. This occasion gave me an opportunity to become acquainted with that remarkable veteran of surgery and his two sons, William and Charles, both graduates of medicine, who assisted him, particularly William, the eldest, who had recently arrived from Vienna after two years of study in the surgical clinics of that great and flourishing center of medical culture.[18]

The patient, a white woman of 55 years, presented a huge ovarian cyst of the gigantic size now never seen, but common enough then, when tumors grew unmolested in patients living in the rural districts, like the trees of a primeval forest which has never known the aggression of the sawyer or of the lumber jack. The patient had been tapped many times and the effects of these tappings were secondary peritoneal reactions followed by general adhesions which completely immobilized the sac. Besides, the tumor was so large that the patient, who was small, thin, and worn by prolonged suffering, seemed to have grown to the tumor rather than the tumor to her. "A very unpromising case" as Dr. Carson and Dr. Schuppert remarked. Under Schuppert's instructions, the patient was kept in bed and given the benefit of all the preliminary examinations and dietetic and hygienic care to fit her as much as possible for the operation. Miserable and discouraged, she begged to have something done regardless of consequences. Accord-

18. I have been unable to identify Dr. William Carson further. William E. Carson (?–1895) and his brother Charles were both practitioners in New Orleans.

ingly, a small operating room was chosen, away from the main theatre to avoid dust and overcrowded audience. The night preceding the operation, the floors were scrubbed and covered over with sheets rinsed in a 5 per cent carbolic acid solution and the walls were also covered with sheets rinsed in the same solution. The tables for instruments and accessories were all draped in the same freshly laundered sheets which had been wrung out in the carbolic solution, the gowns of operators, assistants and nurses alone were exempt from the acid bath. The instruments, previously well scrubbed, were kept immersed in a 5 per cent carbolic solution. Large "elephant ear" marine sponges were kept immersed in the carbolic solution, ready for use in the abdomen.

The wash room was furnished with soap, brushes and a 5 per cent carbolic solution for hand scrubbing and disinfection. There were no caps, no masks, no gloves, as these were unknown at that time (1878). The abdominal surface was prepared in the usual way by applying a thin poultice of green soap, to be followed by a thorough wash of the softened skin with a 5 per cent carbolic water solution, leaving a thin towel wrung out of alcohol over the abdomen until the start of the incision. The drapery of the patient was all freshly laundered.

A hypodermic of morphia was given twenty minutes before the operation and the anesthesia started with chloroform dropped over an open cone. The anesthetist was an undergraduate intern, as it was the custom to give the residents practical experience.

Finally, a large steam atomizer was started to keep a steady spray of a 5 per cent carbolic solution continuously over the operating field.

Finally, the moment for the operation had come but, despite the efforts to reduce the number of spectators they continued to squeeze in always getting nearer the operating table in their street clothes without any over-gown or other pretense of a cover to reduce the risk of contaminating the room, depending only on the spray to shield the field of the operation from air infection. As it was a hot summer day, the combined effect of the spray and the over-crowding of the small room caused the perspiration to start freely on the forehead of the operator (Dr. C.) and his first assistant, Dr. William S., while the senior Dr. Schuppert, as director and counsellor, sat on a stool by the side of the patient with the operating field in excellent view. A nurse was kept busy from the start with a cold wet towel to wipe the perspiration which was streaming from the heads of the operators.

The pathology in the peritoneum was found even worse than anticipated, for the cyst, with thickened walls, contained over six quarts of dark discolored serum, and the cyst was uniformly fixed and bound down by adhesions to the abdominal wall and intestines. In fact, it was only by extreme caution that an adherent coil attached to the abdominal wall immediately under the line of incision escaped injury. After working with great care for over an hour to detach the densely adherent bowels, the cyst was mobilized sufficiently to exteriorize two-thirds of the sac. leaving the last segment sutured to the abdominal incision where it could drain externally through a rubber tube. In the course of the detachment of the bowel from the cyst, the intestinal walls, were so thin in places that they had to be protected by a reinforcing line of sutures, as in some places it was not certain that some gas had not escaped from minute tears. The abdominal incision had to be very much enlarged to deal with the adhesions, requiring much time to close it with the through and through silver wire sutures which were in favor at that time.

In the meantime, the carbolic spray was kept going, much of the atomized vapor settling on the incision and peritoneal cavity. Fine carbolized silk was used for the intestinal sutures and ligatures but the profusion of intestinal clamps and hemostats which we now find so indispensable in present day practice were not there. It is really remarkable, as I think retrospectively, how much good work was done by the two relatively young operators who were tackling, with no previous experience in the abdomen, one of the most formidable surgical problems imaginable, at that time. I was therefore not surprised when I heard Dr. William S. say, in a low voice, "Carson, this is terrible; it is almost inviting the patient to be present at her own autopsy."

The operation had to be hurried in its last stages, as the patient was showing signs of collapse. The abdominal incision was covered with a layer of Lister's protective, parafined gauze and several layers of superimposed carbolated cotton in compact gauze bags were laid over the abdomen, which had retracted into a deep hollow, lined with relaxed skin folds. The dressing was held by strips of adhesive plaster and a snug abdominal binder.

Clinical sphygmomanometry was still unborn, but this was not necessary to tell that the patient was suffering from shock and exhaustion. All that could be done was to put the patient to bed, warm her with hot water cans and give camphor oil and caffein and small doses of strychnia, digitalis, atropin and morphia by needle, with a pint of hot coffee given slowly by rectum.

Fortunately, the patient rallied for the first two days and gave promise of recovery; but, unfortunately, nephritis set in with continued vomiting (not of peritoneal origin, but uremic) and progressive oliguria and, finally, total anuria, edema of the lungs, coma and death on the sixth day. To what extent the prolonged contact of the carbolic spray had to do with the suppression of the renal function, is not certain, but the toxic effect of the carbolic spray on the kidneys (carboluria), in prolonged operations over large peritoneal and raw surfaces had been sufficiently demonstrated to make the substitute of other less toxic antiseptics desirable. This objection with other reasons, well established by Volkmann and Thiersch, finally led to the abandonment of the spray as an obligate part of the Listerian ritual, by Lister himself, in 1887.

It is doubtful that the Listerian dressing in full ritual, of the early period, was ever applied in New Orleans outside of Schuppert's clinic. But surgical cleanliness based upon a clear conception of its germicidal purpose, with special regard to the preoperative care of the surgeon's hands and the shaving, scrubbing and washing of the field of the operation, followed by carbolated compresses, was beginning to tell for the betterment of the surgical and obstetrical services. But even in the eighties, *noli me tangere* was written large on the head, chest and abdomen, and their contained organs were still held as in sanctuaries which no one dared to open with unhallowed hands. Surgery was still largely restricted to such interventions in the visceral cavities which were made compulsory by accidental injuries and imperative vital indications. Apart from fractures, dislocations, and the usual accidents that are common to metropolitan and industrial life, the conditions for surgical treatment did not constitute more than 15 or 20 per cent of the indications that call for surgery at the present time. Peritonitis was treated as a disease without regard to its cause. It was a notable event when Homans,[19] of Boston, on May 4, 1886, actually opened, for the first time an intraperitoneal abscess without identifying the appendix. The mere fact that a nonencysted acute intraperitoneal abscess, presumably caused by a suppurating appendix, had been intentionally sought for and opened by an abdominal incision, was regarded as a very audacious procedure (*Med. Rec.*, New York, May 1, 1886). Operations for hernia were limited strictly to the relief of the strangulation. No laparotomies for perforating wounds of the abdomen were performed and opium was the only and universal remedy.

---

19. John Homans (1836–1903) was a graduate of Harvard Medical School (1858) and a surgeon of Boston. He was a leader in the development of abdominal surgery and performed over six hundred ovariotomies. His book, *Three Hundred and Eighty-Four Laparotomies* (Boston: Nathan Sawyer & Son, 1887), gives a rare picture of abdominal surgery as it was practiced in the early days of the aseptic era.

By 1895, the Listerian ritual had been divested of almost all its formulas, and dry heat and steam sterilization had largely replaced chemical sterilization, except in the preparation of the skin and operating field which could not be subjected to sterilization by heat. At the same time rubber gloves introduced by Halsted,[20] in 1890, had created the equivalent of the "boiled hand" which not only gave infinitely greater security to the manipulations of surgery, but protected surgeons' hands from the harshness and injurious effects of the chemical antiseptics of all sorts, which had been ineffectually tried in infinite ways before the boilable rubber gloves were introduced. All that remained, seemingly, as a source of infection in surgical wounds was the possibility of atmospheric contamination, which had been long since relegated to a secondary plane as a negligible quantity when the spray was abandoned as unnecessary, even by Lister himself. In this way the antiseptic practice of Lister by chemical sterilization had undergone radical modifications, while still retaining the integrity of its fundamental principles, namely, the prevention of infection in clean, uncontaminated surgical wounds and the sterilization of wounds already contaminated or infected, in which chemical sterilization still had its application. Antisepsis had yielded to asepsis, a word which Lister himself had coined to indicate a state free from sepsis or infection.

---

20. William Stewart Halsted (1852–1922); see page 352f.

Hydrochlorate of Cocaine

ROBERT JOSEPH HALL (1852?–1897)

The history of local anesthesia is as fascinating—and as impor-tant—in its own right as is the history of general anesthesia. It begins in Vienna in 1884. There, the neurologist Sigmund Freud (better recog-nized, of course, in later years as a psychiatrist) was experimenting with a little-known drug, the hydrochlorate of cocaine, to treat men-tal illness. Those who were using the drug noted that their tongue be-came numb whenever it was taken by mouth. Freud suggested to his friend Karl Koller, an ophthalmologist, that cocaine might be useful in eye surgery as a surface anesthetic. Koller, in turn, experimented with patients and found that the drug was indeed effective when used in this fashion. His findings were reported to the Ophthalmologic Congress held in Heidelberg, Germany, on September 15th, 1884.

Ophthalmologists immediately made use of Koller's (and Freud's) discovery. Just a month later the New York Medical Record for Octo-ber 18, 1884, reported on the use of cocaine for eye surgery; then, as now, news of miracle drugs spread rapidly. Within a few weeks more articles appeared reporting the effectiveness of cocaine when used as a topical anesthetic on other mucous membranes. Next, on December 6, the selection included here appeared as a letter in the New York Medi-cal Journal (40:643–44, 1884). It described the use of cocaine as a local anesthetic when injected directly into the tissues, and further, it de-

scribed the use of the drug for dental anesthesia, for minor surgery, and for blocking major nerves.

The author of the letter, Robert Joseph Hall, reported experimental work that he and his associate, William Stewart Halsted, (cf p. 352), had carried out together. Hall and Halsted had been friends for at least five years, first while studying together in Europe and then as surgeons on the staff of Roosevelt Hospital in New York City. Both men appeared to be headed for brilliant surgical careers and, in 1885, both were candidates for the vacant chair of surgery at the College of Physicians and Surgeons in New York City. It soon became obvious that both men were hopelessly addicted to cocaine and that neither could be considered for the position. A disorganized letter by Halsted on the use and abuse of cocaine appeared in the New York Medical Journal a year later on September 12, 1885; it is revealing, as it was clearly written by a very sick man.

Halsted, after a lengthy illness, resumed his career in Baltimore, although it is unlikely that he ever conquered his drug addiction. He had turned to opiates, as many do who are addicted to cocaine; he was probably on maintenance doses until his death in 1922 (William Osler in his "Inner History of the Johns Hopkins Hospital" notes that Halsted was taking three grains of morphine a day in 1898 and that he was still dependent some years later).

Hall moved to California, where he practiced successfully, but not before he had endured, as he later wrote to Halsted, "a long period of misery, the causes of which I do not need to describe." He died of a ruptured appendix in 1897. It is ironic that Hall is known today for having carried out the first successful operation for a ruptured appendix. He seldom receives credit, as Halsted does, for his contributions to local anesthesia. The following selection, Hall's letter to the New York Medical Journal, is reprinted here in its entirety.

Hydrochlorate of Cocaine

17 East Forty-ninth Street, November 26, 1884.
To the Editor of the New York Medical Journal:

Sir: Wishing to use the hydrochlorate of cocaine in some small operations at the Roosevelt Hospital Out-door Department, I made some experiments on myself, to determine the best mode of using it. The preparation was four-per-cent. solution made by Parke, Davis & Co.. Injecting subcutaneously six minims on the dorsal surface of the forearm, at the junction of the middle and upper thirds, near the ulnar border, caused complete loss of sensation over an area extending *downward* as far as the lower end of the ulna, from three quarters of an inch wide above, to half an inch wide below, obviously following the distribution of a cutaneous branch of the ulnar nerve. There was no diminution of sensibility above the point at which the needle was introduced. A number of subsequent experiments showed that the anaesthesia extended over the region suppled by the cutaneous nerves near or into which the injection was made. Thus, in a number of experiments made by Dr. Halsted and myself, we have found that, injected subcutaneously into the leg or forearm, not in the neighborhood of any large nerve-trunk, it will cause anesthesia for a distance of two or three inches below the point of injection. An injection of eight minims into my left ulnar nerve at the elbow had no effect. An injection of thirty-two minims into the right ulnar nerve at the elbow caused, in two or three minutes, numbness and tingling down the forearm and little finger, and in five or six minutes anaesthesia extending down the ulnar border of the forearm and hand and over the little finger, with much reduction of the sensibility on the ulnar border of the ring–finger. There was an anaesthetic area over the olecranon and the posterior surface of the external condyle, which we should not expect to be supplied by the ulnar nerve. There was no apparent diminution of muscular power, and no anaesthesia of the skin at the point where the injection was given. We have noticed that, when the needle is thrust into the deeper layers of the subcutaneous connective tissue, there is usually no loss of sensibility at the point where the needle was introduced.

With the anaesthesia, marked constitutional symptoms appeared; about six minutes after the injection there was giddiness, at first slight, then well marked, so that I could not walk without staggering; and finally there was quite severe nausea, which would have been much worse, I think, had not the stomach been empty. At the same time, the skin was covered with cold perspiration, and the pupils were dilated, the nausea passed off with the local anaesthesia, in about twenty minutes, leaving some dizziness for an hour or so longer.

The same evening Dr. Halsted removed a small congenital cystic tumor, situated directly over the outer third of the left supra-orbital ridge, and believed to be a meningocele, the communication of which with the cranial cavity had become shut off. Nineteen minims of the four per-cent. solution were given hypodermically in divided doses, one external to the tumor, and the others close to the supra-orbital notch. In about five minutes the anaesthesia was complete. The incision through the skin and the earlier steps of the operation were not felt at all, but, in consequence of the close adhesions of the sac and its extensive prolongations, especially into the upper lid, the operation was somewhat protracted, and the anaesthesia had passed off to a considerable extent before it was completed. I was informed of a case, occurring on the same day, in which cocaine was injected, preparatory to performing a small plastic operation, in the same region, but no anaesthesia of the field of operation was produced. On inquiry, I was told that the injections had been given *above* the point where the incisions were to be made.

This afternoon, having occasion to have the left first upper incisor tooth filled, and finding that the dentine was extremely sensitive, I induced Dr. Nash, of No. 331 West Thirty-first Street, to try the effects of cocaine. The needle was passed through the mucous membrane of the mouth to a point as close as possible to the infra–orbital foramen, and eight minims were injected. In two minutes there was complete anaesthesia of the left half of the upper lip and of the cheek somewhat beyond the angle of the mouth (as I was in the dentist's chair, I could not determine the exact limits), involving both the cutaneous and the mucous surfaces; also of the left side of the lower border of the septum nasi and of the anterior surface and lower border of the gums, extending from the median line to the first molar tooth. Forcing the teeth apart with a wedge caused no pain except when the wedge impinged on the unaffected mucous membrane of the posterior surface of the gums. Dr. Nash was then able to scrape out the cavity in the tooth, which had previously been so exquisitely sensitive, and to fill it, without my experiencing any sensation whatever. The anaesthesia was complete until twenty-six minutes after the injection, and sensibility was much diminished for ten or fifteen minutes longer. Piercing the mucous membrane with the needle caused pain like the prick of a pin, but its subsequent introduction until it struck the bone and the injection of the solution were not felt. In the same way, the introduction of the needle into the ulnar nerve caused quite severe pain, with tingling down to the little finger, but the injection of the fluid gave rise to no sensation. In the experiment on the teeth, it surprised me that the incisor tooth should be rendered insensitive, as the anterior–superior dental nerve is given off in the infra-orbital canal. I can only suppose that the effect extends some distance along the nerve centrally, or that the fluid travelled along the sheath of the nerve into the canal.

We have already used this mode of administration successfully in a number of cases in the Roosevelt Hospital Out-door Department, and it is obvious that, when the limits of safety have been determined, it may find very wide application. For instance, in addition to the usual application to the conjunctiva, in operations on the eye, an injection

into the orbit, in the neighborhood of the ciliary nerves, would doubt-less diminish the liability to a very grave acident, which, I understand, has already occurred several times in the city—namely, the extrusion of the lens, from blepharospasm, occurring during iridectomy per-formed with the aid of cocaine. We have injected twenty minims a number of times, without causing any constitutional sympotms
Very truly yours,

                                                              R. J. Hall, M.D.

Postscript, December 1st—Since the foregoing was written we have made some additional experiments which seem of interest. Dr. Halsted gave Mr. Locke, a medical student, an injection of nine minims, trying to reach with the point of the needle the inferior dental nerve where it enters the dental canal. In from four to six minutes there was complete anaesthesia of the tongue, on the side where the injection had been given, extending to the median line and backward to the base as far as could be reached with a pointed instrument. There was, fur-ther, complete anaesthesia of the gums, anteriorly and posteriorly, to the median line, and all the teeth on that side were insensitive to blows. The soft palate and the uvula, on the same side, were anaemic and quite insensitive. Mr. Locke thought also that there was some diminution of sensibility in the domain of the auriculo-temporal nerve.

In four or five other cases where the injection was made in the same way, from fifteen to twenty minims being used, the fluid seemed to have come nearer the lingual than the inferior dental. In all, the tongue was affected sooner than the gums; the anaesthesia extended as far back as the epiglottis, and the sense of taste was abolished on the affected side; and the posterior surface of the gums was earlier and more completely anaesthetized than the anterior.

This evening Dr. Halsted gave me an injection of seventeen minims, the needle being introduced along the internal surface of the left ramus until it touched the inferior dental nerve, causing a sharp twinge along the whole line of the lower teeth. In three minutes there was numbness and tingling of the skin, extending from the angle of the mouth to the median line, and also of the left border of the tongue. In six minutes there was complete anaesthesia of the left half of the lower lip, on both the cutaneous and the mucous surfaces, extending from the median line to the angle of the mouth and downward to the inferior border of the jaw. A pin thrust completely through the lip caused no sensation whatever. There was also complete anaesthesia of the pos-terior surface of the gums and of the lower teeth on the left side, exactly to the median line; hard blows upon the teeth with the back of a knife caused no sensation. The anterior surface of the gums was anaesthetic only from the median line to the first bicuspid. There was a small area of complete anaesthesia, about the middle third of the left border of the tongue, not more than an inch in diameter. A slight return of sensation began twenty-five minutes after the injection, and five minutes later no complete anaesthesia remained any where. I should mention that fifteen to twenty minims in this region caused, in two or three cases, slight constitutional symptoms similar to those previously described.

Early Operative Interference in Cases of Disease of the Vermiform Appendix

CHARLES McBURNEY, M.D. (1845–1913)

The following paper (originally an address given before the New York Surgical Society) helped to establish appendectomy as a rational surgical procedure. Its author, Charles McBurney, was the surgeon at New York City's Roosevelt Hospital. Only three years earlier, in 1886, Reginald Heber Fitz (1843–1913), a pathologist of Boston, had shown that appendicitis was a clear-cut clinical entity and that it was frequently fatal. Fitz pleaded for early operative removal of the inflamed organ. This plea was well timed, for surgeons, using Lister's techniques, were finally prepared to enter the peritoneal cavity. McBurney, among others, showed that early operation for appendicitis was indeed practical. He also pointed out the single most important sign in early diagnosis—tenderness localized in the right lower quadrant of the abdomen at "McBurney's point." Five years later he described the popular muscle splitting or "gridiron" incision that also bears his name. Appendectomy soon became the most frequently performed abdominal operation. Its rapid acceptance paved the way for more complicated abdominal procedures, as the abdomen became the "surgeon's playground."

Charles McBurney was born in Roxbury, Massachusetts, on February 17, 1845. He received both an A.B. and an M.A. degree from Harvard and then graduated from New York's College of Phy-

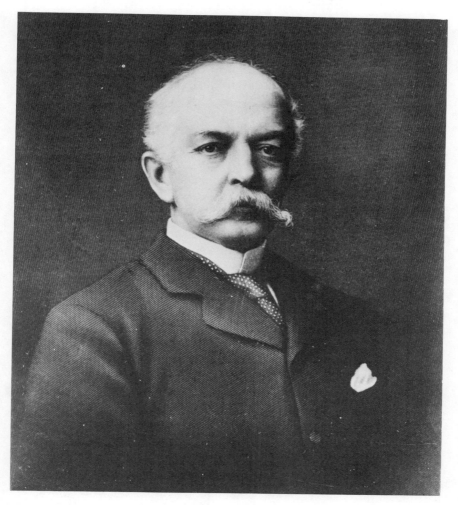

Figure 47. Charles McBurney (1845–1913). (Courtesy National Library of Medicine.)

sicians and Surgeons in 1870. In the custom of his day he traveled
abroad to complete his medical training. McBurney's career in New
York was a distinguished one. He served on the staff of many hospitals,
belonged to many societies, and was a popular teacher. In spite of other
contributions, McBurney's name will always be associated with surgery of the appendix. McBurney retired from active practice in 1907
and died on November 7, 1913, in Brookline, Massachusetts.

The following paper, describing "McBurney's point," is as it appeared in the New York Medical Journal (50:676) in 1889.

Experience with Early Operative Interference in Cases
of Disease of the Vermiform Appendix

I venture to introduce once more a subject that has been so ably
treated by numerous writers, because I have for some time been devot-
ing my attention in suitable cases to a particular line of treatment, and
because I have been fortunate enough to have had recently a considerable number of cases of disease of the appendix under my care. Nearly
two years ago the account of a case of successful laparotomy for perforation of the vermiform appendix was read before this society by our
much-lamented colleague, Dr. Henry B. Sands.[1] The case was a most
brilliant one throughout, and illustrated particularly well the clever-
ness of diagnosis and the rapidity of successful action which we all remember as so characteristic of the reader of that paper. It should not be
forgotten that at the time such action was a very bold step into ground
that was almost unknown. We did not all agree with Dr. Sands in the
views which he expressed in regard to the pathology of perityphlitis,
but these views did not prevent him, when the proper case occurred,
from making, in regard to treatment, a brilliant stride in advance of

---

1. Henry Berton Sands (1830–1888), surgeon of New York City, graduated from the College of Physicians and Surgeons in New York in 1854. He
was a pioneer in the treatment of appendicitis. In his first paper on the subject, in 1880, he advocated operating during the second week of the disease to
drain the abscess that had formed. He felt that "perityphlitis" originated in
the cecum, or possibly in the appendix. With this program he had 24 survivals
out of 26 patients. Fitz's paper in 1886 showed the true nature of appendicitis
(Transactions of the Association of American Physicians, 1:107, 1886). After
the appearance of Fitz's work, Sands was able to diagnose appendicitis pre-
operatively and recognized the need for early surgery. McBurney's contributions were an extension of Sands' and the credit that McBurney extended to
his deceased colleague was quite justified.

others. This case gave an impulse to the study of inflammatory affect-ions of the vermiform appendix from which we shall not recover for a long time. During the following months Dr. Sands devoted much at-tention to this study, and it was my privilege to assist him in a number of successful operations for the removal of the appendix at an early stage of disease. It seemed to me that each one of these operations shed a flood of light upon the pathology of the so-called pericaecal inflamma-tions, and during the summer following, while discussing this subject, he expressed to me views which were far in advance of most surgeons and very different from those which he entertained at the time when he wrote his last paper. If he were here to-night he would, by the results of his own last year's original work, enlighten us upon many points re-specting the pathology of perityphlitis. I feel it a pleasure and a duty to thus refer to Dr. Sands, because, unfortunately, no special record has been kept of his last year's brilliant work, and his sudden death pre-vented him from telling us himself what would have been so valuable. Certainly no other surgeon ever did so much to improve the treatment of a very fatal disease. Beginning with the first suggestions of Dr. Wil-lard Parker,[2] which taught surgeons how to save many lives, although by a slow and often unsatisfactory process, Dr. Sands ended his work in this direction by showing us how we might cut short at its very in-ception a disease that is even to-day responsible for many deaths.

It is not my intention in this paper to attempt to present the subject of pericaecal inflammations in a systematic manner. That has already been done, and very recently, by a large number of writers. I have chosen rather to dwell upon some points in the pathology and treat-ment of these inflammations, which are beginning to be better under-stood and which especially interest us all. The fact that inflammatory affections of the vermiform appendix give rise to a considerable num-ber of the so-called pericaecal inflammations is now accepted in every part of the medical and surgical world, although one still reads of peri-typhlitis and paratyphlitis, and of intraperitoneal and extraperitoneal abscesses. Certainly all of these terms are misleading, inasmuch as each of them, when used without explanation, implies that the particular disease to which it refers is a disease by itself, and fundamentally dif-

---

2. Willard Parker (1800–1884) was a graduate of Harvard Medical School (1830) and a surgeon of the New York Hospital. He was probably the best known surgeon in New York in his day. In 1864 Parker drained a perityphlitic abscess and recognized that the disease had originated in the appendix. He argued that such abscesses should be drained before they pointed on the sur-face. Parker had been antedated by Henry Hancock (1809–1880) of London, who had performed a similar operation in 1848.

ferent from the others. The usual term perityphlitis means, strictly speaking, nothing more than an inflammation of the peritonaeum surrounding the caecum, but it is understood by many to mean often a localized and harmless peritonitis arising from impaction of faeces, by others a fatal septic disease originating in perforation of the appendix. Now it is unquestionably true that every case of inflammation of the appendix is sooner or later accompanied by inflammation of the neighboring peritonaeum, either on the caecum or mesentery or ileum, etc., but if from the whole list of acute inflammatory affections occurring in the right iliac fossa we set aside those originating in the appendix, how many shall we have left? Very rarely will occur a perforation of the caecum by ulcer or foreign body, giving rise to a local peritonitis at this point, and traumatisms from without may accomplish the same result. For all of such causes as compared with inflammations of the appendix, let me hazard the proportion one in one hundred.

How many cases of localized peritonitis or perityphlitis arise from impaction of faeces in the caecum? Some writers would lead us to believe that is a frequent cause, and not long ago it was looked upon as the *most* frequent cause. Is there a *single* observation brought from the dead-house or from the operating-table to support this idea? I have never heard or read of such observation, and I do not believe that any such case ever occurred. Clinically we meet with cases of pain in the right iliac fossa, accompanied by some rise of temperature, and not infrequently in these cases we may detect masses of faeces in the caecum, but no peritonitis exists, and it is no more likely to arise from this cause than from ordinary constipation, which often causes pain and rise of temperature. Correctly speaking, then peritonitis localized in the immediate neighborhood of the caecum and characterized by the well-known symptoms may, with the rare exceptions referred to, be attributed to an inflammation of the vermiform appendix in some one of its numerous stages. This inflammation may be a comparatively mild catarrhal one, affecting little more than the mucous membrane, or it may have rapidly passed through various stages to complete gangrene of the organ. I must therefore prefer to use the term inflammation of the appendix, or appendicitis, and give up, once and for all, the terms perityphlitis, paratyphlitis, extraperitoneal abscess, etc., as misleading and not valuable except in explanation of secondary pathological processes. In regard to the so-called extraperitoneal abscess as a result of inflammation of the appendix, there remains nothing to be said to any one who has read Dr. Weir's[3] admirable paper in the "Medical

3. Robert Fulton Weir (1838–1927); see footnote 15, page 285.

News" for April 27th of this year. The statements and observations which Dr. Weir there makes are perfectly convincing, and I have often confirmed many of them during an operation. As a late result of a much-neglected case, pus may force its way through the lateral or posterior peritoneal lining of the abdomen, but even in very old cases this must be a rare condition, and I have myself never met with such a one. All of these abscesses originating in inflammation of the appendix are intraperitoneal. Inflammatory adhesions, which glue together the adjacent coils of intestine, prevent the contents of the abscess from flowing into the pelvis or among the intestinal folds. At every point the pus is bounded by peritonaeum. All of the operations done by the Willard Parker method require section of the peritonaeum which forms the anterior wall of the abscess. I have dwelt upon this point because it is a very important one, and one's views in regard to it will determine his operative methods. In this connection I must refer to two other terms—extraperitoneal abscess and extraperitoneal incision for the opening of such abscesses. These again are very misleading, and imply that uninflamed peritonaeum can be pushed away from the iliac fossa, the connective tissue broken through, and the abscess evacuated. If these abscesses are, as I have stated, *all* (with possibly a very rare exception) intraperitoneal, then, of course, these terms are false and misleading. The peritonaeum may be pushed back and the abscess incised deep in the iliac fossa by a roundabout and unsurgical method, but when incised the peritonaeum will be cut. In the present state of surgical opinions, it remains with those who claim that they meet with extraperitoneal abscesses and make extraperitoneal explorations to prove their point. In not a single one of the early operations for appendicitis which I have done and seen done has there been the slightest doubt as to the fact that the incipient abscess was entirely within the peritoneal cavity. I mean that this fact has always been demonstrable to the satisfaction of every one present. This one must consider as a valuable piece of evidence, for the observations were made at a period in the disease when there could be no obscurity as to the actual condition present. Weir has clearly shown also, in the paper already referred to, by carefully analyzing the reports of one hundred autopsies, that in no one of them did the abscess originate in the extraperitoneal tissue, and that in only four was pus found there at all. Weir also states, when referring to the difficulty of demonstrating the intraperitoneal origin of these abscesses after a considerable abscess has formed, that in only eight out of twenty-six abscesses opened by him could he "recognize that the inner wall of the abscess was made up of loops of intestine bound together by adhesions." But, as I have already said, *no difficulty* is found in making this demonstration when an operation is done at an early stage of the disease.

In these early operations I have found a very varied condition of the appendix and its surroundings, from a mild catarrhal condition of the mucous membrane accompanied by some infiltrations and thickening of the submucous and other tissues, to the state of complete gangrene of the whole organ, with more or less extensive peritonitis.

In one instance I removed the appendix from a young lady who in the course of little over a year had had no less than twelve attacks of so-called perityphlitis. These attacks had been severe, giving rise to great pain with rise of temperature, and causing alarm not only to the members of her family, but to her medical attendants, two of these at least being as careful observers as exist in New York. The operation was done during a period of complete health and after careful consultation, to prevent recurrence. The appendix was found rigid and swollen, the mucous membrane mildly inflamed, the other tissues of its walls greatly thickened. Not the slightest evidence of peritoneal inflammation or adhesion existed. The appendix was readily removed and the patient made a rapid recovery. The operation was done nine months ago. Since that time the patient has enjoyed unbroken health, has resumed active exercise, and has gained twenty pounds in weight. In another case, also a young lady, attacks of abdominal pain, accompanied by vomiting, exquisite tenderness in the right iliac fossa, and considerable elevations of temperature, had occurred on four different occasions. This patient had also been taken care of by the most competent men. Curiously enough, just at the time of this patient's last attack her sister died without operation from a violent purulent peritonitis caused by perforation of the appendix. Subsequently to this last attack and during a period of complete health I removed the appendix after careful consultation with her physician, Dr. J. W. McLane,[4] to prevent recurrence. A condition of disease somewhat in advance of the case already narrated existed. The appendix was quite firmly bound by old adhesions to the under surface of the intestinal mesentery and to the caecum. The mesentery of the appendix had been nearly obliterated; the organ itself was dark-colored, considerably swollen, but soft. The mucous membrane was very dark-colored and swollen and inclosed some fine faecal grains. Two partial strictures of [narrow] caliber existed which produced retention of a dirty brown fluid. The evidences of

---

4. James Woods McLane (1839–1912), M.D., College of Physicians and Surgeons of New York, 1864; obstetrician and subsequently professor of obstetrics and dean at the college.

former limited peritonitis existed on the neighboring portion of the caecum. This patient also made a rapid recovery, being out of bed at the end of two weeks, with a wound completely healed. The operation was done over four months ago, and the patient has remained in perfect health, having gained largely in weight and having resumed active exercise from which she had been entirely debarred. These two cases are quoted at this point to show that comparatively slight conditions of inflammatory disease in the appendix may give rise to threatening illness, which by some would be described as resolving perityphlitis without further explanation. There can be little doubt that both of these cases were preparing for abscess or general peritonitis.

In other cases—all in an acute state of inflammation—and which will be quoted later, the conditions found have been these: In one the appendix formed a considerable cyst containing nearly an ounce of dark-brown pus. No communication with the caecum existed.

In several the appendix was swollen, discolored, diseased throughout, but gangrenous only at one or two points were perforation had occurred, and in these cases one or more faecal concretions existed, either within or just outside of the appendix.

In several the appendix was in general only moderately diseased, but perforation had occurred, and quite firm recent adhesions had tied the appendix to some adjacent part, doubling it upon itself and so inclosing a small collection of pus with or without concretion.

In two cases the appendix was thick, but flattened so as to be with difficulty recognized, and very firmly bound to the under side of the caecum, and in two cases the appendix was completely gangrenous. In all of these acute cases peritonitis existed—usually a plastic peritonitis of greater or less extent—always involving the caecum and generally the adjacent intestinal coils and abdominal walls. In one case the omentum was quite extensively involved, partly enveloping the appendix. In *no* case was the appendix more than lightly attached by adhesion to the peritonaeum covering the iliac muscles, and in none was *extra*peritoneal inflammation observed, excepting sometimes in the anterior abdominal wall. In most cases some pus was found more or less confined by adhesions within a limited area, and in one absolutely no adhesion of any kind existed, though the appendix was perforated by concretion, an very foul pus filled the pelvis and ran freely upward beside the colon.

The pathological conditions of the appendix, as compared with the symptoms in my own cases, most positively show that one can not with accuracy determine from the symptoms the extent and severity of the disease. I therefore doubt the safety of the advice given by several recent writers, to watch the symptoms and to be guided by their violence in determining the method of treatment. This will appear more clearly in the histories of the cases. I should like now to refer to some of the special symptoms *the weight and value of which have been subsequently determined by an immediate operation*, for it is in this manner that we shall mostly advance our knowledge of the pathology of appendicitis. By autopsy we can not learn very much more in this direction, if one may judge by the length of time it required to learn the important single fact that abscesses originating in the appendix are almost invariably intraperitoneal. Pain to a greater or less extent is present in all cases of appendicitis, but many a mistake has been made and a golden opportunity lost by looking for pain in the iliac fossa and an *absence* of pain in other parts of the abdomen. General abdominal pain is often all that the patient will complain of during the first few hours of his attack, and in many cases it requires a careful and pointed examination to determine that the cause of the pain is situated in the iliac fossa. But after the first few hours it becomes more and more evident that the chief seat of pain is at that point, and the general pain then usually subsides. The epigastric region is frequently the point first complained of. One patient, who died on the third day from violent septic peritonitis from perforation, complained of comparatively little pain even when the iliac fossa was firmly compressed. The *exact* locality of the greatest sensitiveness to pressure has seemed to me to be usually one of importance. Whatever may be the position of the healthy appendix as found in the dead-house—and I am well aware that its position when uninflamed varies greatly—I have found in all of my operations that it lay, either thickened, shortened, or adherent, very close to its point of attachment to the caecum. This of course, must, in early stages of the disease, determine the seat of greatest pain *on pressure*. And I believe that in every case the seat of greatest pain, *determined by the pressure of one finger,* has been very exactly between an inch and a half and two inches from the anterior spinous process of the ilium on a straight line drawn from that process to the umbilicus. This may appear to be an affectation of accuracy, but so far as my experience goes, the observation is correct.

Chill and vomiting are frequent, but so often absent as to be in no sense of much diagnostic value. Fever to some extent is present in all cases, but very different in degree, some severe cases having a temperature on the first day of less than 100.5°, others rapidly reaching a temperature of 103.5°. But, as nearly excluding non-inflammatory pains, the presence of this symptom is certainly of importance. Rigidity in the abdominal muscles, generally much more marked on the affected side than on the other, I have found very constant, and I believe to be a sign of value.

Abdominal distension by tympanites varies greatly, and its degree by no means measures the severity of the diseased process. It may be very decided during the very first hours of a mild case, and also entirely absent in the worst form of sudden perforation. It must, of course, be influenced greatly by the condition of the patient's bowels, the ease with which the intestine in each individual is brought to a state of paresis, and by many other causes. But when the gut has been found during the operation to be overdistended, the portion of gut so affected has always been the large intestine. Probably paresis from the local peritonitis is here a large factor.

Tumor of greater or less size I have usually been able to detect at a very early stage, but the composition of this tumor, as shown during operation, has varied greatly. In one case the tumor consisted of the distended unruptured appendix, which was partly wrapped in an inflamed and thickened omentum. In another it was formed of a mass of intestinal coils swollen and glued together by recent plastic exudation. This tumor was large, quite firm, and gave one the impression that a large quantity of pus was present; but only a very minute abscess was found, and that was situated quite beneath the caecum. But under ether some tumor can invariably be detected; and this agent will, I think, be found to be a valuable help to diagnosis in some doubtful cases. The tumor may be dull on percussion, as when pus has formed and lies against the anterior abdominal wall; but I have more than once found a small deep tumor containing pus, which was so completely covered in front by intestines that the percussion note, before ether was given, was purely tympanitic. The pulse during the onset of appendicitis is usually rapid and irritable. The patient prefers to have the right thigh elevated, and objects to its overextension. Rectal examination at the onset I have not found of any value.

The combination of symptoms present will usually render a correct diagnosis as to the seat of the disease quite easy, but in reference to the stage which the disease has reached—that is, whether pus has formed or not, whether the appendix is already perforated or not, even sometimes whether already general septic peritonitis exists or not—the diagnosis is often very doubtful. I remember one case where Dr. Sands performed a beautiful operation and saved the patient's life. At the consultation held before operation four gentlemen were present. Three of them had certainly seen many cases of appendicitis. Three quite different opinions were expressed. Dr. Sands thought that the appendix was perforated, and that pus had formed. One of the others thought there was probably appendicitis, but advised an extraperitoneal incision. Another thought the case so mild that it should be treated without operation. Dr. Sands operated by an incision along the right edge of the rectus muscle, opened an intraperitoneal abscess just in the middle of his incision, and removed a perforated and sloughing appendix. The patient rapidly recovered. This case occurred very shortly after Dr. Sands read his last paper before this society. I mention it simply to show that the diagnosis of the exact condition in such cases is not easy. A means of diagnosis lauded by some, permitted by others, and totally condemned by a few, is the exploring needle. I believe that the use of this instrument will become less and less frequent as we know more of the disease. While perhaps occasionally permissible at a late stage of the disease, it is certainly totally to be condemned at its beginning. The discovery of pus with the syringe is, to be sure, gratifying to a hesitating operator, but the withdrawal of an injected needle through several layers of peritonaeum, which it may have passed during its introduction, can totally nullify a good subsequent operation. And, if the needle does *not* discover pus, which has often happened even when that fluid has been present in considerable quantity, then the man who pinned his faith on a needle is induced to underestimate the importance of the case and its mode of treatment.

Some years ago I went a long distance into the country prepared to operate upon a nine-days-old abscess, the result of appendicitis. There existed a large fluctuating tumor, and the case was plain and needed just one cut. But the family physician was very conservative, and said the time had not come, and that there was no pus. I was in despair, for the journey took many hours. Fortunately, I had a good hypodermic syringe with me. The doctor said rather superciliously that the thing was harmless anywhere. So he permitted its introduction; and when the barrel filled with pus he yielded to an operation, and treated me afterward with great respect. But to search for pus with a needle, first in one direction and then in another, at the risk of doing harm, and with no certainty of acquiring any real information, is a practice as unsurgical as it is unnecessary.

I think that there is still much misapprehension in the minds of many practitioners as to be the symptoms produced by perforation of the appendix. Many associate with this condition, and with no other, a very violent onset of the disease with quite well-marked symptoms, as compared with the less severe commencement of a slowly forming abscess. The truth is that, in the early stages, no accurate diagnosis can be made as to whether the appendix is perforated or not, excepting in those cases where comparatively mild symptoms *suddenly* become much aggravated, when perforation or the rupture of an abscess may be inferred. Perforation often occurs with but few symptoms at the very beginning of the disease, but, being preceded by the formation of more or less plastic adhesion of the appendix, no sudden increase in the severity of the disease occurs at all. An abcess slowly forms, which may increase to a considerable size without being discovered, and then force its way, or proceed by infection, in the most dangerous directions. The comment might fairly be made upon this description of the early symptoms of appendicitis that the diagnosis of the disease is very obscure and uncertain. To the careful observer it is not difficult, however, to determine as to the existence of the disease. The only real difficulty lies in determining within the first few hours what the future progress of the disease is to be in deciding whether firm adhesions are forming, which will effectually exclude pus from the general peritoneal cavity, and so provide for subsequent safe evacuation of abscess, or whether no such protecting wall exists, and an overdistended appendix threatens to instantly set up a fatal peritonitis. If this difficulty could be set aside by a more careful study of symptoms, and without losing valuable time, our course would be clear, and we should no longer helplessly hesitate as to when to operate and when to stand aside. There is no reason to think, however, that diagnosis from symptoms alone will ever reach that perfection. We need some further aid to diagnosis; some positive and rapid means of determining what method of treatment we are apt to adopt. We have reached a point where we can never be satisfied with the mortality that attends an expectant treatment. What we wish to accomplish in the treatment of appendicitis is, not to save half of our cases, nor four cases our of five, but *all of them;* and how is this end to be attained except by improved methods of diagnosis at the very earliest stage of the disease? I hope that I may never again go every day to visit a threatening case, waiting for the authority of a clearly defined general peritonitis before I dare take action. I do not mean to deny that many very ugly-looking cases of appendicitis go on to the formation of abscess which may be safely opened and end in complete recovery; we have all of us seen many such. I am well aware that numerous cases have presented all the symptoms of the disease, have become very ill, and have finally recovered without any operation. Within two years I have seen two cases, in one of which the patient was so ill that I refused to operate, and in the other case I strongly urged operation and was refused permission. Both of these patients recovered after long illness without operation of any kind. Probably the abscesses emptied themselves at some point into the intestine. But such unexpected recoveries, and the frequent formation of abscesses which can be opened safely at a later stage, even the many cases which quite rapidly terminate, at least temporarily, without suppuration, do not console us for the heavy mortality caused by appendicitis. What this mortality has been we shall of course never know. We do know that the cases which are recognized and which die are numerous, and it is safe to assert that a very large number of fatal cases of peritonitis commence with an unrecognized inflammation of the vermiform appendix. No one will dispute that if we could so improve our methods of diagnosis that we could recognize within the first few hours the serious nature of many cases, we would operate in these cases at once, willingly preferring to incur the risks of an operation rather than face the certainty of death that septic peritonitis implies. How may we improve our methods of diagnosis? At present I see no clearer road than the exploratory incision permitting a direct inspection of the parts and a complete study of the disease. If it can be shown by future experience with improved methods of operation, and with more perfect antiseptic precautions, that the exploratory incision for inspection of the diseased appendix is much more free from danger than the expectant treatment, then there could be but one answer to the question, What is the best treatment? The firm conviction that very early operation for the cure of appendicitis can, with proper care, be done with very slight risk, has induced me to subject a considerable number of these cases to the earliest operation possible, and my chief purpose to-night is to present to you the results of my work in this direction. It is proper to state that no case of appendicitis has been refused operation, and that all the cases operated upon in the early stage of the disease are here reported:

CASE I

E. M. P., a young gentleman nineteen years of age, complained of general abdominal pain at 11 A. M. on May 21, 1888. The pain was regarded as due to indigestion, and was treated with family remedies. In the afternoon the patient fainted, and by four o'clock his pain had greatly increased in severity. He received a little morphine and hot applications were applied. At 5 P.M. his mouth temperature was 98.4°, his pulse 100. During the night and the following day the patient complained sometimes of severe pain, and occasionally felt much better; he took a considerable quantity of milk, and at 8 P. M. his temperature was only 100°. During the second night he suffered much pain, and at 5 A. M. on the 23rd it was noted that his pain was chiefly in the right iliac fossa. At 5:30 he had a severe chill and his temperature rose to 103°, his pulse to 120. At this time he was visited by his physicians, Dr. Fessenden N. Otis[5] and Dr. William K. Otis,[6] who diagnosticated at once acute appendicitis, and requested me to see the patient. This I did at about 8:30. I found the pulse and temperature as stated, and the following condition: Great rigidity of right abdominal muscles; exquisite tenderness on pressure at a point just two inches internal to the anterior spine of the ilium, in the direction of the umbilicus. Beneath the finger at this point could be felt a small resisting mass, less than one inch in diameter. No dullness on percussion anywhere. General appearance excellent. The diagnosis of appendicitis already made by Dr. Otis was confirmed by myself, and an hour later by Dr. Sands. Immediate operation advised and accepted.

General appearance of patient excellent. It should be noted that at 11:30 the temperature had fallen to 101°.

Operation at 12 o'clock, just forty-nine hours from the first pain. Present, Dr. F. N. Otis, Dr. William K. Otis, Dr. L. R. Morris,[7] and Dr. Tuttle.[8]

Ether anaesthesia. A slightly oblique incision four inches and a half long, the center of this incision being two inches from the anterior iliac spine toward the umbilicus. Tissues of abdominal wall quite markedly oedematous, particularly near the peritonaeum. On opening the peritonaeum freely, the appendix came at once into view. It was larger than a man's thumb, dark-brown in color, tense, evidently full of fluid, and at no point gangrenous, but its wall evidently nearly as thin as paper. A tail of omentum partly enveloped it, and this was much inflamed and freshly adherent. Everywhere else the peritonaeum was healthy, and not an indication of the formation of any bounding wall of adhesions existed. Coils of small intestine surrounded this full-to-bursting sac. The omentum was gently separated and the inflamed portion ligated and cut away. The mesentery of the appendix was carefully tied in sections, and the base of the appendix dislodged from an inverted pouch of caecum, ligated at its base, and cut away. It proved to contain at least half an ounce of very foul brown pus, but no concretion. Its communication with the caecum was closed by stricture, so that the unbroken, purulent, acutely inflamed cyst was removed entire. The

---

5. Fessenden Nott Otis (1825–1900), M.D., New York Medical College, 1852; urologist and syphilologist of New York City.

6. William K. Otis (1870–1906), M.D., Columbia, 1885; the son of F. N. Otis and also a urologist.

7. Lewis Rutherford Morris (1862–1936), M.D., Bellevue Hospital Medical College, 1884; practitioner of New York City.

8. "Dr. Tuttle" was probably George Montgomery Tuttle (1856–1912), M.D., Columbia, 1880; professor of gynecology at Columbia.

stump was disinfected with 1-to-1,000 bichloride solution. Two silver-wire sutures passing through the whole thickness of the abdominal walls closed the upper part of the wound, and one similar suture the lower part. The central portion was loosely packed with iodoform gauze down to the ligated stump. Dressing of iodoform and bichloride gauze over all.

At 6:40 P. M., less than six hours after the operation, patient's temperature was 99.8° and pulse 80. A small quantity of morphine was given for wound pain. The dressings were changed on the third day, and a perfectly aseptic condition of wound found. This patient made a rapid and absolutely unbroken recovery, and is to-day perfectly well.

This is, I believe, the first recorded case where an acutely inflamed unruptured appendix has been removed full of pus. Who can doubt what the result would have been in this particular case had the cyst rup-tured, and the operation been delayed a few hours? Would not the op-portunity for recovery have been lost had the advice so often and so recently given been followed—to delay operation until symptoms of spreading peritonitis appeared?

CASE II

John S., ten years of age, was admitted to my care at the Roose-velt Hospital on August 19, 1889. He gave no history of previous at-tacks. A week ago he became ill, and complained of general abdominal pain. He went to bed, and says that since that time he has been feverish and has not been free from pain. Four days ago the chief seat of pain is said to have been in the right side and low down. On admission his pulse was 110, his temperature 103.4°, and he was nauseated. Between the umbilicus and the right iliac spine was noted a considerable tumor, which was markedly tender on pressure. The percussion note over the tumor, which was markedly tender on pressure. The percussion note over the tumor was dull. No tympanites existed. The general appear-ance of the patient was that of severe illness. I operated on the same day. The usual incision was made, and the tissues found in a normal condition down to the peritonaeum. The anterior peritonaeum itself was perfectly uninflamed, and uninflamed small intestine covered the anterior face of the tumor. When these were drawn toward the median line, a mass of adherent intestines was disclosed, which inclosed a small indurated tumor.

The intestinal coils were gently separated on the anterior face of the tumor, and several drachms of faecal pus at once escaped, empty-ing a cavity somewhat tubular in shape and large enough to admit the finger. The appendix lay in this cavity, congested, much swollen, and infiltrated with pus. No perforation existed, and no concretions were found. The appendix was tied off with silk and removed. A rubber drain was introduced, the cavity packed with iodoform gauze beside the drain, and a full antiseptic dressing applied.

On the following day, August 20th, the boy's temperature was 99.6° as against 103.4° of the day before, a reduction in less than twenty-four hours of nearly four degrees. This patient recovered rapidly and completely, and on September 25th his wound was entirely healed.

CASE III

W. K., a male, sixteen years of age, was admitted to my care at the Roosevelt Hospital on July 26, 1889. Previous history negative. Forty-eight hours before admission first felt pain in the right iliac fossa. On the next day diarrhoea set in; abdominal pain was quite general, though more distinctly localized in the right iliac fossa than elsewhere, and this increased up to the time of admission to the hospital. The patient's temperature was then 102°, his pulse 110. The abdomen was slightly distended and tympanitic. In the right iliac fossa was found a small, very tender non-fluctuating tumor, which lay just inside of the anterior iliac spine. Diagnosis, acute appendicitis.

Operation at 3:30, July 26th. The usual incision was made. Beneath the incision were found normal non-inflamed intestines. These were drawn toward the median line, when the appendix was found projecting stiffly forward and slightly upward by the inner side of the caput coli.

It curled around the end of the caecum and then turned upward and forward. Slight recent adhesions tied the appendix at its base only to the caecum. At other points it floated freely among non-inflamed intestines. The adhesions were broken down and the appendix ligated at its base and removed. It was six inches and a quarter long, oedematous, and much thickened and inflamed throughout. Minute foci of pus were scattered through its substance, but there was no concretion and no perforation. On its removal the seat of the operation was left perfectly clean, but, to insure safety, a rubber drain was passed through the loin directly to the base of the stump, and the anterior wound was partly closed and partly packed with iodoform gauze. The next day patient's temperature was 100°. His wound was inspected, but not dressed completely until July 30th. No pus was found. This patient made an unbroken recovery without incident, and his wounds were completely healed on August 19th.

CASE IV

Annie O., eighteen years of age, was admitted to the medical wards of the Roosevelt Hospital on May 29, 1888. Six years ago she had an attack similar to the present one from which she entirely recovered without operation. Two days ago she was seized with severe epigastric pain accompanied by fever and headache, and tenderness on pressure in the right iliac fossa. On admission, the abdomen was tense, tympanitic, tender on pressure at all points, but more especially in the right iliac fossa. Here a small tumor is distinctly felt. I saw this patient for the first time on May 30th, and, having expressed the opinion that she should be operated upon at once, she was transferred to my care. At this time her symptoms had become much more threatening; abdominal distension was extreme. Her temperature was low, 100.4°, pulse 100, respiration 36. I operated at once, making the usual incision. The tissues of the abdominal wall were oedematous and the deeper ones much fused together. Beneath the center of the incision the distal end of the appendix was readily found. It was much enlarged and thickened, and greatly discolored. At first no pus was seen, but, on gently separating the end of the appendix from adjacent parts, a small cavity was found beneath it containing less than one ounce of pus. The cavity was cleansed with hot water and it was then seen that the appendix was perforated at about its middle and lying in the perforation was a large faecal concretion. The whole appendix was then removed after ligating the base, the cavity was swabbed with 1-to-1,000 bichloride solution, two rubber drains introduced, and the cavity packed with iodoform gauze. A complete antiseptic dressing was applied. On June 1st the patient's temperature was 99°, pulse 100, respiration 18. Abdomen free from pain or distension.

This patient made an unbroken recovery, being out of bed on June 23d, with a small superficial, flat ulcer still to heal.

CASE V

Charles E. A., twenty-five years of age, was admitted to the Roosevelt Hospital on September 1, 1889. Patient gives a history of probable appendicitis occurring five months ago.

Two days ago, after several weeks of abdominal discomfort, the patient was seized with severe abdominal pain, nausea, vomiting, and fever.

On admission, his temperature was 102°. Internal to the anterior iliac spine, on the right side, some resistance and tenderness on pressure were noted. Diagnosis, appendicitis.

On September 2d, under ether narcosis, the usual incision was made, the tissues of the abdominal wall being found very oedematous. Marked adhesions and thickening of the peritonaeum were found over a large area, indicating clearly the existence at some previous time of a quite extensive peritonitis. This probably occurred during the attack referred to above. The appendix was found, after some difficulty, hanging over the edge of the pelvis, greatly thickened and hardened. After being freed from adhesions, it was ligated close to its base and removed. The immediate neighborhood of the stump was cleansed and the space packed with iodoform gauze. The upper portion of the abdominal wound was closed by suture. With the exception that a slight superficial abscess developed beneath the suture line, this patient made an easy recovery, and was discharged, with a wound completely healed, on October 17th. This patient was operated upon by Dr. Frank Hartley,[9] my first assistant at the hospital.

CASE VI

Miss E. C., twenty-five years of age, a patient of Dr. W. T. Alexander,[10] of this city, had complained of a sense of uneasiness and discomfort in the right abdominal region, low down, for two or three weeks. She had, however, gone about as usual, and walked several miles daily. On June 18, 1889, in the evening, she was seized with severe general abdominal pain, most severe in the epigastrium, and was nauseated. She went to bed, and was then first seen by Dr. Alexander, who diagnosticated appendicitis, and ordered hot applications and a little morphine, with complete rest in bed. On the following day Dr. Alexander asked me to visit the patient. This I did in the afternoon. The patient's temperature was then 101°, and her pulse 100. She had a very ill look, and complained bitterly of the slightest pressure over the right iliac fossa and of some tenderness all over the abdomen. I advised immediate operation. There were present at the operation Dr. W. T. Alexander, Dr. G. T. Jackson,[11] and Dr. R. P. O'Neill,[12] and these gentlemen assisted me.

---

9. Frank Hartley (1856–1913), M.D., Columbia, 1880; clinical professor of surgery at Columbia and best known for his operation on the trigeminal ganglion intracranially for the treatment of tic douloureux.

10. Welcome Taylor Alexander (1848–1922), M.D., Bellevue Hospital Medical College, 1870; surgeon of New York City with a special interest in dermatology (!).

11. George Thomas Jackson (1852–1916), M.D., Columbia; and subsequently professor of dermatology there.

12. Roger Power O'Neill (b. 1856), M.D., Jefferson, 1883; practitioner of New York.

I made the usual incision. The tissues of the abdominal wall were normal, and within the peritoneal cavity scarcely the slightest trace of adhesions was found. The appendix, nearly completely gangrenous, as large as one's middle finger, lay just outside of the caput coli, not perforated, but containing two large faecal concretions, just ready to escape through very soft gangrenous tissue. A little purulent fibrin lay beneath the appendix. No limiting wall of any kind existed and reddened small intestine lay above and below. The mesentery of the appendix was carefully and with some difficulty tied off, the appendix ligated at its base and removed. The immediate neighborhood was then thoroughly cleansed with 1-to-1,000 bichloride solution, dusted with iodoform, and packed with gauze. A rubber drainage-tube was introduced beside the gauze down to the stump. The upper part of the incision was closed with two sutures. The patient suffered from nausea and tympanites for two or three days, when her temperature fell to normal and remained so. On the seventh day the wound discharges were decidely faecal, and continued to have this character for about a week. The wound then became perfectly healthy and rapidly healed. This patient has gained greatly in health and weight, and has been, up to date, perfectly well.

CASE VII

Edgar C. B., a stalwart young man, twenty-one years old, complained of pain in the lower part of the abdomen during the evening of January 13, 1889. The next morning, when he had gone to work, this pain spread through the whole abdominal cavity and became very severe. He reached home with difficulty and went to bed. During the afternoon of the 14th—that is, at the end of about twenty hours—the pain localized itself chiefly in the right iliac and lumbar regions. At noon on the 15th he had a chill, and, feeling very ill, came to the Roosevelt Hospital in the evening. His temperature was then 101.6°, pulse and respiration about normal. The abdominal muscles on the right abdominal half were rigid, and very acute tenderness was complained of when pressure was made over the right iliac fossa about two inches inside of the anterior iliac spine. No tumor could be felt. The diagnosis of acute appendicitis was made, and I determined on an immediate operation. This was done at 11 P. M., as nearly as possible forty-eight hours after the first symptom. The usual incision was made. The tissues of the abdominal wall were found in a normal condition. Beneath the line of incision were coils of noninflamed small intestine. These were pushed inward, exposing a mass of small intestines matted together by adhesions and quite free from the iliac fascia. After a short search, and after breaking down some of these adhesions, the appendix was found, passing backward and inward from the caecum, then doubling back upon itself. It was closely tied by adhesion to the caecum and adjacent mesentery. The adhesions were broken down, the mesentery of the appendix tied off in sections, and the appendix itself ligated at its base with catgut and removed. The appendix was much diseased, thickened, and distorted but not ruptured. On section I found within it some black, semi-fluid material. The mucous membrane was gangrenous throughout, and the wall of the appendix at one point gangrenous *as far as the peritoneal coat*. The stump was sponged with 1-to-1,000 bichloride solution. The upper part of the wound was closed with silver stitches, a rubber drainage-tube passed down to the stump, and the open wound packed with iodoform gauze. During the next hours considerable pain was experienced, and for a few days constipation was obstinate. On the morning of the 17th the temperature became normal and remained so throughout convalescence, which was unbroken and entirely completed by February 11th. A small superficial ulcer was completely healed on February 21st.

CASE VIII

C. G. McK., a young gentleman twenty-three years old. First attack of pain in right iliac fossa two years ago. Second attack in May last, when he was confined to bed five days with fever and severe pain and tenderness in the same region. On Thursday morning, October 17th, he had a sudden attack of severe pain in region of appendix, went to bed, and his temperature was noted to be 99°. In the evening his temperature rose to 100°. Pain and tenderness steadily increased. Friday he remained in the same condition, and was seen by me, at the request of Dr. E. E. Swift,[13] later at night. The patient was haggard and looked ill. Tenderness on pressure about two inches inside of the iliac spine was very marked. An ill-defined tumor existed, and decided distension of abdomen. Operation was advised, but the circumstances were such that it was postponed until twelve o'clock on the following day.

Operation October 19, 1889. Ether anaesthesia. The usual incision was made. On opening the peritonaeum, an enormously distended caput coli filled the wound and rendered the search for the appendix

13. Edwin E. Swift (1855–1933), M.D., medical school of the University of New York, 1880; practitioner of New York City with a special interest in neurology.

extremely difficult, forcing me to handle the intestines far more than
was to be desired. The appendix was at last found, flat, wide, and so
firmly adherent to the under surface of the caecum as to be identified
with great difficulty, and numerous firm old adhesions prevented the
free movement of intestines and at one point formed a nearly constricting band. An indurated mass beneath the center of the appendix was
opened with the finger by separating adhesions which, however, were
very strong, and many of them evidently old. From this mass about a
drachm of foul faecal pus escaped and was sponged away. The difficulty of dissecting away the appendix was so great that I was finally
obliged to desist and to be satisfied with removing only that portion of
it which formed the wall of the abscess. The cavity was very thoroughly
cleansed, and an attempt made to return the prolapsed large intestine
and close the wound. This was found to be exceedingly difficult, own-
ing to the very excessive distension of the gut, and much time was ex-
pended and much handling of gut necessitated. Finally the wound was
closed as in other cases, the lower part being packed and drained. The
patient recovered well from the effects of the operation, but at the end
of twenty-four hours his temperature rose to 102°, and the abdominal
distension increased. He was bright and looked fairly well, however,
and I did not expect serious illness. His temperature, however, continued to rise, symptoms of peritonitis developed, complete paresis of
bowel persisted, and the patient died at the end of four days, of peritonitis. No autopsy could be obtained.

Whether the difficult and unusual handling of the intestines was
the chief cause of peritonitis, or whether constricting bands, formed by
old adhesions, caused actual obstruction, I am unable to say. No
movement of the bowels could be obtained and no flatus passed after
the operation excepting by the aid of a long rectal tube. Certainly the
peritonitis was not septic, and such was the opinion of Dr. Delafield[14]
and Dr. Swift, who visited the patient with me. Moreover, when, on
the second day, I removed the packing, I found a perfectly healthy
wound, without the slightest sign of infection. One thing is clear—that,
had the operation been done during the patient's first attack two years
ago, none of the great difficulties which I met with would have been encountered.

I stated at the beginning of this paper that I did not here intend to
review the treatment of appendicitis in a systematic manner, but I
should not do justice to the real subject of this writing were I to drop

---

14. Francis Delafield (1841–1915), M.D., Columbia, 1863; a leading
physician and pioneer pathologist of New York City.

the matter at this point. I must, in the first place, as accurately as possible, define the class of cases of appendicitis to which I have applied the method of treatment described; and then I wish to devote a few minutes to a description of the technique of the operations. I have presented eight cases of appendicitis operated upon at an early stage of *acute* inflammatory process. These eight cases include *all* of those operated upon since May 20, 1888, to date. Previous to May 20, 1888, I had never operated upon a case except by the older methods. During this period of eighteen months I have seen and operated upon a much larger number of cases of appendicitis at late stages in the disease— that is, when extensive abscess has existed, and in some cases of early general septic peritonitis due to appendicitis. Such cases are excluded from the list given, as belonging to an entirely different category. I have measured the stage of the disease, not by the number of hours or even days that it has existed, but by the character and extent of the inflammatory process, all cases being included in the list excepting those where it was clear that large, comparatively safe abscess was forming, or where general septic peritonitis was already established. I should, moreover, state that in every case operation has been done as soon as possible after being seen, excepting that in the fatal case various circumstances, contrary to my wish, necessitated a delay of about twelve hours. In no case has a diagnosis of appendicitis been made which has been subsequently proved by operation to be incorrect. To those who have been in doubt as to whether the operation or the disease carries with it the most danger, I think these cases, although limited in number, must be convincing in favor of the operation. All will acknowledge that every case of appendicitis may, so far as the cleverest observer can tell, have to pass by many very dangerous obstacles before reaching the smooth water of a comfortable abscess. For my part, I would endeavor to insure safety early, before reaching the rapids, rather than trust to finding my way with my eyes blindfolded through a dangerous passage. I am familiar with the good-natured jest that the surgeon is now ready to cut every one who has a stomach-ache. The death-rate from appendicitis within the professional circle of New York alone is a sufficient answer to that criticism.

But I should be much misunderstood if I should give the impression that, while I believe the operation to be less dangerous than the disease, I also believe the operation to be simple and easy of execution. I look upon it as often an exceedingly difficult one, and one which requires as much care and patience and attention to detail as any with which I am familar. Moreover, I have never seen two cases of appendicitis operated upon in which the pathological conditions, the position of adhesions, the relation of surrounding parts, etc., were very nearly alike. Every case presents some new problems, and in every case there is large opportunity for the excercise of careful judgment as to how best to meet this or that difficulty. Of course there must be pioneers, as Sands was, and such may be the most succesful, but my strong feeling is that it is well worth while for any one who may have to do this operation to see it done, at least once, first.

Before describing the steps of the operation, I refer again to the important aid to diagnosis of which I have already spoken—namely, the ascertaining, by the pressure of a single finger-tip, that the point of greatest tenderness is, in the average adult, almost exactly two inches from the anterior iliac spine, on a line drawn from this process through the umbilicus. Much greater tenderness at this point than at others, taken in connection with the history of the case and the other well-known signs. I look upon as almost pathognomonic of appendicitis. This point indicates the situation of the base of the appendix, where it arises from the caecum, but does not by any means demonstrate, as one might conclude, that the chief point of disease is there. The abscess, or concretion, or cyst may be at quite a little distance, but the greatest pain, on pressure with one finger, will be felt at the point described.

The incision should be a liberal one, for much room may be required, and a five-inch cut in the adult is not too much. It should follow as nearly as possible the right edge of the rectus muscle, and the center of the incision should lie opposite to or a little below the anterior iliac spine, on a line drawn to the umbilicus.[15] When the external oblique aponeurosis is cut through by this incision, the aponeurotic structure, in which the other abdominal muscles end, comes into view, and is easily divided without cutting muscular fiber. Then the fascia transversalis, the subperitoneal fat, and the peritonaeum are cut in succession. If pus has formed close against the anterior abdominal wall, these last-mentioned tissues will be found infiltrated with serum, and even thickened so as to look like cheesy tubercle. Otherwise these parts may appear perfectly normal. On opening the peritonaeum the appendix may at once be seen, or adhesions and inflammatory exudations may have so distorted the parts that a careful and difficult search may be required to find the appendix at all. It may be flattened out and glued firmly to the inflamed surface of the caecum by old and recent adhesions, or it may be coiled upon itself and buried out of view in a mass

---

15. McBurney subsequently devised the muscle-splitting "McBurney incision" and published a description of this in 1894.

of lymph. The finger is often quicker than the eye to detect the appendix in these conditions, as it is very certain to be found where the greatest thickening, as felt by the finger, exists. More than once I have had to turn the caecum out of the wound and examine carefully the usual region of origin of the appendix before I could identify it. Usually then with the finger or a dull-pointed instrument the adhesions can be broken down or tied off, as may seem required by vascularity. If the appendix has been thus separated, I have usually tied it off with silk or catgut close to the caecum and cut it away, and generally between two ligatures. Careful disinfection of the stump should be made. I have scraped its interior and disinfected with 1-to-1,000 bichloride solution, and then rubbed in iodoform. Once where it looked dangerous, I tied with silver wire, and then used the fine-pointed cautery to disinfect. If thoroughly cleansed, it seems to be unnecessary to lose time in sewing the peritonaeum over the stump, as recommended by Treves.[16] When the appendix has been removed nothing remains to be done but to disinfect the whole neighborhood, insert a drain, and pack the small space with iodoform gauze. The upper half of the wound may perfectly well be tightly closed with stout sutures, which should include the whole thickness of the abdominal wall–peritonaeum as well. In some cases I believe it to be good practice to introduce a large drain by a separate opening well above and behind the iliac spine, for in some cases the region of disease may extend especially in that direction. But the question may fairly arise in any case as to whether it is wise to attempt to dissect out the appendix and remove it. If the difficulties of dissection would evidently be very great, I think it is better to open the abscess if there is one, cleanse the cavity, and, leaving the appendix *in situ*, pack and drain the wound. The packing I have usually removed on the third day and replaced it with less, and the cavity has rapidly granulated. If, at the time of operation, one introduces sutures throughout the whole length of the wound, leaving the central and lower ones loose, these can subsequently, after one or two dressings, be tied, and the wound thus rapidly narrowed. Over the whole wound, of course, a complete dressing is applied, and good bandaging is better than any binder, to prevent the possibility of extrusion of gut by either vomiting or intestinal distension. None of my patients have developed a hernia at the site of the operation. I have kept them all in bed for four weeks or more.

---

16. Sir Frederick Treves (1853–1923), a surgeon of the London Hospital. He described the "bloodless fold of Treves" connecting the appendix and the ileum. He is also famous for the successful drainage of an appendiceal abscess on King Edward VII in 1902.

None have had any recurrence of inflammatory action of any kind.

A few more words, Mr. President, and I have finished. Are there any contra-indications to this operation in a clear case of appendicitis? I think there are. Very great abdominal distension, which might in a given case probably be relieved by a few hours' treatment, would lead me to delay the operation, for expulsion of intestine is a very serious obstacle to the proper completion of the operation without risk. Unusual obesity I should regard as a good reason for a more expectant method of treatment. But the most important contra-indication of all is the absence of any one of the necessary safeguards and aids, such as the best assistance, the best light, and the best appliance for performing a perfectly aseptic operation.

Cholecysto-Intestinal Anastomosis Without Suture

and

Arterial Resection with End-to-End Suture

JOHN BENJAMIN MURPHY, M.D. (1857–1916)

Toward the end of the nineteenth century a few surgeons recognized that the ability to operate without incurring septic complications presented almost unlimited opportunities to extend the scope of surgery. J. B. Murphy of Chicago was such a man. The best known of his many surgical contributions—the Murphy button—is described in the first of the following selections. This small device revolutionized surgery of the gastrointestinal tract by proving that it was feasible to join portions of the intestine and that it was within the scope of any competent surgeon to do so. Once this was recognized, Murphy's device gradually fell into disuse, and suture techniques were substituted.

Murphy was also interested in surgery of the blood vessels, and the second selection, a case report, is the description of the first successful suture of the divided ends of a major artery in a human subject. Unfortunately, the concept of working with open blood vessels was too daring to be widely accepted in Murphy's day. Reconstructive vascular surgery did not come into full flower for another half century.

John Benjamin Murphy was born in Appleton, Wisconsin, on December 21, 1857. Both his parents were immigrants from Ireland. Murphy worked his way through Rush Medical College, graduated in 1879, and then went on to interne at Cook County Hospital in Chicago. He practiced for a while in Chicago and then went to Vienna, at that

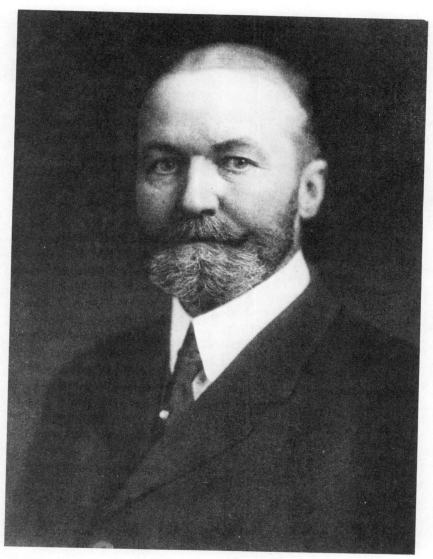

Figure 48. John Benjamin Murphy (1857–1916). (Courtesy National Library of Medicine.)

time the world's leading medical center, where he completed his train-
ing. Murphy returned to Chicago and embarked on his distinguished
surgical career.

J. B. Murphy was one of America's most dynamic surgeons, a tire-
less researcher and teacher. Although his primary interest was always
centered on the abdominal cavity, he also made significant contribu-
tions to thoracic, vascular, and bone surgery. His famed Murphy
Clinics, first relatively informal surgical teaching sessions, later be-
came highly formal. They continue today as the popular Surgical
Clinics of North America. *Murphy died on August 11, 1916, while va-*
cationing on Mackinac Island, Michigan.

The first of the following selections appeared in much longer form
in the Medical Record *(42:665) in 1892. The second was abstracted*
from the same journal (51:73, 1897).

Cholecysto-Intestinal Anastomosis Without Suture

Intestinal surgery occupies a very advanced place in the category
of great surgical questions of the present day. Medical literature teems
with reports of successful cases operated on, and not a few of the disas-
ters are also placed on record. All over the world investigators are
trying to solve the many perplexing problems that accident and disease
of the gastro-intestinal tract present to them for consideration. That
this subject has had such exhaustive consideration during the last
decade, and that it is still a theme for spirited controversy and discussion, carries with it the implication that many vital points are yet un-
settled and need further investigation, experimental and clinical. The
results of experiments on lower animals have been conducive to great
improvement, both in principle and technique of treatment of intestinal lesions in the human subject. Fair results are obtained in the treatment of bullet wounds of the intestines at present. At least an effort is
made by the surgeon to repair the injury.

The question above all others on which the profession is divided
is, "What are the best means and methods of producing agglutination
of surfaces and preventing subsequent contraction at the point of adhesion?" If means can be devised—1, to hold the surfaces in contact; 2,
while in contact, to produce a speedy and permanent adhesion of the
surfaces; 3, to keep an opening sufficiently large for the free passage of
intestinal contents; 4, to produce, as a result, a cicatrix that will not
contract to any great extent, and by the contraction produce complete
or partial obstruction—we will have overcome the great barriers that
still remain between us and ideal success in intestinal surgery.

The marvellous ingenuity displayed in plans devised for intestinal approximation and anastomosis is worthy of the greatest success, and that success would have been realized were it not that some of the following complications occurred: "The suture was imperfectly applied; the bowel sloughed through at line of suture; the induced invagination increased after the operation until complete obstruction was produced; openings in the bone-plates[1] and disks were not in apposition; the ends of the bone-plates caused pressure, atrophy, and perforation; the catgut sutures were too rapidly absorbed; lastly, and with appalling frequency, prolonged operation produced fatal shock," and many other well-known obstacles, not necessary to mention here, intervened.

To overcome these obstacles and thus lessen the risk to the life of the patient, I have devised a mechanical means to dispense with the need of sutures, the necessity of invagination, the possibility of non-apposition, the sloughing through of disks, the digestion of the catgut, the almost insurmountable difficulties of technique of operation, the prolonged and fatal exposure of the abdominal contents and the protracted anaesthesia. How much I have accomplished by my labor I desire you to be the judges, after I have demonstrated to you the results of my experiments, and performed for you a gastro-enterostomy and an end-to-end approximation of intestine by means of the device I here present to you, to be known as the Anastomosis Button.

The buttons are made in three sizes. A button consists of two small circular bowls; size No. 2 measures as follows: Diameter, 23 mm; depth, 8 mm. There is "sweated" into a circular opening, 12 mm. in diameter, at the bottom of one bowl, a cylinder 15 mm in length, with female screw thread on its entire inner surface. The cylinder extends perpendicularly from bottom of bowl. There is an opening in the male bowl in which is "sweated" a similar and smaller cylinder of a size to easily slip into the female cylinder. There are two brass springs sol-

---

1. Bone plates were used by Nicholas Senn (1844–1908), the professor of surgery at Rush Medical College in Chicago. Senn was a Swiss-born and American-trained surgeon and pathologist. He received his degree in medicine from the Chicago Medical College in 1868. Senn was a prolific writer and an ingenious experimenter: his books on *Surgical Bacteriology, Intestinal Surgery,* and *Experimental Surgery* (all published in 1889) were among the first on these subjects.

Senn used decalcified plates, or disks, of bone fashioned with a central hole. These were inserted, one in each end of a divided length of bowel, and then sutured so as to oppose each other. The bowel healed and the plates were either digested or passed. Senn's bone plates were the forerunners of Murphy's button, but in practice they were more cumbersome and far less dependable than Murphy's device.

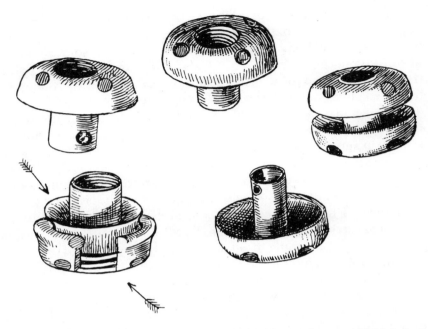

Figure 49. The Murphy button. This is the illustration used in Murphy's original paper.

dered on either side of the inner surface of the lower end of the male cylinder, which extend almost to the top, where small points of them protrude through openings in the cylinder; these points are designed to catch the screw-thread, when the male cylinder is pressed into the female cylinder, and thus hold the bowls together at any point desired. To separate them again they are simply unscrewed. A small brass ring, with a thin though not cutting edge, to which is attached a wire spring, is placed in the male bowl and retained in position, projecting one-eighth of an inch above the edge of the bowl. This is held up by the wire spring, and is there for the purpose of keeping up continuous pressure until the entire tissue between the edges of the bowls is cut off. This spring attachment is absolutely necessary only when the stomach is operated on. There are four openings, 5 mm. in diameter, in the side of each bowl, for the purpose of drainage. By this, it will be seen, we have two hemispherical bodies held together by invaginating cylinders. These hemispheres of the button are inserted in slits or ends of the viscera to be operated on. A running thread is placed around the slit in the viscus, so that when it is tied it will draw the cut edges within the clasp of the bowl. A similar running thread is applied to the slit in the viscus into which the other half of the button is inserted, and the bowls are then pressed together. The pressure atrophy at the edge of the bowl is produced by the brass ring supported by the wire spring. The opening left after the button has liberated itself is the size of the button.

This differs from all other previous devices in the following particulars or combinations thereof: 1, It retains its position automatically; 2, it is entirely independent of sutures; 3, it produces a pressure atrophy and adhesion of surfaces at the line of atrophy; 4, it insures a perfect apposition of surfaces without the danger of displacement; 5, it is applicable to the lateral as well as to the end-to-end approximation; 6, it produces a linear cicatrix and thus insures a minimum of contraction; and 7, in the extreme simplicity of its technique, which makes it a specially safe instrument in the hands of the everyday practitioner as well as the more dexterous specialist. We will now consider its application.

While reading of the great difficulties experienced by the operators mentioned in performing this operation, I realized that the profession was sorely in need of some more simple and perfect means for the approximation of the gall-bladder and the intestine; and after trying several devices, I succeeded in producing and perfecting this anastomosis button, which I think fulfils all of the indications. The button is inserted in the following manner:

An incision is made from the edge of the rib, two inches to the right of, and parallel to, the median line, extending downward three inches. The gall-bladder is drawn into the wound, also the duodenum. The duodenum is cleared of its contents by gentle pressure with finger. My short intestinal compression forceps are placed upon the duodenum to prevent the escape of gas and fluids after the incision is made. A needle with fifteen inches of silk thread is inserted in the duodenum, directly opposite its mesentery and at a point near the head of the pancreas. A stitch is taken through the entire wall of bowel, one-third the length of the incision to be made. The needle is again inserted one-third the length of the incision from its outlet, in a line with the first, and brought out again, embracing the same amount of tissue as the first. A loop three inches long is held here, and the needle is inserted in a similar manner, making two stitches, parallel to the first, in the reverse direction, and one-eighth of an inch from it, coming out at a point near the original insertion of the needle. This forms a running thread, which, when tightened, draws the incised edge of the bowel within the cup of the button. In the gall-bladder a similar running thread is inserted. An incision is now made in the intestine, two-thirds the length of the diameter of the button used. The button is slipped in, the running string tied, and the button held with the forceps. The contents of the gall-

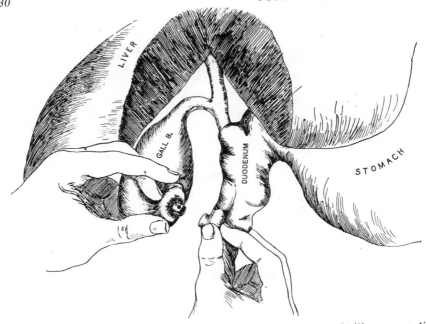

Figure 50. The Murphy button used in the treatment of biliary tract disease. An illustration from Murphy's original paper. (Courtesy National Library of Medicine.)

bladder are withdrawn with an aspirator. An incision is then made in the gall-bladder the same length, and between rows of sutures, the button is inserted in a similar manner, and the running string tied. The serous surfaces to be approximated are scraped with the edge of a scalpel. The forceps are removed and the button is held between the fingers and pressed together. A sufficient degree of pressure must be used to bring the serous surfaces of the gall-bladder and intestine firmly in contact and compress the tissues. The elastic pressure of the spring cup of the button produces a pressure atrophy of the tissue embraced within the cup, and leaves an opening as large as the button, the button dropping into the bowel and being passed through the intestines.

It takes about as long to describe the operation as to perform it. The time occupied with the first lady on whom I operated was eleven minutes, from the entering of the peritoneal cavity until the closing of the same.

REPORT OF CASES

Case I

A.Q ————, aged thirty-five, female; admitted to the medical department of Cook County Hospital, May 27, 1892. Transferred to the surgical division of the hospital, June 10, 1892, and came under my care. Gave the following history: During the last fifteen years has had stomach troubles; pain and tenderness in the epigastrium; the attack would last from two to four days, was almost always accompanied by vomiting, never by jaundice. Had pain in back since childbirth; suffered from chronic constipation. One of these attacks was accompanied by jaundice for the first time, December 14, 1891. At that time had constant and intense pain for twelve hours, and an aching pain and tenderness in the epigastrium for two months following it. Jaundice cleared in about two months. During the past few months the attack of stomach trouble would last from twelve to twenty-four hours. In February the present attack began, accompanied by jaundice and severe pruritus, which has been constant from that time up to date. These symptoms increased in severity up to the time she was admitted into the hospital. While in the medical department her jaundice was constant; her mental condition became very much impaired and her emaciation rapidly increased. *Condition when Admitted to the Surgical Department.*—The patient intensely jaundiced; very much emaciated; has a point of tenderness in the right hypochondriac region just below the margin of the rib; no tumor to be felt. The urine contains a large quantity of bile, no albumin. The patient suffers from considerable mental derangement, very slight elevation of temperature.

June 11th.—I decided to perform cholecysto-enterostomy by means of my anastomosis button, which I had used for the first time on a dog six days previous. An incision three inches long was made, three inches to the right of the median line, extending directly downward. The gall-bladder was found distended, non-adherent, and contained a large number of small calculi. Duodenum and gall-bladder were both drawn into the wound; an incision was made in the duodenum and half of the button inserted. A running thread was put in the gall-bladder, an incision made, and the other half of the button inserted. The gall stones were not removed. There was considerable escape of gall, as gall-bladder was not aspirated before putting in the button. The button was then pressed together without any difficulty, and the mass dropped into the abdominal cavity. Time from the opening of the peritoneum until the closing of same, eleven minutes. After the operation the patient showed no unpleasant symptoms; temperature at no time exceeded 100° F., and in fourteen days from the operation she was allowed to walk about the ward. The jaundice rapidly disappeared, and three weeks after the operation there was no trace of bile in the urine. The patient was of a very hysterical temperament after her mental condition improved; she noticed that she was an object for observation and became so erratic that we could not control her at the hospital and were compelled to discharge her five weeks after the operation. Up to that time she states that "she has not passed the button." She was apparently well in every particular.

October 28th.—Patient was examined by Dr. H. R. Wittwer.[2] He found the jaundice had not returned; there was no bile in the urine, and the patient was in excellent health. He could not ascertain whether she had passed the button or not.

Case II

Mrs. B ———, aged thirty-eight, widow, has three children. Parents are still alive, aged seventy-six and seventy-four respectively. Brothers and sisters well; no history of any hereditary disease.

Dr. Hoelscher[3] saw the patient for the first time October 7, 1892, and found her as follows: "Healthy, well nourished appearance; pain of sudden onset in the epigastric region, and from this point it gradually extended over the whole abdomen. She had vomited the contents of the stomach and some bile on two occasions after the seizure with pain. Bowels were constipated and had been in this condition two or three days before the seizure. Vesical tenesmus and diminished quantity of urine. Gave no history of any previous pain, gastric disturbance, jaundice, or colics."

On examination found a tumor in right hypochondriac region, extending downward into the iliac region and terminating in a rounded smooth end; could be distinctly felt in lumbar region, was moveable and tender on pressure; there appeared to be a deep fissure between the tumor and the liver, no fluctuation apparent, bowel or colon not overlying the tumor. The diagnosis could not be determined, but it was presumed to be some lesion of the kidney, so it was decided to make an exploratory laparotomy.

October 19th.—I made an incision three inches long, from the edge of the tenth rib directly downward toward the border of the ilium. The tumor was exposed and found to be a very much enlarged gallbladder with large calculi within. The viscus was very oedematous, red, and thickened. It was decided to make a cholecysto-enterostomy with my anastomosis button. The gall-bladder was aspirated, and the running thread inserted. The running thread was then inserted into the

---

2. Herman R. Wittwer (?–1895) graduated from Rush Medical College in 1888. He was Murphy's assistant and then apparently went into private practice in 1893. I have been unable to identify him further.

3. Julius H. Hoelscher (1864–1926). M.D., Northwestern University Medical School (Chicago Medical College), 1885; prominent internist in Chicago.

duodenum and the intestine incised and the male half of the button inserted, the female half was then inserted in the gall-bladder through a slit made between the running thread, and the button closed. The gall-bladder measured at least 1 ctm. in thickness and was very oedematous. There was no difficulty in inserting the button. The gall-stones were allowed to remain, as I do not consider it necessary to remove them unless they are larger than the button. They will pass out after the button escapes.

October 20th.—Temperature, 101° F.; pulse, 96. Vomited considerably during the night and complained of headache, which seemed to be effects of the anaesthetic. There was no pain nor abdominal tenderness.

October 21st.—At 5 P.M. yesterday the vomiting ceased, and the patient is feeling very well this morning.

October 27th.—The patient has had no unpleasant symptoms since October 20th. This morning in the stool were found two large gall-stones. The larger one weighed 117 grains (7.8 gm.); its longest diameter 1 inch, its shortest ⅞ inch. The second stone 102 grains (6.8 gm.); its longest diameter ⅞ inch, its shortest ¾ inch. It will be noticed that the shortest diameter of the larger stone measures exactly the same as the diameter of button used. The patient is feeling very well and is sitting up in bed. Complete primary union. Button passed eighteen days after operation.

Case III

Cholecysto-enterostomy with Button No. 1.—This case was referred to me by Dr. J. H. Hoelscher, who gave me the following history: Mrs. Z. ———, aged thirty-six, married, six children. Enjoyed perfect health until twenty-two years of age; at that time, three months after childbirth, had an attack, of short duration, of severe epigastric pain and vomiting. It was not accompanied or followed by jaundice. Ever since that attack she has had digestive disturbances, as distress following certain kinds of food, eructations of gas, constipation, loss of appetite. Four years ago she had a similar attack of pain in the epigastrium, accompanied by vomiting. From that time on the pain returned every five or six weeks, up to five months ago, when she noticed a constant aching pain and tenderness in the right hypochondriac region, that persisted until the present time. The pain and soreness were very much increased after working in a stooping posture. She has suffered much from general debility, and complains of slight and frequent chills. Throughout the entire progress of her disease jaundice was never present. The urine was tested several times for her with negative results. She does not give a distinct history of having had "hepatic colic."

About three months ago she found small particles, the size of mustard-seeds, in the faeces, which someone told her were gall-stones. There is no positive evidence that she ever passed a gall-stone. Physical examination revealed a heart and lungs normal; liver not increased in size. Manipulation reveals a pear-shaped, hard tumor in the region of the gall-bladder, measuring about three inches in length, and two in width. It moves synchronously with the diaphragm in respiration. On pressure considerable pain is produced, and a slight crackling sensation is felt by the fingers.

It can be separated from the kidney, and can be moved considerably from side to side. The diagnosis of gall-stone was made by Dr. Hoelscher, and the case was referred to me for operation.

Operation, November 23, 1892, assisted by Drs. Hoelscher and Lee,[4] in the presence of Dr. Nicholas Senn, who expressed a desire to see my method used, Dr. Dunn,[5] of Minneapolis, and Dr. Mayo,[6] of Rochester, Minn. The incision was made the same as in Case II; contracted gall-bladder packed full of gall-stones slipped into the wound.

A little difficulty was experienced in drawing the duodenum forward, as some old adhesions existed. The running threads were inserted in gall-bladder and duodenum; male half of button placed in duodenum, and held by assistant. An incision was made in the gall-bladder, which was found so full of gall-stones that half of the button could not be inserted without removing some of them. A dozen were quickly picked out with the dissecting forceps. About twice as many were allowed to remain. The female half of the button was inserted in the gall-bladder and the running thread tied. Button pressed together. Toilet of field of operation was made with dry sponge and the viscera dropped back into abdomen. Deep and superficial layer of sutures in abdominal wall. Time for entire operation, twenty-one minutes. The time for inserting the button was not taken. Patient rallied rapidly from

---

4. Edward W. Lee (1841–1907), M.D., University of Dublin, 1862; came to Chicago in 1864 and specialized in surgery. Murphy was greatly influenced by Dr. Lee, who was an attending surgeon at Cook County Hospital. Lee subsequently chose Murphy to be his assistant for several years. Lee was also one of the first surgeons in Chicago to operate for appendicitis and for gallbladder disease.

5. James Henry Dunn (1853–1904), M.D., University of New York, 1853–1904), M.D., University of New York, 1878; a surgeon and urologist of Minneapolis. Subsequently he became a professor and head of the department of surgery at the University of Minnesota.

6. "Dr. Mayo" was, of course, either William (1861–1939) or Charles (1865–1939) of the famed Mayo Clinic.

the anaesthetic. Pulse after operation, 70. Temperature, normal. Neither nausea nor vomiting.

November 25th.—Pulse, 78. Temperature, 100.5° F. Patient complains of slight pain at seat of operation. No tympanites nor abdominal tenderness.

November 28th.—Patient expresses herself as feeling very well. At no time since the operation has patient's temperature exceeded 100.5° F. She is allowed to take a quantity of liquid nourishment, but not sufficient to satisfy the appetite. I consider her now out of danger. The ease and rapidity with which this operation was performed satisfied those who witnessed it, as well as myself, that the operation of cholecysto-enterostomy by this means is relieved of many of its dangers and all of its difficulties.

Arterial Resection with End-to-End Suture

H. V ———, Italian, peddler, aged twenty-nine. He was shot at eleven o'clock September 19th, and was brought to the hospital two hours later.

Clinical history: The patient was shot twice, one bullet passing into the abdominal wall just above the great curvature of the stomach without penetrating the abdomen; the other entered Scarpa's triangle below Poupart's ligament. There was no bruit at this point or increased pulsation noticed at the time the patient was admitted to the hospital. I saw the patient first October 4th; examination revealed a loud bruit; it could be heard with the ear placed six inches from the thigh. There was no tumor and but slight increase in pulsation. The pulsation in the popliteal, dorsalis pedis, and posterior tibial arteries was scarcely perceptible. I examined the case again on October 6th and demonstrated it to a class of students. A thrill could be felt and a bruit could be heard. The latter was the loudest to which I had ever listened. The pulsation though very feeble could now be felt in the dorsalis pedis, but not in the posterior tibial.

Diagnosis: Penetrating wound of the common femoral artery about one and one-half inches below Poupart's ligament. It was decided to cut down and expose the artery, and if a penetrating wound of more than one-half the circumference was found to make a resection and unite end-to-end.

Operation, October 7, 1896. An incision five inches long was made from Poupart's ligament along the course of the femoral artery. The artery was readily exposed about one inch below Poupart's ligament; it

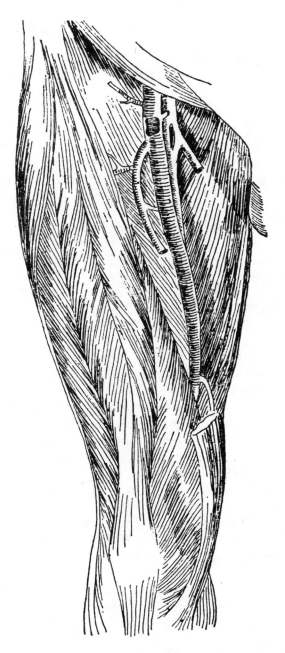

Figure 51. Arterial injury before repair. Murphy's illustration to show the site of the bullet wound before the repair was carried out. (Courtesy National Library of Medicine.)

was separated from its sheath and a provisional ligature thrown around it but not tied. A careful dissection was then made down along the wall of the vessel to the pulsating clot. The artery was exposed one inch below that point and a ligature thrown around it but not tied; a careful dissection was made upward to the point of the clot. The artery was then closed above and below with gentle compression clamps and was elevated, at which time there was profuse hemorrhage from an opening in the vein. A cavity, about the size of a filbert, was found posterior to the artery communicating with its calibre, the aneurismal pocket. A small aneurismal sac about the same size was found on the anterior surface of the artery over the point of perforation. The hemorrhage from the vein was very profuse and was controlled by digital compression. It was found that one-eighth of an inch of the arterial wall on the outer side of the opening remained, and on the inner side of the perforation only a band of one-sixteenth of an inch of the adventitia was intact. The bullet had passed through the centre of the artery, carried away all its wall except the strands described above, and passed downward and backward, making a large hole in the vein in its posterior and external side just above the junction of the vena profunda. Great difficulty was experienced in controlling the hemorrhage from the vein. After dissecting the vein above and below the point of laceration and placing a temporary ligature on the vena profunda, the hemorrhage was controlled so that the vein could be sutured. At the point of suture the vein was greatly diminished in size, but when the clamps were removed it dilated about one-third the normal diameter, or one-third the diameter of the vein above and below. There was no bleeding from the vein when the clamps were removed. Our attention was then turned to the artery. Two inches of it had been exposed and freed from all surroundings. The opening in the artery was three-eighths of an inch in length; one-half inch was resected and the proximal end was invaginated into the distal for one-third of an inch with four double-needled threads which penetrated all the walls of the artery. The adventitia was peeled off the invaginated portion for a distance of one-third inch; a row of sutures was placed around the edge of the overlapping sistal end, the sutures penetrating only the media of the proximal portion; the adventitia was then drawn over the line of union and sutured. The clamps were removed. Not a drop of blood escaped at the line of suture. Pulsation was immediately restored in the artery below the line of approximation, and it could be felt feebly in the posterior tibial and dorsalis pedis. The sheath and connective tissue around the artery were then approximated at the position of suture with catgut, so as to sup-

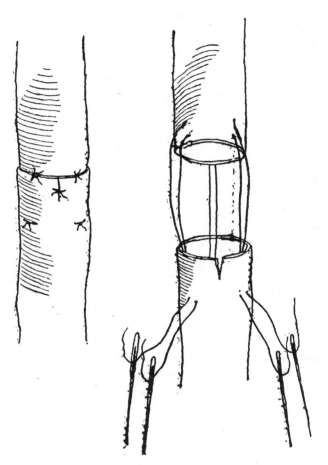

Figure 52. Murphy's method of arterial repair. This method of blood vessel anastomosis consisted of invaginating one end into the other. It has since been supplanted, of course, by direct end-to-end suture as described by Alexis Carrel (1873–1944) in 1902. (Courtesy National Library of Medicine.)

port the wall of the artery. The whole cavity was washed out with a five-per-cent solution of carbolic acid and the edges of the wound were accurately approximated with silkworm-gut sutures. No drainage.

The time for the operation was approximately two and one-half hours, most of that time being consumed in suturing the vein. The artery was easily secured and sutured, and the hemorrhage from it readily controlled. The patient was placed in bed, with the leg elevated and wrapped in cotton.

A pulsation could be felt in the dorsalis pedis on October 11th, four days after the operation. There were no oedema of the leg and no pain. The circulation was good continuously from the time of operation. The wound suppurated; drainage was inserted, but at no time did the patient's temperature exceed 100.8° F. December 8, 1896, the circulation is perfect, the wound has healed with the exception of a small superficial ulcer, one-third of an inch in diameter. The patient has not had an unpleasant symptom since the operation. January 4th, patient is walking about the ward of the hospital, has no oedema and no disturbance of the circulation.[1]

---

1. I am unable to locate any case of successful repair of a divided artery in a human that antedates this one of Murphy's. C. C. Guthrie, a pioneer in experimental vascular surgery, reviewed the history of blood vessel repair up to 1912. He mentioned Murphy's work in this field without assigning priority, and quotes Dörfler as stating that only nine successful repairs had been carried out in man as of 1900. (C. C. Guthrie, *Blood Vessel Surgery,* 1912, reprinted in 1959 by the University of Pittsburgh Press.)

The Surgical Operations on President Cleveland in 1893

WILLIAM WILLIAMS KEEN, M.D. (1837–1932)

Stephen Grover Cleveland (1837–1908), the only president to serve two nonconsecutive terms, was elected for the second time in 1892. The United States was then on the brink of one of the cyclic depressions that have occurred throughout its history, which led the following year to the panic of 1893. A brief historical note is indicated at this point, because the nation's problems directly influenced the way in which President Cleveland's operations were performed.

The panic of 1893 was precipitated partly by trade imbalances that required the exportation of great sums of gold to pay overseas debts and partly by the Sherman Silver Act, which committed the government to heavy purchases of silver. An alarming decline of treasury gold reserves resulted from these expenditures. The possibility that the nation would be forced to abandon the gold standard was discussed sensationally in the press and led to great popular concern and unrest. Bank runs and bank failures were common. The immediate repeal of the Sherman Act appeared to be the one means by which financial stability might be restored, but this was a step that Western silver interests strongly opposed.

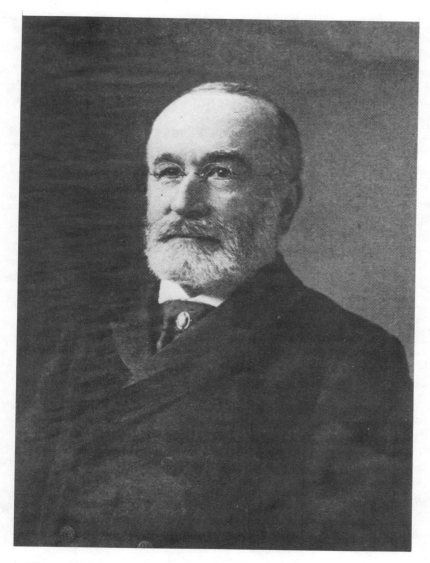

Figure 53. William Williams Keen (1837–1932).

A strong leader was needed to force repeal of the Sherman Act through Congress. Cleveland had the strength and the support that was necessary; but, in the meantime, his visible presence was required to prevent a complete financial collapse. At this point, early in June of 1893, the president was found to have a malignant intraoral tumor. The cancer needed to be treated, but both Cleveland and his advisers felt that this had to be done secretly in order not to precipitate further panic.

Miraculously, the events surrounding the president's operation were kept secret until they were reported 24 years later by Dr. William Keen, one of the attending surgeons, in an account published first in the Saturday Evening Post *(September 22, 1917) and then in a small volume entitled* The Surgical Operations on President Cleveland in 1893 *(Philadelphia: J. B. Lippincott, 1917, republished 1928).*

William Williams Keen was one of this country's most illustrious surgeons. His medical career began with his enrollment in Jefferson Medical College in 1861. He then volunteered, while still a medical student, to act as an assistant surgeon in the Union Army during the difficult early days of the war, and he served during the disastrous first Battle of Bull Run. He returned to Jefferson and graduated in 1862. Keen served in the army during the remainder of the war; at the second Bull Run, at Antietam, and then in various hospitals. He had the good fortune to be assigned in 1863 to work in Philadelphia with neurologist Silas Weir Mitchell (1829–1914) on wards set aside for the treatment of patients with peripheral nerve injuries.

In 1864, Gunshot Wounds and Other Injuries of Nerves *by S. Weir Mitchell, M.D., George R. Morehouse, M.D., and William W. Keen, M.D. (Philadelphia: J. B. Lippincott) was published. Keen, a coauthor, was only 27 when this monograph, a medical classic, appeared. He went abroad for two years (obligatory in those days for anyone with an academic interest) when his wartime service was completed, and then returned to Philadelphia to practice and to teach anatomy and surgical pathology. He retained an interest in surgery of the nervous system and apparently was first in the United States to operate successfully for intracranial tumor. Keen was professor of surgery at Jefferson when he was summoned to assist with President Cleveland's surgery. His prestige was such, both in this country and abroad, that he could have weathered the storm if the president had not survived his surgery. Fortunately, all went well. The following selection has been edited from Keen's account of these historic operations.*

The Surgical Operations on President Cleveland in 1893

THE HISTORY PRECEDING THE FIRST OPERATION

On Sunday, June eighteenth, 1893, Dr. R. M. O'Reilly[1]—later Surgeon-General of the United States Army—the official medical attendant on officers of the Government in Washington, examined a rough place of the roof of Mr. Cleveland's mouth. He found an ulcer as large as a quarter of a dollar, extending from the bicuspid teeth to within one-third of an inch of the soft palate, and some diseased bone. The pathologist at the Army Medical Museum—who was kept in ignorance, of course, of the name of the patient—after examining the small fragment which Doctor O'Reilly had removed, reported that it was strongly indicative of malignancy.

Doctor O'Reilly, foreseeing the need for an operation, advised Mr. Cleveland to consult Dr. Joseph D. Bryant,[2] long his medical attendant and intimate friend. Doctor Bryant quickly went to Washington and confirmed the diagnosis. The President, after the examination, with no apparent concern, inquired: "What do you think it is, doctor?"

To which Doctor Bryant replied: "Were it in my mouth I would have it removed at once." This answer settled the matter.

During the discussion as to what arrangements could be made, the President would not under any circumstances consent to a time and place that would not give the best opportunity of avoiding disclosure, and even a suspicion that anything of significance had happened to him. The strong desire to avoid notoriety was dwarfed by the fear he had of the effect on the public of a knowledge of his affliction, and on

---

1. Robert Maitland O'Reilly (1845–1912) served as a medical cadet in the Civil War and graduated from the University of Pennsylvania School of Medicine in 1867. He chose to remain in the army. He served on the frontier, in Washington, and at a number of other posts. He also served in Cuba during the Spanish–American War. O'Reilly was an influential and competent surgeon–general of the army from 1902 to 1909.

2. Joseph Decatur Bryant (1845–1914), M.D., Bellevue Hospital Medical College, 1866; served on the Bellevue staff for his entire professional life, was professor of surgery from 1897 until his death, and authored a two-volume text, *Operative Surgery*. Although he was close to the Cleveland family, it was not publicly known during Bryant's lifetime that he had operated on the president.

the financial questions of the time. He decided that July first was the earliest suitable date. Colonel Lamont,[3] the Secretary of War, and a close personal friend, was then informed of the facts, and it was soon arranged that to secure secrecy the operation should be done aboard Commodore Benedict's[4] yacht, the 'Oneida'.

The next question was as to how soon after the operation the President could probably safely return to Washington. August seventh was decided on.

Meantime Doctor Bryant had written me, asking for a consultation "in a very important matter." As I was about to go to New England I suggested that I should go to New York at noon and that we meet at three-fifteen on the deserted deck of the Fall River boat, which did not leave till 6 P.M. There, without any interruption, we laid all necessary plans. The living rooms on the 'Oneida' were prepared and disinfected; an operating table and all the necessary instruments, drugs, dressings, and so on, were sent on board. Arrangements were made with Dr. Ferdinand Hasbrouck,[5] a dentist accustomed to giving nitrous oxid, to assist.

My own family were kept in entire ignorance of the facts. To explain my absence I simply said that I was called to a distance for an important operation and would probably be absent for some days.

On June thirtieth I reached New York City in the evening, went

---

3. Daniel Scott Lamont (1851–1905) was active in business and politics in New York State. He went with Cleveland to the White House, where he served as a personal secretary to the president. Lamont was appointed secretary of war in 1893 and served creditably.

4. Commodore Elias Cornelius Benedict (1834–1920) was an intimate (and obviously wealthy) friend of Grover Cleveland. I have been unable to identify him further.

5. Ferdinand Hasbrouck, dentist, told the entire story of the president's operation to professional acquaintances, and then repeated it, completely and accurately, in an interview with E. J. Edwards, a New York correspondent for the Philadelphia *Press*. The story, with all details substantially correct, was published on August 29, 1893; it was denied vehemently and categorically by every official who had access to the president and by Dr. Bryant. This, plus the president's normal voice and normal appearance during the special session of Congress in July, caused other papers to brand the story a "cancer fake," and it was discounted. (For further information on this and other aspects of the Cleveland operations, see W. W. Keen's *The Surgical Operations on President Cleveland in 1893*, (1917) and C. L. Morreels, Jr., "New historical information on the Cleveland operations," *Surgery* 62:542–51, 1967. The latter citation is of special interest, as it contains previously unpublished material from W. W. Keen's scrapbook. It is also the most comprehensive article available on Cleveland's operations.)

to Pier A, and was taken over to the yacht, which was lying at anchor at a considerable distance from the Battery. Dr. E. G. Janeway,[6] of New York; Doctor O'Reilly; Dr. John F. Erdmann,[7] Doctor Bryant's assistant; and Dr. Hasbrouck had also secretly gone to the yacht. The President, Doctor Bryant and Secretary Lamont, at a later hour arrived from Washington, openly drove to Pier A, whence they were taken to the yacht.

At the time when he left Washington, on June thirtieth, Mr. Cleveland issued a call for a special session of Congress on August seventh, with the object of averting the financial danger by the repeal of the silver clause of the Sherman Act.

On arriving on the yacht the President lighted a cigar, and we sat on deck smoking and chatting until near midnight. Once he burst out with "Oh, Doctor Keen, those office-seekers! Those office-seekers! They haunt me even in my dreams!" I had never met him before; but during that hour or more of conversation I was deeply impressed by his splendid personality and his lofty patriotism. I do not believe there was a more devoted patriot living.

He passed a good night, sleeping well without any sleeping medicine. Before he dressed, Doctor Janeway made a most careful examination of his chest and found nothing wrong. There was little if any arteriosclerosis. His pulse was ninety. His kidneys were almost entirely normal. I then examined him myself. He stated that he was sure the rough place was of recent origin; that it was not there on March fourth, when he was inaugurated, but had been first observed about six or eight weeks before July first. There were no perceptibly enlarged glands. I confirmed the facts as to the ulcer and deemed the growth to be unquestionably malignant. During the morning his mouth was repeatedly cleansed and disinfected.

---

6. Edward Gamaliel Janeway (1841–1911) graduated in 1864 from New York's College of Physicians and Surgeons after serving as a medical cadet during wartime. He then joined the faculty of Bellevue, where he held chairs first in pathological anatomy and then in the principles and practice of medicine: later he became dean of the combined Bellevue–New York University School of Medicine (1898–1905). Janeway was first a pathologist and later a physician. He wrote very little but had a superb reputation as a teacher and diagnostician.

7. John Frederick Erdmann (1864–1954) graduated from Bellevue Hospital Medical College in 1887. He enjoyed a long and distinguished career as a surgeon in New York City, and held a number of academic appointments. Erdmann was professor of surgery and director at the Post–Graduate Medical School and the Hospital of Columbia University from 1908–34.

The anesthetic troubled us. Our anxiety related not so much to the operation itself as to the anesthetic and its possible dangers. These might easily arise in connection with the respiration, the heart, or the function of the kidneys, etc., dangers which are met with not infrequently as a result of administering an anesthetic, especially in a man of Mr. Cleveland's age and physical condition. The patient was 56 years of age, very corpulent, with short thick neck, just the build and age for a possible apoplexy—an incident which had actually occurred to one of my own patients. He was also worn out mentally and physically by four months of exacting labor and the officeseekers' importunities. Twenty-four years ago we had not the refined methods of diagnosis, nor had we the greatly improved methods of anesthesia which we have to-day. After canvassing the whole matter we decided to perform at least the earlier steps of the operation under nitrous oxid, and the later, if necessary under ether. Doctor Hasbrouck was of opinion that we could not keep the patient well anesthetized with nitrous oxid long enough to complete the operation satisfactorily.

Dr. Bryant and Secretary Lamont had spent the night at their homes, but returned to the yacht the next morning—July first. The yacht then proceeded up the East River at half speed while the operation was performed. So careful were we to elude observation that Doctor Bryant and all of us doctors, who might have been recognized by some of the staff of Bellevue Hospital, deserted the deck for the cabin while were steaming through the East River in sight of the Hospital at Twenty-sixth Street.

THE FIRST OPERATION

Commodore Benedict and Secretary Lamont remained on deck during the operation, which was performed in the cabin. The steward was the only other person present, to fetch and carry. I have always thought that due credit was not given to him, and to the captain and the crew, for their never betraying what had taken place. It is curious also that the alert and ubiquitous reporters seem never to have thought of interviewing the captain and crew of the 'Oneida'. The captain and crew knew Mr. Cleveland very well, for he had already traveled over fifty thousand miles on the yacht and his mere presence was no novelty. Any curiosity as to the evidently unusual occurences was apparently allayed by the statement that the President had to have two very badly ulcerated teeth removed and that fresh, pure air, and disinfected quarters and skilled doctors, all had to be provided, lest blood poisoning should set in—a very serious matter when the patient was the just-inaugurated President of the United States.

Dr. Hasbrouck first extracted the two left upper bicuspid teeth under nitrous oxid. Doctor Bryant then made the necessary incisions in the roof of the mouth, also under nitrous oxid.

At one-fourteen P.M. ether was given by Doctor O'Reilly. During the entire operation Doctor Janeway kept close watch upon the patient's pulse and general condition. Doctor Bryant performed the operation, assisted by myself and Doctor Erdmann.

The entire left upper jaw was removed from the first bicuspid tooth to just beyond the last molar, and nearly up to the middle line. The floor of the orbit—the cavity in the skull containing the eye-ball—was not removed, as it had not yet been attacked. A small portion of the soft palate was removed. This extensive operation was decided upon because we found that the antrum—the large hollow cavity in the upper jaw—was partly filled by a gelatinous mass, evidently a sarcoma. This diagnosis was later confirmed by Dr. William H. Welch,[8] of the Johns Hopkins Hospital, who had also examined the former specimens.

The entire operation was done within the mouth, without any external incision, by means of a cheek retractor, the most useful instrument I have ever seen for such an operation (Figure 54). This retractor I had brought back with me from Paris in 1866. The retention of the floor of the orbit prevented any displacement of the eyeball. This normal appearance of the eye, the normal voice, and especially

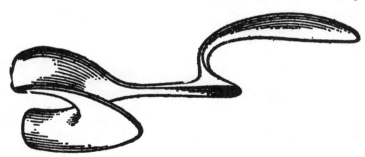

Figure 54. W. W. Keen's Luer cheek retractor, from *The Surgical Operations on President Cleveland in 1893* by W. W. Keen. (Courtesy Lippincott/Harper & Row.)

---

8. William Henry Welch (1850–1934); dean and professor of pathology at Johns Hopkins University School of Medicine. See also footnote 7, page 379.

the absence of any external scar, which was the most important evidence of all, greatly aided in keeping the operation an entire secret.

Only one blood vessel was tied. Pressure, hot water, and at one point the galvanocautery,[9] checked the bleeding. The hemorrhage was not large, probably about six ounces—say a tumblerful—in all. At the close of the operation, at one–fifty–five P.M., the pulse was only eighty. The large cavity was packed with gauze to arrest the subsequent moderate oozing of blood. At two-fifty-five P.M. a hypodermic of one-sixth of a grain of morphine was given—the only narcotic administered at any time.[10]

What a sigh of intense relief we surgeons breathed when the patient was once more safe in bed can hardly be imagined!

Mr. Cleveland's temperature after the operation was 100.8 degrees Fahrenheit, and never thereafter rose above 100 degrees. His pulse

---

9. An electric cautery introduced in 1876 by the French surgeon Claude Andre Paquelin (1836–1905). It is of interest here because of the risk of using it with ether, an explosive anesthetic.

10. Keen kept notes, as did all of those involved in the care of the president. These and other materials pertaining to the Cleveland operations were gathered into a scrapbook, which is held by the Philadelphia College of Physicians. Keen's original description (which follows) as reported in C. L. Morreels's article (see footnote 5 above), was rather more detailed than the published account:

The cheek was dissected loose the hemorrhage was arrested by hot water pressure and the ligature of one vessel. The front of the jaw was then chiseled loose from the first bicuspid to the posterior extremity of the bone. By the bone forceps the palatal process was then divided from the alveolar border to the median line. By the lion forceps, the loosened bone was removed, a few shreds of tissue being divided by the scissors. Examination of the part removed during the arrest of hemorrhage by pressure, showed that the disease had begun around the roots of the molar teeth and had extended into the antrum from its floor. The growth into the antrum was a gelatinous mass, apparently a myxosarcoma, and totally different in appearance from the typical epithelioma of the roof of the mouth. The question of removal of the entire upper jaw had been thoroughly discussed, but as the disease seems so localized partial removal had been deemed to be indicated. But on finding the invasion of the antrum it was determined to remove all the jaw except the floor of the orbit and the intermaxillary portion, which were clearly free from invasion. This was effected from within the mouth and without external incision with little hemorrhage.... All loose shreds of tissue and some small fragments of bone having been removed, the cavity was disinfected with Theirsch's solution [boric and salicylic acid in water] and packed with iodoform gauze.

was usually ninety or a little over. With the packing in the cavity his speech was labored but intelligible; without the packing it was wholly unintelligible, resembling the worst imaginable case of cleft palate. Had this not been so admirably remedied by Doctor Gibson[11] secrecy later would have been out of the question.

In turn with the others, I sat by Mr. Cleveland's bedside much of the time that evening and the next day, reading to him at times to help pass the time. Doctor Bryant's and my own full notes say nothing about any stimulant. They would have recorded the stimulant if any had been administered. My recollection, also, is clear that none was given. Our notes do not record the exact day when Mr. Cleveland was able to get out of bed, but my recollection is that it was late on July second. That he was up and about on July third is certain, for I saw in Commodore Benedict's guest register of the 'Oneida' the signatures of the President, Secretary Lamont and Doctor Bryant on July third, two days after this very serious operation.

Doctor Hasbrouck had been landed at New London on July second. I left the yacht at Sag Harbor early on July fourth and came directly home. On July fifth, in the evening, the yacht reached Gray Gables and the President walked from the launch to his residence with but little apparent effort.

THE SECOND OPERATION

During such an operation, especially in operations on bone, with the parts quickly bathed in blood after withdrawing the sponge, it is often impossible at the operation to judge accurately whether all the diseased tissue has certainly been removed. When, later, he could see clearly the condition of the parts, Doctor Bryant was not quite satisfied with the appearance at one point. At his request, Doctors Janeway, Erdmann and I (and undoubtedly Dr. O'Reilly, though neither Dr. Bryant nor my own notes record his name) again boarded the 'Oneida'. We went by train to Greenwich, Commodore Benedict's

---

11. Dr. Kasson C. Gibson was a New York prosthodontist who went to Gray Gables, the president's summer home on Cape Cod, Massachusetts, where he made a temporary prosthesis of vulcanized rubber. This enabled Cleveland to return to Washington on August 5 for the scheduled special session of Congress. His speech and appearance were apparently normal. The casts that Gibson made of the president's mouth were later donated to the New York Academy of Medicine; they are pictured in Morreels's article (see footnote 5 above).

home, and there, secure from discovery, went on board. Mr. Cleveland joined us on the yacht at Gray Gables; and on July sevententh Dr. Bryant, with our assistance, removed all the suspicious tissue and cauterized the entire surface with the galvanocautery. This operation was brief and the President recovered quickly. On July nineteenth, again the second day after the operation, the same three signatures appear in Commodore Benedict's register. This second operation has never been disclosed before.

[Grover Cleveland returned to Washington on August 5 to attend the special session of Congress that he had—rather optimistically, it would seem—called before boarding the Oneida for his surgery. A temporary prosthesis had been made at Gray Gables, the president's summer home. This served him well by supporting his cheek and permitting him to speak normally. After examining the president in Washington on September 1, Dr. Bryant noted tersely that the wound was "All healed." A new, permanent, and more comfortable prosthesis was made for him in October; by that time the president had apparently completely recovered from his ordeal. The nation was also, slowly, recovering from financial depression; the Sherman Silver Act, responsible in part for the financial panic of 1893, was repealed that autumn. Keen continued to follow the president's condition. He wrote; "I went to Washington at intervals several times afterward to examine Mr. Cleveland's mouth and never found anything wrong.... Mr. Cleveland died June 24, 1908, fifteen years after our operations. That he should have survived after the removal of a sarcoma[12] of the jaw without local recurrence for so unusually long a period was a great satisfaction to Doctor Bryant and his colleagues."]

---

12. The pathologic specimen that was removed is in the Mutter Museum of the College of Physicians of Philadelphia. The college has refused to permit microscopic examination of the specimen on the grounds that this "will contribute nothing pathologically or historically." I do not agree and feel that it would be of great interest to know the cell type. It is likely that it was a low-grade sarcoma, as Welch and the other pathologists believed. This diagnosis would be consistent with the president's subsequent course.

The Results of Operations for the Cure of Cancer of the Breast

and

The Training of the Surgeon

WILLIAM STEWART HALSTED, M.D. (1852–1922)

William Stewart Halsted was born in New York City on September 23, 1852. He graduated from Yale College in 1874 and then entered the College of Physicians and Surgeons of New York, choosing as his preceptor Henry B. Sands (1830–1888), a prominent surgeon of that city (see footnote 1, page 300). After his graduation in 1877. Halsted traveled and studied in Europe for three years. He then returned to New York where he soon became known as a promising surgeon and popular teacher. His early career in New York then came to an abrupt end; he was almost hopelessly addicted to cocaine (cf pp. 292–93).

Halsted was hospitalized in 1886 for the treatment of his addiction. He went to Baltimore later that year at the suggestion of his friend William Welch, the professor of pathology at Johns Hopkins University Medical School (Welch's was a premature appointment, for the hospital and medical school were yet to be built). Halsted worked in Welch's laboratory for some months, but then, still troubled by his addiction, was again hospitalized in 1887. He returned to Baltimore the following year, now well enough to accept an appointment as acting surgeon in the newly completed Johns Hopkins Hospital. Finally, on the basis of demonstrated ability, Halsted was named professor of surgery at Johns Hopkins in 1892.

William Stewart Halsted made many significant contributions to his specialty, particuliarly to surgery for hernia, and breast cancer and

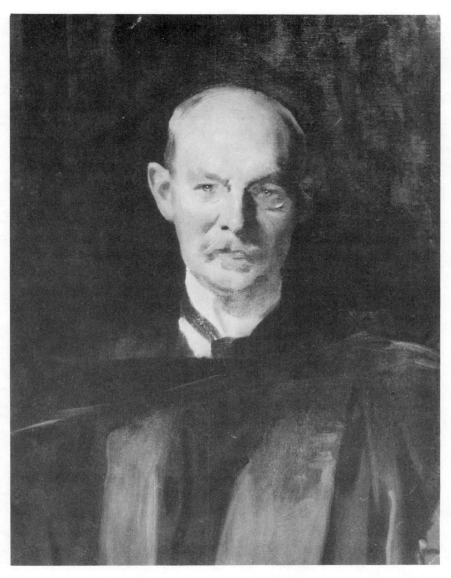

Figure 55. William Stewart Halsted (1852–1922). Detail from John Singer Sargent's famous portrait of the four professors of Johns Hopkins Medical School. (Courtesy National Library of Medicine.)

to surgery of the thyroid and of the blood vessels. He developed the meticulous surgical technique that was a hallmark of his school and his pupils. He also introduced a surgical residency program with gradually increasing responsibility for the surgeons-in-training. In time, Halsted's residents, many of whom became professors and heads of departments, spread throughout the United States to lay the foundations of the surgery that we practice today. Halsted did more than any other American surgeon to advance his specialty. He died in the Johns Hopkins Hospital on September 7, 1922.

*Halsted's collected writings fill two volumes (*Surgical Papers of William Stewart Halsted, *edited by William C. Burket [Baltimore: The Johns Hopkins Press, 1924]), and there is much in them that is worthy of inclusion in an anthology of American surgery. I have elected to include the two papers that I feel are most important. The first, "The Results of Operations for the Cure of Cancer of the Breast," has influenced the practice of surgery for almost a century. The second, "The Training of the Surgeon," takes us into the twentieth century; here is Halsted's entire philosophy of surgical teaching.*

The first selection, on cancer of the breast, is for many reasons one of the most important articles ever written by an American surgeon. First, it presents a rationale for the surgical treatment of cancer of the breast, carefully thought out and logically based on all the evidence then available. It has taken almost a century for surgeons to realize that Halsted's premises were not entirely correct. His "cures" were not cures; he did not alter the life expectancy at all for those women that he was operating on with far-advanced disease. Nevertheless, his operation was of great importance; for the first time the most distressing symptom of breast cancer, the local disease, was effectively controlled.

Second, this paper spelled out in careful detail the method of performing an operation of considerable magnitude and complexity, particularly for the era in which it was introduced. Halsted's operation, modified only by the retention of the pectoral muscles, continues today to be the cornerstone of surgical treatment of carcinoma of the breast.

Third, Halsted's article, and those that followed, did much to sanctify the concept of radical en bloc resection for the treatment of all localized cancer. Halsted was sure (on the basis of inadequate follow-up) that his operation cured cancer of the breast. His enthusiasm was communicated to the entire surgical world; it seemed possible that all cancer could be cured by similiar operations. With improvement in surgical care, increasingly radical and superradical procedures could be carried out—on the head and neck, in the chest, and in the abdomen and pelvis. Gradually, however, in recent years, it has become apparent that the limits of surgical efficacy have been reached.

Fourth, in this paper Halsted explained his surgical techniques ("if no blood is lost, there is no perceptible shock . . . "). This large, carefully documented series of major operations associated with minimal morbidity and no mortality was most impressive. Halsted had no antibiotics, no anesthesia machines, no monitors, and no intravenous or intensive-care therapy. Surgical masks had not yet been thought of. Rubber gloves were first introduced and were just starting to be used by Halsted's team at Hopkins in 1894, the year this paper appeared (close inspection of Figure 58 shows the operator, possibly Halsted, wearing a rubber finger cot, but only over the right index and middle fingers). Meticulous tissue-sparing surgical technique was responsible for Halsted's results. There was then—and there still is—a lesson here for surgeons.

Fifth, Halsted presented his own statistical results as well as those from a number of European centers. This was in marked contrast to the anecdotal presentations that Americans surgeons contributed to their journals and at their meetings. Halsted had studied in Vienna. He traveled abroad almost yearly. He knew and visited many of the surgeons whose work he cited in this article. He recognized the superiority of European surgery, and—most importantly—he saw the need to introduce it to America.

Halsted's original paper on the treatment of carcinoma of the breast has been shortened. I have omitted a few long paragraphs of text and a number of lengthy tables that gave the results, patient by patient, of the European surgeons whom he cited. I have also left out the 50 individual case reports of his own patients. With these exceptions, however, this paper is as it appeared in the Annals of Surgery (20:497–555, 1894).

Halsted read the second selection, "The Training of the Surgeon," as an annual address in medicine at Yale University in 1904. This paper gave formal notice that a new surgery was born and accurately predicted its great future. The coming of the new surgery was, of course, gradual; its coming extended from many years earlier and was to extend for many years after the turn of the century. Yet the future could be predicted, as Halsted did with remarkable prescience. He was unable in that year to see all the directions in which surgery would advance, but he was able to see how these advances would come. The surgeons of the present century were trained in programs patterned after Halsted's; these are the men who have carried surgery forward. It is of interest to

contrast Halsted's paper with John Jones's Introductory Remarks,
*given almost a century and a half earlier. Correct surgical philosophy
changes little; surgery itself changes much. "The Training of the Surgeon" first appeared in* American Medicine *(8:69–75), in 1904. It has
been shortened slightly—by leaving out material that could only be of
interest to Yale alumni—for inclusion here.*

The Results of Operations for the Cure of Cancer of the Breast Performed at the Johns Hopkins Hospital from June, 1889, to January, 1894

In 50 cases operated upon by what we call the complete method,
we have been able to trace only three local recurrences.

Local recurrence is a return of the disease in the field of operation—in the apparent or buried scar. The more extensive, therefore, the
operation the more liberal our interpretation of local recurrence. Until
it became the custom to remove in every case the contents of the axilla,
a local recurrence was understood to be a return of the cancer in the
apparent scar; but now that we regularly clean out the infraclavicular
and usually the supraclavicular region and remove a part, at least, of
the pectoralis major muscle, a return of the disease in any part of the
explored regions should be considered a local recurrence.

Thanks to the most persistent efforts of my house-surgeon, Dr.
Joseph C. Bloodgood[1], the result of the operation has been ascertained
in all but two cases. The two unheard-from cases were classed at
the time of the operation with the most favorable ones. Only those who
have tried it can know what an amount of labor it represents to have
traced in this country, and in this part of it, the subsequent histories
of such a large percentage of so many cases.

Only one of the three local recurrences was inoperable. In one,
suspicious granulations excised one month after the operation were on
microscopical examination pronounced carcinomatous. The patient is
now perfectly well, without local or regionary recurrence, 2 years and

---

1. Joseph Colt Bloodgood (1867–1935) M.D., University of Pennsylvania, 1891, was Halsted's fourth resident surgeon (1892–1897). Bloodgood
was probably the first surgeon to wear rubber gloves routinely in surgery.
After completing his surgical training Bloodgood functioned at Hopkins in
two capacities, as surgeon and as surgical pathologist with a particular interest in oncology. He was an excellent surgeon and a popular teacher who became known internationally as an authority on malignant disease.

3 months after the second operation. The third case developed internal metastases prior to the local recurrence, which latter appeared 2 years after the operation.

In eight cases there has been regionary recurrence [Halsted uses this term for regional recurrences outside of the actual field, or scar, of the original operation]. Four of these cases are living and four are dead. Of the dead, one (cancer of both breasts) had an inoperable recurrence. Two were operated on successfully so far as the regionary recurrence was concerned. The fourth case developed cancer of the pleura prior to the regionary recurrence, which latter did not appear until 2 years and 4 months after the operation. Of the four living, three have been operated upon for their regionary recurrences and are now well and without recurrence 1 year and 3 months, 11 months, and 3 months respectively after the second operation. One case has operable skin metastases, but has an inoperable carcinoma of the femur.

So far as local and regionary recurrence is concerned the result is known in all but five cases. In 34 (73 per cent) of these there has never been a local or regionary recurrence. Twenty-four are living and 10 are dead. In 43 of the 46 cases (93 per cent) there has been no true local recurrence. In other words, there has, as I have said, been a local recurrence in only three cases (6 per cent). These statistics are so remarkably good that we are encouraged to hope for a much brighter, if not a very bright, future for operations for cancer of the breast.

The prognosis at the time of the operation was recorded as hopeless or unfavorable in 27 of the 50 cases of complete operation. In every one of the 50 cases some or all of the axillary glands were cancerous. It is stated in the histories of 17 cases that the highest infraclavicular gland was involved. In only seven cases is it recorded that the highest glands were not involved. In half of the cases, unfortunately, the historian has neglected to give precise information as to the extent of the involvement of the axillary glands. The supraclavicular glands were cancerous in at least five (10 per cent) of the cases.

The pectoral muscles may be involved and the prognosis still be good. Volkmann[2] many years ago, noted the great difference, prognostically, between involvement of the muscle by simple extension of the growth and invasion of the muscle by metastases.

---

2. Richard van Volkmann (1830–1889), professor of surgery at Halle, an early advocate of antiseptic surgery and one of Germany's most notable surgeons. He described the eponymic "Volkmanns contracture" in 1881. Volkmann was also noted as a writer and poet ("Richard Leander") whom Halsted quotes in his "Training of the Surgeon."

[Halsted next wrote, at some length and with a number of citations, on the importance of the underlying muscle as a barrier to spread of cancer; a barrier that ceased to be effective once invasion occurred. There then follows an extremely lengthy, detailed, and tabulated review of the literature on carcinoma of the breast, which served to show how few cures resulted from surgery as it was then practiced for this disease. He summarized this in the following paragraph.]

Bergmann[3] had local recurrence in at least 51 per cent, and not improbably in 60 per cent of 114 cases operated upon between the autumn of 1882 and May, 1887. I venture to say *not improbably*, because of nineteen patients nothing is known except that they are dead. Eight patients whom I have tabulated as having no local recurrence survived the operation only seven and a half months (average time p.o.). Six cases died in from nine days to two months after the operation.

Billroth[4] had local recurences in 85 per cent of 170 cases, from 1867 to 1876.

Czerny, in 62 per cent of 102 cases, from 1877 to 1886.

Fischer, in 75 per cent of 147 cases, from 1871 to 1878.

Gussenbauer, in 64 per cent of 154 cases, from 1878 to 1886.

Konig, in from 58 to 62 per cent of 152 cases, from 1875 to 1885.

Kuster, in 50 per cent of 228 cases, from May, 1871, to December, 1885.

Lucke, in 66 per cent of 110 cases, from 1881 to 1890.

Volkmann, in 59 per cent of 131 cases, from 1874 to 1878.

---

3. Ernst von Bergmann (1836–1907); see footnote 7, page 276.

4. The following European surgeons range from famous to obscure. A note is included on those who are well known or are listed in standard biographical sources.

Theodore Billroth (1829–1894), pupil of Langenbeck. Billroth became Europe's leading surgeon and surgical teacher, professor first at Zurich and then at Vienna (1867–1894). One of the first surgeons to grasp the importance of bacterial sepsis, with Lister, Billroth was noted, first, for heroic resectional surgery (esophagus, stomach, intestine, larynx, and other organs) and, second for his pupils, who included many of Europe's great surgeons.

Vincenz Czerny (1842–1916), pupil of Billroth's who became professor of surgery at Freiburg and then at Heidelberg (1887). Noted for pioneer tumor resections.

Georg Fischer (1836–1921).

Karl Gussenbauer (1842–1903), pupil and associate of Billroth's in Vienna.

Konig has not been identified.

Ernst Georg Ferdinand von Kuster (1839–1930), associate of Bergmann.

I believe that this is a fair exposition of the best work that has been done in the treatment of cancer of the breast. Many of these cases were operated upon before it had become a universal rule to systematically clean out the axilla. But each of the distinguished surgeons whose results I have tabulated recognized the fact that the axillary glands were usually involved, even when they could not be felt, and had made for himself a rule to explore the axilla in almost every case. Volkmann and Gussenbauer were perhaps the first to suggest that it might be well to explore the axilla in every case, but Kuster was the first to advocate the systematic cleaning out of the axilla.

Every one knows how dreadful the results were before the cleaning out of the axilla became recognized as an essential part of the operation. Most of us have heard our teachers in surgery admit that they have never cured a case of cancer of the breast. The younger Gross[5] did not save one case in his first hundred. Hayes Agnew[6] stated in a lecture a very short time before his death that he operated on breast cancers solely for the moral effect on the patients, that he believed the operation shortened rather than prolonged life. H.B. Sands[7] once said to me that he could not boast of having cured more than a single case, and in this case a microscopical examination of the tumor had not been made. There are undoubtedly many surgeons still in active practice who have never cured a cancer of the breast. But occasional cures of breast cancer have in all times been observed by reliable surgeons. C. V. Siebold[8] removed the breast and susequently the contents of the axilla for cancer, and for many years after the second operation had opportunities to see his patient and to convince himself that there was no recurrence of the disease.

Nelaton[9] reports several permanent cures after operation for breast cancer.

Velpeau[10] from 187 women operated upon for breast cancer, knew of seven who had lived for from 5 to 20 years after the operation.

---

5. Samuel Weissell Gross (1837–1889) M.D., Jefferson, 1857. Eldest son of S.D. Gross and very much in his prominent father's shadow. He wrote a number of surgical treatises including one on cancer of the breast; see also footnote 4, page 281.

6. David Hayes Agnew (1818–1892); see footnote 6, page 281.

7. Henry Barton Sands (1830–1888), surgeon, teacher, and popular preceptor of many noted pupils, including Halsted; see also footnote 1, page 300.

8. Possibly Carl Theodor Ernst von Siebold (1804–1885).

9. Auguste Nelaton (1807–73); see footnote 2, page 261.

10. Alfred-Armand-Louis-Marie Velpeau (1795–1867), Parisian surgeon and author of several excellent texts, including one on surgical anatomy and a massive and popular three–volume *Operative Surgery* (1847, edited

Pauli[11] excised first one breast and then the other for cancer and saw his patient 18 years later.

Encouraged by these rare but positive cures, German surgeons led by Volkmann have for many years been earnestly at work on this problem. But no positive advance in the pathology of breast cancer and no essential improvement in the operation for its cure has been made since Volkmann's contribution in 1875. Indeed, with one or two uncertain exceptions, there have been no results better than his so far as local recurrence is concerned.

As to ultimate results—permanent cures effected by the operation—we again look to Volkmann and accept, as every one does, but with some modifications, his views as to what shall be called a radical cure. I must quote again the lines which have so often been quoted: "I unhesitatingly make this statement for all cancers, that when a whole year has passed and the most careful examination can detect neither a local recurrence nor swollen glands, nor any symptoms of internal disease, one may begin to hope that a permanent cure may be effected; but after two years usually, and after three years almost without exception, one may feel sure of the result."

Billroth thought that Volkmann expressed himself too cautiously and said: "I think that one may express himself more boldly and may declare that if the careful examination of an experienced surgeon detects no recurrence when one year has passed since the operation, one may be sure that there will be neither a local nor glandular recurrence and may pronounce the patient as radically cured." Volkmann prophesied truer, for recurrences after one year are very common. Most surgeons have accepted Volkmann's views and do not consider the disease as radically cured unless three years have passed since the operation. The best results after three years are as follows:

Bergmann, 30. 2 per cent; Billroth, 4.7 per cent; Fischer, 9 per cent; Gussenbauer, 16.7 per cent; Konig, 22.5 per cent; Kuster, 21.5 per cent, Lucke, 16.2 per cent; Volkmann, 14 per cent.

Volkmann's statistics seem to have some bearing on the question as to the advisability of removing in all cases the pectoralis major muscle. He excised the pectoralis major and with it sometimes the minor in 38 cases. These were his worst cases, cases in which one or both muscles were involved. They were sometimes hopeless and always more or less desperate. In only 11 of these cases was there recurrence

---

in this country by Valentine Mott). Velpeau's *Diseases of the Breast* (1854) was the best book written on the subject up to that time.

11. Pauli has not been identified.

in the scar; in seven there was regionary recurrence, and in 13 there was neither local nor regionary recurrence. Four died from the effects of the operation. In three cases the result was unknown. Excluding deaths and unknown results (seven cases in all), there was a true local recurrence in only 35 per cent of the cases in which the pectoralis major or major and minor muscles were removed. And in only 58 per cent was there either local or regionary recurrence. Comparing these results with the 60 per cent of local and regionary recurrences in the cases in which the pectoralis muscle was not removed (the milder cases), we are at a loss to explain them unless it be true that the excision of the pectoral muscle or muscles means altogether a more complete operation—a more thorough removal of the fascia at the lower edges of the muscles and between the muscles, and a more radical cleaning out of the infra-clavicular region. A large proportion of the recurrences occurred in hopeless cases. The comparatively large percentage of nonrecurrence in such desperate cases is remarkable. I wish that there were time to consider the cases in detail. Any one interested in this subject would be rewarded for his labor if he should study these cases in the original.

If we may judge from the incomplete description of the operations, Volkmann is the only one, Billroth perhaps excepted, of the surgeons whose work we have considered who occasionally removed the pectoral muscle. I am at a loss to know how to explain this, for I operate not infrequently on cases in which the disease has involved at least the fat and areolar tissue between the muscles, if not one or both of the pectoral muscles.

Surely no one will question the fact that the comparatively good results in the operative treatment of breast cancer which the Germans are now getting are to be attributed to the systematic and comparatively thorough operation which they perform. But, excluding the great body of surgeons who, the world over, are improving their methods day by day and occasionally curing cases of breast cancer, a thing which they had never done before, the results of today are not very much better than Volkmann's were 20 years ago, if we base our calculations solely on the cases in which at the outset he performed the typical cleaning out of the axilla.

But Volkmann's operation is manifestly an imperfect one. It admits of the frequent division of tissues which are cancerous and it does not give the disease a sufficiently wide berth.

Even if it were always possible to dissect a delicate layer of fascia (the so-called sheath) from the anterior surface of the pectoralis major muscle, it is surely a dangerous as well as an incomplete procedure whether the sheath is infiltrated with cancer or not. The manipulation of the tissues necessary for this nice dissection must often express cancer cells from the alveoli and lymphatic vessels even if one should be so fortunate as not to cut through the diseased tissues.

Why should we shave the under surface of the cancer so narrowly if the pectoralis major muscle or a part of it can be removed without danger and without causing subsequent disability, and if there are positive indications for its removal?

The pectoralis major muscle, entire or all except its clavicular portion, should be excised in every case of cancer of the breast, because the operator is enabled thereby to remove in one piece all of the suspected tissues.

The suspected tissues should be removed in one piece (1) lest the wound become infected by the division of tissues invaded by the disease, or of lymphatic vessels containing cancer cells, and (2) because shreds or pieces of cancerous tissue might readily be overlooked in a piecemeal extirpation.

The operation which has been attended with such surprisingly good results in our hands is performed as follows:

1. The skin incision is carried at once and everywhere through the fat.

2. The triangular flap of skin, ABC, plate 1 [Figure 56], is reflected back to its base line, CA. There is nothing but skin in this flap. The fat which lined it is dissected back to the lower edge of the pectoralis major muscle where it is continuous with the fat of the axilla.

3. The costal insertions of the pectoralis major muscle are severed, and the splitting of the muscle, usually between its clavicular and costal portions, is begun, and continued to a point about opposite the scalenus tubercle on the clavicle.

4. At this point the clavicular portion of the pectoralis major muscle and the skin overlying it are cut through hard up to the clavicle. This cut exposes the apex of the axilla.

5. The loose tissue under the clavicular portion (the portion usually left behind) of the pectoralis major is carefully dissected from this muscle as the latter is drawn upwards by a broad, sharp retractor. This tissue is rich in lymphatics, and is sometimes infiltrated with cancer (an important fact).

6. The splitting of the muscle is continued out to the humerus, and the part of the muscle to be removed is now cut through close to its humeral attachment.

7. The whole mass, skin, breast, areolar tissue and fat, circumscribed by the original skin incision is raised up with some force, to put the submuscular fascia on the stretch as it is stripped from the thorax

close to the ribs and pectoralis minor muscle. It is well to include the delicate sheath of the minor muscle when this is practicable.

8. The lower outer border of the minor muscle having been passed and clearly exposed, this muscle is divided at right angles to its fibres and at a point a little below its middle.

9. The tissue, more or less rich in lymphatics and often cancerous, over the minor muscle near its coracoid insertion is divided as far out as possible and then reflected inwards in order to liberate or prepare for the reflection upwards of this part of the minor muscle.

10. The upper, outer portion of the minor muscle is drawn upward, plate 2 [Figure 57], with a broad sharp retractor. This liberates the retractor which until now has been holding back the clavicular portion of the pectoralis major muscle.

11. The small blood vessels (chiefly veins) under the minor muscle near its insertion must be separated from the muscle with the greatest care. These are imbedded in loose connective tissue which seems to be rich in lymphatics and contains more or less fat. This fat is often infiltrated with cancer. These blood vessel should be dissected out very clean and immediately ligated close to the axillary vein. The ligation of these very delicate vessels should not be postponed, for the clamps occluding them might of their own weight drop off or accidentally be pulled off; or the vessels themselves might be torn away by the clamps, Furthermore, the clamps, so many of them, if left on the veins, would be in the way of the operator.

12. Having exposed the subclavian vein at the highest possible subclavicular point, the contents of the axilla are dissected away with scrupulous care, also with the sharpest possible knife. The glands and fat should not be pulled out with the fingers, as advised, I am sorry to say, in modern textbooks and as practised very often by operators. The axillary vein should be stripped absolutely clean. Not a particle of extraneous tissue should be included in the ligatures which are applied to the branches, sometimes very minute, of the axillary vessels. In liberating the vein from the tissues to be removed it is best to push the vein away from the tissues rather than, holding the vein, to push the tissues away from it. It may not always be necessary to expose the artery, but I think that it is well to do this. For sometimes, not usually, the tissue above the large vessels is infiltrated. And we should not trust our eyes and fingers to decide this point. It is best to err on the safe side and to remove in all cases the loose tissue above the vessels and about the axillary plexus of nerves.

13. Having cleaned the vessels, we may proceed more rapidly to strip the axilliary contents from the inner wall of axilla—the lateral

wall of the thorax. We must grasp the mass to be removed firmly with left hand and pull it outwards and slightly upwards with sufficient force to put on the stretch the delicate fascia which still binds it to the chest. This fascia is cut away close to the ribs and serratus magnus muscle.

14. When we have reached the junction of the posterior and lateral walls of the axilla, or a little sooner, an assistant takes hold of the triangular flap of skin and draws it outward, to assist in spreading out the tissues which lie on the subscapularis, teres major and latissimus dorsi muscles. The operator having taken a different hold of the tumor, cleans from within outwards the posterior wall of the axilla. Proceeding in this way, we make easy and bloodless a part of the operation which used to be troublesome and bloody. The subscapular vessels become nicely exposed and caught before they are divided. The subscapular nerves may or may not be removed, at the discretion of the operator. Kuster lays great stress upon the importance of these for the subsequent usefulness of the arm. We have not as yet decided this point to our entire satisfaction, but I think that they may often be spared to the patient with safety.

15. Having passed these nerves, the operator has only to turn the mass back into its natural position and to sever its connection with the body of the patient by a stroke of the knife from *b* to *c*, repeating the first cut through the skin.

All that has been removed is in one piece, (*vide* plates I–IV) [Figures 56-59]. There are no small pieces nor shreds of tissue. I believe that

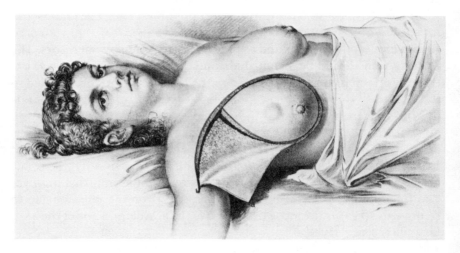

Figure 56 (Plate I). Diagram showing mastectomy skin incisions, triangular flap of skin, *abc*, and triangular flap of fat.

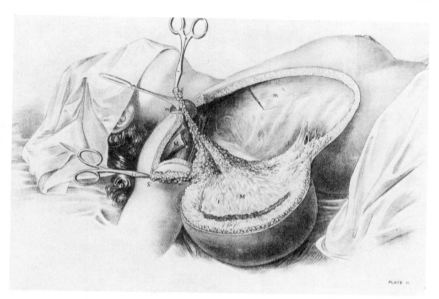

Figures 57 (Plate II). Diagram to elucidate Figure 58. *M*, major pectoral muscle; *m*, minor pectoral muscle; *S*, apex of infraclavicular fat below the subclavian vessels; *S*, apex of fat above the vessels.

we should never cut through cancerous tissues, when operating, if it is possible to avoid doing so. The wound might become infected with cancer either by the knife which has passed through diseased tissue and perhaps carries everywhere the cancer–producing agents, or by the simple liberation of the cancer cells from their alveoli or from the lymphatic vessels. The division of one lymphatic vessel and the liberation of one cell may be enough to start a new cancer.

[Halsted goes into some detail at this point, speculating on the nature of cancer recurrence and its possible relationship with tumor inoculation at the time of surgery.]

The operation, as we perform it, is literally an almost bloodless one. From the first to the last each bleeding point is stopped with an artery forceps as quickly as possible. When practicable the vessels are clamped before they are divided. If no blood is lost there is no perceptible shock from the operation. This is true of almost every operation. The symptoms which are so often ascribed to shock are due almost invariably to loss of blood. I have performed this operation for breast cancer on patients whose pulse before the operation was so feeble that the anaesthetizer and bystanders have pronounced it barely perceptible. As a rule the pulse is little if any feebler after the operation than it was before it.

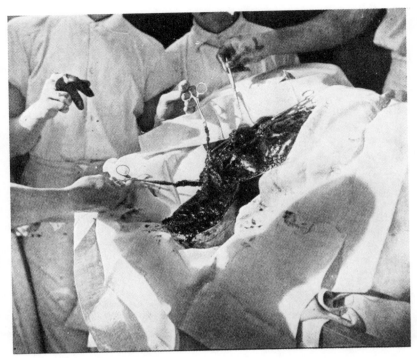

Figure 58 (Plate III). Photograph of field of operation, taken just before the final cut, which severs from the body the mass that has been extirpated.

The edges of the wound are approximated by a buried, purse–string suture of strong silk. Of the triangular flap of skin (abc) only the base is included in this suture. The rest of this flap is used as a lining for the fornix of the axilla. The apex of this flap is consequently shifted to a new and lower position. The axilla is never drained and invariably heals by first intention. The uncovered wound often heals by the so-called organization of the blood clot.

Seventy–six operations (complete and incomplete) for breast cancer have been performed in the hospital, and not one death has resulted from the operation.

Twenty–six incomplete operations have been performed. Seven were incomplete because of the small size and recent appearance of the tumor. Four of these are living, one with a local recurrence. Two died with metastases—one, and perhaps both, with local recurrence. The seven incomplete operations probably furnished as many (3) local recurrences as the 50 complete operations.

Nineteen operations were incomplete because of the magnitude of the growth and the hopelessness of the case. These operations were

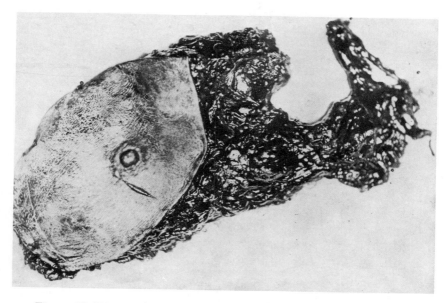

Figure 59 (Plate IV). Photograph of the excised mass. The cancer was very small, and the glands, although involved, could not be felt before the operation.

undertaken for the moral effect upon the patient, and were usually little more than an ablation of the greater part of the new growth.

As to the disability produced by the operation, it has in some cases been so slight as to be absolutely inappreciable. In most cases the arm of the side operated upon has been quite as useful as before the operation. Some of the patients when questioned complain that they cannot dress their back hair. This disability is due to the loss of skin and not to the loss of muscle. The cicatrix sometimes prevents the patients from raising the arm high enough to dress the back of the head. We have twice relieved this trouble by skin grafting. In no case that I know of has the disability of which the patient complained been due to the excision of the muscle or muscles. Occasionally there has been temporary swelling of the extremity.

If we permitted the arm to become glued to the side—and this would often happen if we did nothing to prevent it—there would be disability from fixation. We are careful, therefore, to secure a high axillary fornix. This is accomplished by means of the triangular flap of skin (abc) which is devoted almost entirely to this purpose, and which is held in place by a carefully applied dressing. After all, disability, ever so great, is a matter of very little importance as compared with the life of the patient.

Furthermore, these patients are old. Their average age is nearly 55 years They are no longer very active members of society. We should, perhaps, sacrifice many lives if we were to consider the disability which might result from removing a little more tissue here and there.

I sometimes ask physicians who regularly consult us why they never send us cancers of the breast. They reply, as a rule, that they see many such cases but supposed that they were incurable. We rarely meet a physician or surgeon who can testify to a single instance of positive cure of breast cancer. The conscientious physician could not under the circumstances advise his patient to be operated upon, and he was justified in treating her with salves and internal remedies. But now we can state positively that cancer of the breast is a curable disease if operated upon properly and in time. I cannot emphasize too strongly the fact that internal metastases occur very early in cancer of the breast, and this is an additional reason for not losing a day in discussing the propriety of an operation.

Surgeons should practise this operation on the cadaver. It is not an operation that can be properly performed after two or three trials. We operate for cancer of the breast better now than we did last year, and we operated better last year than five years ago. I have not had a local recurrence for more than three years.

Now that surgery is specialized to such an extent, surgeons have plenty of time to drill themselves in operating. They should not cast about for easy operations—for operations that any one can do at any time and in any place. I think that surgeons will some day contemplate with astonishment some of the handy, happy-go-lucky methods for intestinal suture which are now so much in vogue.

[Fifty case reports follow—all of those cases in which the "complete" operation was carried out. As mentioned in Halsted's article, the combined local (6 per cent) and "regionary" (16 per cent) recurrence rate was 22 per cent. It must be mentioned, however, that his follow–up time was very short, only a few months for several of the patients. Most of Halsted's cases were very unfavorable (as he recognized himself, and mentioned in a number of the reports), with large tumors and palpable axillary nodes. Most of his patients would not be considered today as candidates for mastectomy. It must be noted, however, that control of the local disease was impressive, as most of his patients died of systemic spread without evidence of local recurrence. This in itself made the Halsted mastectomy a significant advance.]

The Training of the Surgeon

Pain, haemorrhage, infection, the three great evils which had always embittered the practice of surgery and checked its progress, were, in a moment, in a quarter of a century (1846–1873) robbed of their terrors. A new era had dawned; and in the 30 years which have elapsed since the graduation of the class of 1874 from Yale, probably more has been accomplished to place surgery on a truly scientific basis than in all the centuries which had preceded this wondrous period. The *macula levis notae*[1] clung to surgeons the world over until the beginning of the nineteenth century, although distinguished and scholarly men, as well as charlatans and barbers, have practised the art in almost unbroken succession from the time of Hippocrates (460–375 B.C.) to the present day. A warning for all time against satisfaction with present achievement and blindness to the possibilities of future development is the imperishable prophecy of the famous French surgeon, Baron Boyer, who over a hundred years ago declared that surgery had then reached almost, if not actually, the highest degree of perfection of which it was capable.

Could Boyer, we ask, have been satisfied with the status of surgery when anesthesia was undiscovered, when haemorrhage was awkwardly and insufficiently controlled, when infection of wounds was not understood and could not be prevented? And yet I might quote from the writings of distinguished men of our time to show that even today some think that surgery is almost complete. Anesthesia, one of the greatest blessings, is at the same time one of our greatest reproaches, haemorrhage is still awkwardly checked, and of surgical infection once started we have often little control and then mainly by means of the knife. We have reason to hope that the day will come when haemorrhage will be controlled by a quicker procedure than the awkward, time-consuming ligature; when infections will be controlled by specific products of the laboratory; and when pain will be prevented by a drug which will have an affinity only for the definite sensory cells which it is desirable it should affect. The first of these may be last and the last first. Let us trust that it may, as Gross expresses it, "be a long time before the laws of this department of the healing art will be as immutable as those of the Medes and Persians."

---

1. "Macula levis notae"—roughly, "suggestion of disrepute."

"Literature," said Horace Walpole, "has many revolutions; if an author could rise from the dead after a hundred years what would be his surprise at the adventures of his work." Gross recognized, not altogether without regret, that this was particularly true of scientific works however erudite they may be. "Few survive their authors."

Tempted to belittle by comparisons the performances of our progenitors, we should remember that the condition of surgery has at all times reflected the knowledge and thought of the ablest minds in the profession. We may well recall the admonition so gently given by the highly talented von Volkmann, who was also a popular poet, writing under the pseudonym of Richard Leander.

> "Hoch aufhebt Schnee-schimmernd das Haupt in die
>   Wolken die Jungfrau,
> Aber sie deckt mit dem Fuss ein unendliches Land."[2]

Surgery, like other branches of the healing art, has followed in its progress zigzag paths, often difficult to trace. Now it has seemed to advance by orderly steps or through the influence of some master mind even by bounds; again it has stumbled apparently only from error to error, or has even receded; often there has appeared some invention or discovery for which the time was not ripe and which had to await for its fruitful application or perhaps its rediscovery a more favorable period, it might be centuries later.

There is a most intimate interdependence of physiology, pathology and surgery. Without progress in physiology and pathology, surgery could advance but little, and surgery has paid this debt by contributing much to the knowledge of the pathologist and physiologist, never more than at the present time. Harvey's immortal discovery marks an epoch for surgery, as it does for all medicine, for without knowledge of the circulation of the blood only the most primitive kind of surgery is thinkable. And yet there is abundant proof that the ligation of vessels, with the introduction of which Ambrose Pare' (1517–1590) has until recently been accredited, was known to the school of Alexandria; carried, it is said, to Rome by Euelpistus, it is mentioned by nearly all surgical writers of importance, from Celsus to the Renaissance. The brilliant Fallopius (1523–62), Pare"s contemporary, alas a very short-lived one, wrote much about the use of the ligature for the

---

2. Snow–glistening, the Jungfrau lifts up her head
     high into the clouds,
   Yet with her foot she covers an infinite land."

arrest of haemorrhage. Nevertheless, until Harvey demonstrated (1628) the true course of the blood, the principles underlying the control of bleeding by the ligature could not be understood, and surgeons studiously avoided operations which entailed haemorrhage and necessitated its control.

We can hardly understand in these days that surgeons who were at the same time anatomists and physiologists could have accepted for so many centuries, almost without remonstrance, Galen's views. Our inability to comprehend their state of mind with reference to this problem illustrates particularly well the difficulty experienced when we attempt to transport ourselves to other times, to obtain the point of view which subjugated our forefathers of centuries ago. It is now, as it was then and as it may ever be; conceptions from the past blind us to facts which almost slap us in the face. The blood which spurted from the divided artery was believed to come not from the left heart, but in some mysterious and indirect way from the veins, in which it was supposed to flow and ebb to and from the right heart. Harvey knew nothing of the paths by which the arterial and venous system communicate, and his discovery was not made complete until Malpighi in 1661 demonstrated by the microscope the capillaries.

How bewildering haemorrhage must have been when a wound suddenly filled with blood from a source unknown, and when sometimes, with little bleeding, a patient suddenly died from aspiration of air into the veins! What more natural than to pack quickly the wound, as Heliodorus and others were wont to do, with compresses of lint or sponge, to ligate large masses of tissue by circumvection, to draw the bleeding edges of a wound tightly together by stitches, as is still sometimes done, or to sear the bleeding surfaces with the cautery or with boiling oil! Imagine the terror and suffering of the patient, the desperation and haste of the surgeon, conditions not suited to the tranquil pursuit of physiological knowledge.

In all times, even to the present day, the surgeon's chief concern during an operation has been the management of the blood vessels. The fear of death on the table from haemorrhage has deterred many a charlatan and incompetent surgeon from performing otherwise perilous operations. The care exercised in the control of haemorrhage may constitute the chief difference between a rapid and a slow operator. This was eminently the case in the days within my experience when two or three artery clamps were considered abundant for operations which now require one or even two hundred.

The five things declared by Pare, usually designated as the father of French surgery, as proper to the duty of a surgeon may serve to indicate how restricted was the field of surgery before the course travelled by the blood was determined:

1. To take away that which is superfluous, as in amputation.

2. To restore to their places such things as are displaced, as in hernias.

3. To separate those things which are joined together, as in parts rendered adherent by burns.

4. To join parts which are separated, as in stitching up a wound.

5. To supply the defects of nature, as in setting an eye, an ear, a nose, or one or more teeth; filling up the hollowness of a defective palate with a gold or silver plate.

The studies of Hunter, born just 100 years after Harvey published (1628) his demonstration of the circulation of the blood, and about 70 years after Malpighi discovered the capillaries, on the healing of wounds, on inflammation, on the ligation of arteries, were made possible by the discoveries of these great investigators. John Hunter's (1728–1793) name is eclipsed by that of no other surgeon, and for the fame of his contributions, particularly to biology and physiology, an inextinguishable lamp will forever burn. Let us remain with him, if only for a moment, for he is an inspiration and a teacher for us all, as great perhaps for his time as the world has seen or will ever see again.

How fascinating to follow the groping in the dark and the searching for the light of a great mind! How refreshing and what a lesson is his honest doubt! "I am not able under such circumstances," he writes, "decidedly to say which is the best practice, whether to leave the slough to separate, or to make a small opening and allow the blood to escape slowly from the cavity." And again, speaking of that common class of injuries in which the wound communicates externally and the blood has formed a scab over the breach, he says: "But this operation of nature reduces the injury to the state of a mere superficial wound, and the blood which is continued from the scab to the more deeply seated parts, *retaining its living principle* (italics mine), just as the natural parts do at the bottom of a superficial wound, the skin is formed under the scab in the one case as in the other; yet if the scab should either irritate or a part underneath lose its uniting powers, then inflammation and even sometimes suppuration may be produced." Here Hunter recognizes facts which have been fully appreciated only in recent years, that there is a power for good in the blood, that the blood clot has a value and should be undisturbed, and that the dry scab usually desirable is sometimes harmful.

Under the conditions existing until the time of Hunter near the end of the eighteenth century, it was doubtless right that the practising surgeon should have been sharply differentiated in social position and professional standing from the physician proper, the latter being equipped with all the academic knowledge of the time, the former an apprentice of the barber shops. "The reasoning of the army surgeons endured as butter in the sun," wrote Abraham a Gehema in 1690, and the army commanded the services of the best surgeons. Nevertheless, it is often refreshing to find records of sound personal observations in the writings of the old surgeons, who, rude and unlettered though they might be, were dealing with realities at a time when the minds of physicians were buried in scholastic subtleties and fruitless speculations. In the German universities, when chairs of surgery were first created, it was considered beneath the dignity of the physician who taught the doctrines of this art actually to practise it. Thus Haller (1708–1777) about the middle of the eighteenth century taught, among other things, surgery both in Goettingen and Berne, but never demeaned himself to perform an operation. Billroth, commenting on this arrangement, says: "That Albrecht von Haller in Berne should for many years have lectured on surgery without ever having touched a single human creature with the knife is for us, in these days, hard to comprehend." How different apparently from Haller's was the attitude of mind at that time of John Hunter (1728–1793) in England, whose practice yielded a yearly income of 6000 guineas; and yet in spirit perhaps not so different after all, as exemplified by the remark to an assistant, "Well, Lynn, I must go and earn this damn guinea, or I shall be sure to want it tomorrow."

Even in America a little more than a hundred years ago a definite stigma still adhered to the exercise of the surgeon's art. Thus writes the eminent Dr. John Morgan, founder of the Medical Department of the College of Philadelphia, later the University of Pennsylvania, in a letter from London, November 10, 1764, to Dr. Cullen, after a long period of study abroad: "I am now preparing for America to see whether, after 14 years of devotion to medicine, I can get my living without turning apothecary or practitioner of surgery."

It was not until the year 1800 that the Royal College of Surgeons received its charter, and then only with great difficulty. Parliament had again and again refused to grant a new charter to the disbanded "Company of Surgeons." Lord Thurlow is reported to have said in the House of Lords when the bill had passed the Commons: "There is no more science in surgery than in butchering," and it was only when the Court of Examiners, a body still in existence, decided to appeal to the Crown, to King George III, that the charter was ultimately obtained. From the days of the great Hohenstaufen, Frederick II, who in 1231 commanded the teachers at Salernum diligently to cultivate the art of dissection, up to the present time medicine has repeatedly been aided and advanced by the enlightened intervention of kings and rulers. When Maria Theresa brought Gerhard van Swieten from Leyden to Vienna in the face of great opposition from the profession, she laid the foundations of the fame of the medical school of Vienna and she placed to her credit an achievement from which Austria and Germany still profit. In Prussia medicine has enjoyed the support of the Crown without interruption from the time of Frederick I to the present day. The splendid new equipment of the surgical department of the University of Berlin is largely the result of Emperor William II's wisdom and liberality. "A king or a privileged class," writes President Hadley,[3] "ruling in accordance with traditions and trying to act for the interests of the people, will give a much larger measure of real freedom than is possible under a democracy whose members have no respect for the past and no higher aim than their own selfish advancement."

The founding of the Academy of Surgery in Paris, 1731, has been referred to as the turning stake in the history of surgery, as the starting line of its scientific labors and of its true career, and the French regard the five anatomical demonstrations made a few years before by the surgeon La Peyronie in the College of St. Come as the inauguration of the new epoch. Von Bergmann reminds us that a Theatrum Anatomicum for students of surgery was erected in Berlin in 1713, but this exerted no such wide influence as the Paris Academy. The development of clinical teaching can be traced by unbroken tradition directly to Boerhaave, professor at the University of Leyden in the early part of the eighteenth century, and a teacher of unsurpassed influence and renown. His pupils carried the new methods to Austria, to Germany, to Edinburgh, and their decendants in the faith were the founders of the early medical schools in this country. In its influence upon the development of medical teaching the University of Leyden occupies historically the first position.

The relation of surgery to general medicine at the end of the eighteenth century was in Germany much less satisfactory than in Great Britian and in France. Under the teacher of clinical medicine was a surgeon who demonstrated the surgical cases. When Reil was called from Halle to Berlin in 1810 as professor of medicine, he naturally expected that the customary relations would be preserved and that

---

3. Arthur Twining Hadley (1856–1930), president of Yale from 1899 to 1921.

Carl Ferdinand Graefe, a young protégé of Wilhelm v. Humboldt, would operate under his direction. But by a mandate from the throne the independence of Graefe and of surgery was established. Graefe was given a responsible post as army surgeon, and his services in war were of such a high order and so greatly esteemed by the King that an independent surgical clinic was soon established and entrusted to him. The first equipment of this clinic was a very modest one, conforming to the straitened condition of the state's exchequer. Five times in the first nine years of its existence his hospital of 10 beds was obliged to seek new quarters, but in 1818 it was located at the site of the present surgical clinic of the University of Berlin. Phillipp v. Walther, his illustrious contemporary, gives his impressions of Graefe's clinic, which he visited in 1834: "a remarkable, splendid spectacle, conducted in a dauntless and highly gifted manner is Graefe's clinic in Berlin; we have no prototype of it either in France, England, North Italy or Holland. Its disposition is entirely national, purely German." "What changes have taken place in a single generation," writes von Bergmann, "changes brought about by the same indefatigable activity of the German clinical teachers and by their absolute devotion to their work, the devotion springing from inner-most convictions which made it possible for Graefe after 15 years of clinical toil to win such testimonials from his fellows."

In the year 1876, the year when I first walked the wards of Bellevue Hospital, New York, the dawn of modern surgery in America had hardly begun, and it may be of interest to note some of its characteristics at that time. The discovery of ether was not so old as to have obliterated all traces of the old surgical rule, "Cito, tuto, jucunde,"[4] but the rapid method of operating was gradually giving place to the safer one. Conservative surgery was made possible by general anaesthesia, as was illustrated particularly well in the exsection of joints and the subperiosteal resection of bone. The discovery of the ophthalmoscope, an invention of incalculable importance, had led to the establishment of the specialized eye surgeon, and it soon proved a great boon to general surgery, leading as it did to the adoption of innumerable specula and mirrors for the examination of hitherto unexplored regions. As a result of a reaction against bleeding and against the reckless waste of blood at operations, there developed a fondness, almost a mania, for bloodless operations, for styptics and the actual cautery, for

---

4. "Cito, tuto, jucunde"—"swiftly, safely, pleasantly."

ecrasement lineaire[5] (Chassaignac), for galvano-puncture and electro-lysis. To the employment of galvano-puncture in the treatment of arterial angiomata is due the introduction by Pravaz of the hypoder-mic syringe, which it is interesting to note was originally designed solely for the purpose of conveying to these growths a substance (solu-tion of chloride of iron) capable of producing coagulation. This little instrument, destined soon to play a part so useful, so indispensable, entitles its inventor to the lasting gratitude of mankind.

None of these methods for the bloodless division of tissues was destined to supplant the knife, so that surgeons became interested in devising better means for the prevention of loss of blood. In 1873, at the German Congress of Surgeons, in Berlin, von Esmarch gave to the world his method of producing artificial bloodlessness ("die kunstliche Blutlehre").

> Von Esmarch is one of the very few surgeons living who, even as a student, can recall the days before anaesthesia. He maintains that he who was not a participant of those times cannot picture to himself the enthu-siasm which took possession of every physician, and particularly of the students in the surgical clinic. Whereas before the introduction of ether, the operating rooms were filled with the groans and shrieks of the unfor-tunate victims, the appalling spectacle causing many students to faint, now, of a sudden, absolute quiet reigns, a stillness almost supernatural, broken occasionally by the senseless chattering or joyous singing of the patient.
>
> Familiarity with the use of cocaine in surgery has robbed somewhat the preanaesthesia days of their interest to the surgeon. We used to admire and wonder at the courage of the old-day surgeons who could inflict such torture for such small rewards, but we know now that certain operations can be performed with very little pain even without the em-ployment of a local anaesthetic. It is often unnecessary to do more than anaesthetize the skin to perform a very considerable operation, in the neck for example. From cocaine we learned in one year (1885) more about the relative sensitiveness of the various tissues and organs than from all the literature of our forefathers. The skin being anaesthetized and incised, we were surprised to find that the underlying parts were

---

5. Ecrasement lineaire. The *ecraseur* was an instrument made popular by the French surgeon Edouard Pierre Marie Chassaignac (1804–1879); see also footnote 1 on page 235. The instrument consisted of a chainlike cable that was tightened slowly over any organ or tumor to be removed. In theory, the compressed tissue in the remaining pedicle did not bleed. This instrument was in vogue during the midnineteenth century and was used for the amputation of limbs, breast, tongue, hemorrhoids, or any other organ or tissue that it could contain.

comparatively insensitive to handling and for the most part, even to cutting. The accidental cutting or crushing of nerves caused the most exquisite pain, and we noticed that the nerve supply of the blood vessels is so abundant that the severing or clasping of even very small bleeding points usually startled a cry of some sort of remonstrance from the patient; and now after many years of experience with cocaine we interpret an unexpected moan as signifying an insult to some small unseen blood vessel or nerve. These facts learned, I say, in one year, perhaps in six months of experimentation with cocaine, were not clearly revealed by all the previous ages of surgery. The explanation undoubtedly lies in the facts that in olden times the first cut through the skin so unnerved the patient and perhaps the surgeon that differentiation was impossible, and that the operation was performed in such haste as to preclude careful observation. I fear that so much practice with cocaine as an anaesthetic has obtunded to some extent our sensitiveness to pain in others. Formerly it taxed one severely to employ cocaine in certain operations which we now perform with equanimity; we are in danger perhaps of acquiring the kind of immunity (it is not indifference) which it seems to me dentists possess or have cultivated to such a high degree. Briefly, then, the story of the surgery of preanaesthesia days has become less interesting because it has been robbed of its terrors by the lessons which cocaine has taught us. If the surgeon of the past could only have known what it seems to the modern surgeon he should have known better than all else, namely, the relative sensitiveness of the various tissues, he could hardly have failed to discover methods of producing anaesthesia of the skin. That one could deliberately divide a nerve of the size of the sciatic or ulnar or even the minutest filaments visible without exhausting his ingenuity to find something to deaden the exquisite or agonizing pain seems inconceivable. How blind we are and how blind we ever shall be.

But no truly great and essential progress in fundamental surgical principles had been made since Hunter's time, until the monumental labors of Pasteur opened the vista through which for a time only the eyes of Lister could peer. It is hard to realize that 40 years have passed since Lister and Pasteur made to surgery a contribution rivalled only by Harvey's in importance. It was in 1867 that Lister first made known the almost incredible results of his experiments with carbolic acid in the treatment of wounds. The great merit of Lister lies in his clear recognition of the significance of Pasteur's discoveries in revealing the underlying causes of the infection of wounds and in the adoption of measures fitted to prevent and combat such infection. This merit will remain whatever changes may be made in the details of antiseptic and aseptic surgical procedures.

It was not, however, until 1875 that even in Germany Listerism obtained a substantial foothold. How I should like to tell the true story of this period in this country and abroad, to do full justice to Lister and his few faithful disciples in the United States and Great Britian, who for nearly 20 years contended with prejudice and parried the almost venomous thrusts of the skeptical and the envious.

Why was Germany the country first to adopt antiseptic surgery? Why did almost every surgeon in every German university eagerly embrace Lister's system almost at the same moment and as soon as it was clearly presented? The answers to these questions are, I believe, to be sought in Germany, and it is especially upon the question of the training of surgeons that I wish to dwell in the remainder of this address. What I shall have to say relates not so much to the mere teaching of surgery in the undergraduate curriculum, as to the requirements for the training of those who desire to fit themselves for a career in surgery.

Thirty years ago as I sat upon the benches, often seven hours a day, listening to medical lectures, I was so impressed with the characters and lives of some of my teachers that I believed they represented all that was most advanced in medicine. But a day in Halle, at the clinic of Volkmann, was a revelation to me. There I heard by one of the young assistants at the early morning clinic an impromptu discourse on epithelioma at which I marvelled. At home the whole subject of tumors had been treated of in one lecture, in one hour, in the "tumor lecture." Attending the Congress of German surgeons, which each year takes place at Eastertide in Berlin, I heard the subject of hip joint tuberculosis discussed. One surgeon alone reported on 600 cases, more or less, some of which he had observed 20 years or longer and most of which he had been able to follow. His methods of observation were new to me; his knowledge was inspiring; I was thrilled by his masterful exposition. Within two weeks, by a strange coincidence, I found myself attending in America a meeting of a very superior "surgical society" in one of our large cities, at which the same subject, "morbus coxarius," was under consideration. Only one of the surgeons had had an experience of as many as 28 cases, and of the subsequent history of most of these he knew very little. The contrast was not only in the knowledge and presentation of and interest in the subject, but in the audience. The Deutsche Gesellschaft für Chirurgie admits to its fellowship any reputable surgeon of any country of the world, and its halls at each Congress are filled and overflowing. The membership of the select "surgical society" was limited to 20 and the average attendance was less than this number.

It may be that the rise and multiplication of proprietary schools of medicine without organic connection with a university was a necessary incident in the rapid growth of a new country, but it is absurd to expect them to yield results in the education of physicians and in the advancement of knowledge comparable with those of the well-supported medical departments of European universities.[6] It is difficult to free either the educated public or our universities from the reproach that they remained so long indifferent to the needs of higher medical education. The times are changing, and we have learned in our own time, indeed within a decade, how superior in all respects is the endowed university medical school to the old-time proprietary school. Who would have believed that one or two well-utilized endowments could have achieved in so short a time so much? It was not only because some of the best men in this country were attracted to the university medical schools, fortunate enough to be so endowed, that the great progress was made; it was also because the further development of these men was made possible by the opportunities which they proffered and the atmosphere which they developed. The influence of these men, comparatively little before, almost at once, under the new auspices, was felt, not only in this country, but abroad. The growth of these men and of these schools has been so great that they are already well known and honored in all civilized countries. Much of what Welch foretold here in 1888 and in Cleveland in 1894 has already come to pass.[7]

Although we now have in the United States several (five or six) moderately well-endowed medical schools with a university connection, the problem of the education of our surgeons is still unsolved. Our present methods do not by any means suffice for their training. Do we require stronger proof of the inadequacy of these methods in producing young surgeons than is presented by the so-called sacrifices which our young men today are willing, nay, most eager, to make in order to obtain a training which seems even to them not only desirable but absolutely essential for success of a high order? Here I may be permitted to instance conditions which have evolved in a natural way at The Johns Hopkins Hospital, where the plan of organization of the staff differs from that which obtains elsewhere in this country.

---

6. Halsted's opinion of proprietary medical schools foreshadows the findings of the famed Flexner Report *(Medical Education in the United States and Canada,* Bulletin no. 4, Abraham Flexner [New York: Carnegie Foundation, 1910]). As a result of this report, medical education slowly improved in America and many of the substandard proprietary schools died out.

7. William Henry Welch (1850–1934), "the dean of American medicine," graduated from New York's College of Physicians and Surgeons in 1875. Welch was a brillian pathologist and a pioneer bacteriologist who was appointed the first dean of Johns Hopkins Medical School, as well as the professor of pathology there. He recognized Halsted's ability, helped him struggle with his addiction, and then brought him to Baltimore as the professor of surgery in the new medical school. Welch spoke often and well on medical education and did much to shape its reform in America.

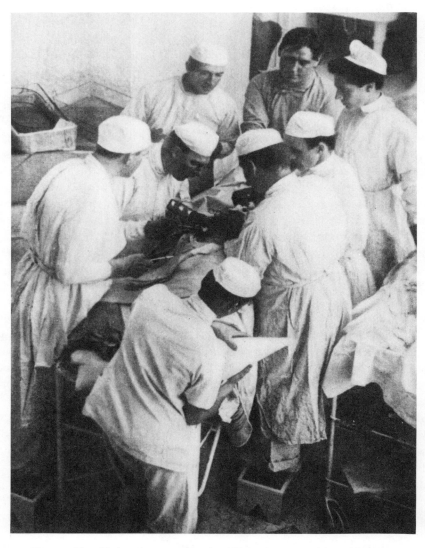

Figure 60. Halsted operating in 1904, the year this address was delivered. Harvey Cushing (1869-1939), also a Yale graduate, stands opposite Halsted as an assistant. From *William Stewart Halsted: Surgeon* by W.G. MacCallum.(Courtesy Johns Hopkins University Press.)

The surgical staff consists of nine men, eight internes, and one externe. The externe is an assistant in surgical pathology; he attends operations whenever it seems desirable in order to do with a clearer understanding the pathological work, to take charge of and describe the pathological material obtained at operations and to keep in touch, for his own benefit, as well as for the sake of the surgical department, with the clinical work. Four of the interns serve for one year, only the honor men of each class at graduation being entitled to these positions; but the *permanent staff*, so-called, consists of four men, the house surgeon and three in line of preferment. Men from any part of the country, if they have had the proper training, are eligible for the permanent positions. Great care is exercised in the filling of the vacancy on the permanent staff, which occurs once in two or three years, and advancement is not guaranteed to the appointee. The House Surgeon's term of service is still optional. He receives a salary; the other assistants are not paid. The assistants are expected in addition to their ward and operating room duties, to prosecute original investigations and to keep in close touch with the work in surgical pathology, bacteriology and, so far as possible, physiology.

The average term of service for the interne on the surgical side who succeeds to the house surgeonship in this hospital is at present eight years—six years as assistant, in preparation for the position, and two years of service as actual house surgeon. Adding to these the four years in the medical school and the junior and senior years in college, which in some colleges may well in considerable part be devoted to branches introductory to the study of medicine, the prospective house surgeon has to contemplate 12 or 14 years of hard work, very hard work, in order to secure this prize to which in this country of necessity only a very few at present attain. Thus far the success of the three or four men who have received, approximately, this training is so convincing that the very best graduates of our own and other schools are eager for the opportunity to be tested as to their fitness to rise to the position; and I know from applications which have been made to me this year that men of the desired quality would gladly serve 10 years on the surgical staff in order to obtain the experience which the house surgeonship and the training leading to it affords. The number of years which an interne who has become house surgeon is expected to serve with us is not and never has been prescribed.

It will be objected that this is too long an apprenticeship, that the young surgeon will be stale, his enthusiasm gone before he has completed his arduous term of service. These positions are not for those who so soon weary of the study of their profession, and it is a fact that the zeal and industry of these young assistants seem to increase as they advance in years and as their knowledge and responsibilities become greater. Nowhere certainly can a surgeon in a given period acquire so much, mature so rapidly, as in a hospital with an active and properly-conducted service. The times devoted to the training in surgery of those who hope to be teachers should not be curtailed, but young men contemplating the study of surgery should as early in life as possible seek to acquire knowledge of the subject fundamental to the study of their profession.

It was our intention originally to adopt as closely as feasible the German plan, which, in the main, is the same for all the principal clinics of the German universities. The house surgeon, or first assistant, as he is called in Germany, is selected, after several years of service, from a number of well-tried assistants. There is no regular advancement from the bottom to the top of the staff of resident assistants. Only a small proportion of these venture to entertain the hope of becoming first assistant. Occasionally an assistant from another clinic may immediately, or almost at once after transfer, succeed to this position over the heads of those who have served many years. This admirable system, which undoubtedly has its disadvantages, is possible only in a country where like conditions prevail and a close affiliation exists between the universities or where some great inducement exists for the making of assistants of the highest possible order. The professor of surgery, or the surgical chief, desires to secure as his first assistant or chief of staff a man of great promise, not only because of the obvious immediate advantage to the clinic, but because such an assistant is likely to have tendered him, ultimately, the chair of surgery in some smaller university. It is a matter of great satisfaction and pride to a professor of surgery to have supplied from his staff one or more university chairs. So, too, it is a great disappointment and sometimes a keen sorrow to the professor of surgery when his scholarly, highly-trained and devoted first assistant after a service with him of eight or nine years is compelled to resign himself to an instructorship, to content himself with the title "Privat-Docent." This occurs often, in fact is usually the case, because there are so many more retiring first assistants than there are vacant chairs of surgery in the 20 German universities. Whenever, consequently, there occurs by the death or voluntary retirement of a professor of surgery, a vacancy in a university, there are possibly 20 first assistants and perhaps as many Privat-Docents hoping for promotion, not necessarily to this particular university, for the vacancy, unless it is in one of the smallest universities, is usually filled by the professor in a still smaller one.

What are the inducements which make it worth while for the young men in Germany to devote so many years to preparation for the practice of surgery, what the careers to which they aspire, and what manner of men are they who furnish by their example and by their achievements the great stimulus?

Not only the first assistants but all the members of the surgical staff of one of the great university clinics in Germany enjoy almost ideal facilities for learning surgery and for prosecuting researches. The amount of clinical material is great. The operative work begins early in the morning and often does not cease till late in the afternoon. The outpatient department is controlled by the chief surgeon and is conducted by his assistants; a patient when discharged is consequently not referred to some dispensary or other and lost sight of. The pathological material obtained at operation is carefully worked up in the special laboratories for surgery and, if need be, is preserved in the museum, which should always be an important feature of the surgical department of a university. Every facility and the greatest encouragement is given each member of the staff to do work of research.

Although during the eight to twelve years of hospital service as assistant in some large university clinic he has laid the foundation of his reputation, the real life work of a German surgeon begins when he is invited to fill a professorial chair. He now longs to prove himself worthy of the new position, he has the incentive to inspire others to achieve, he measures himself by a new standard, and there is born in him the desire to rise higher, to sow the seed which will produce a bloom worthy of the greatest universities, possibly even of Berlin. In European countries no effort, no amount of time, few sacrifices would be considered too great if thereby the chair of surgery in a university might be secured. In Germany the prestige of the position is something that we in the United States who have not lived abroad cannot truly comprehend. In each university the chair has its imperishable traditions, its long line of famous surgeons, whose names are cherished and revered for their services to science, to their universities, to their country and to their fellows. In the nineteenth century, to mention only some of those who have passed to the majority, in the University of Berlin, were v. Graefe, Dieffenbach, v. Langenbeck; in Vienna, Vincenz v. Kern, Billroth, Albert; in Heidelberg, v. Chelius, Carl Otto Weber, Gustav Simon; in my student days there were in Leipzig, Thiersch; in Halle, v. Volkmann; in Bonn, Busch; in Tubingen, Victor v. Bruns; in Munich, v. Nussbaum; in Strasbourg, Lucke; men of great renown, every one. To enroll one's name with such as these, to inherit something of their skill, their knowledge, their zeal, their honor, their sense of duty, is not this worth while? The professor of surgery in Germany is usually a man of great influence and power. His affiliations, his responsibilities, his knowledge of surgery and the allied sciences, and often of art, of music, of literature and of the world's affairs, produce a type of man which his country may well contemplate with pride.

America, too, in spite of discouraging circumstances, has produced great surgeons, but it is to be deplored that here conditions prevail which hitherto have not encouraged, if they have not actually prohibited, such special development as I have outlined. I have known professorial chairs in one of the principal medical schools of this country to go actually a-begging—a-begging, of course, only of men who would adorn the position. Recently I asked a prominent surgeon, to whom a chair in one of our chief universities had been offered, why he had not accepted it. He replied that his practice was a large and lucrative one and that he had neither the time nor the inclination to perpare and deliver 100 lectures, more or less, a year. Young men are naturally only too glad and eager to secure a professorship which would insure a good living and a certain distinction, but older men who are already well known and with an assured income have no inclination to undertake teaching of a prescribed kind for which they are not trained and for which the rewards are not in their opinion proportionate to the labor. Even to those who have held the chairs of surgery for years the work sometimes becomes so irksome that they seek to abandon it as soon as directly or indirectly it ceases to yield a sufficient return.

The faults of our system of educating surgeons begin almost at the bottom and continue to the very top. I am considering only the training of the best men, those who aspire to the higher career in surgery. On graduation they become hospital internes, but their term in the hospital is only one and a half, occasionally two years, only a little longer than the term of hospital service required in Germany of every applicant for the medical degree and not so long, on the average, as that required of each medical graduate of the University of Tokio. The interne suffers not only from inexperience, but also from over-experience. He has in his short term of service responsibilities which are too great for him; he becomes accustomed to act without preparation, and he acquires a confidence in himself and a self-complacency which may be useful in time of emergency, but which tend to blind him to his inadequacy and to warp his career. A surgeon should find his greatest stimulus and support in his assistants with whom he spends or should spend many hours a day; but this is only possible when they have had opportunities for sufficient development.

Think of the labor of breaking in two new house surgeons each year and of the incompleteness of their work. "I thought I had instructed you to examine the vocal chords after every goitre operation," complains the attending surgeon; "No, it must have been my predecessor or some other house surgeon whom you so enjoined," replies the interne. It is a grave mistake, it is a shame to check suddenly the advance of these superior young men who are tense with enthusiasm, who rejoice in the work to which they hope to be able to dedicate their lives. It is from these men, we must not forget, that our teachers of surgery are made.

But much as the interne suffers from the brevity of his hospital experience, the hospital suffers more and the surgeon most. Every important hospital should have on its resident staff of surgeons at least one who is well able to deal not only with any emergency that may arise and to perform any operation known to surgery, but also to recognize the gross appearances of all the ordinary pathological tissues and lesions.

But the interne leaves the hospital unequipped; eventually, it may be, he secures the position of attending surgeon to some hospital and then he is expected to teach others to perform operations which he himself has not learned to do, and to pronounce at the operating table upon conditions with which he is not familiar and which possibly he has never seen nor heard of.

We need a system, and we shall surely have it, which will produce not only surgeons but surgeons of the highest type, men who will stimulate the first youths of our country to study surgery and to devote their energies and their lives to raising the standard of surgical science. Reforms, the need of which must be apparent to every teacher of surgery in this country, must come on the side both of the hospital and of the university, and it is natural to look to our newer institutions, unhampered by traditions and provided with adequate endowment, for the inception of such reforms. It is eminently desirable, if not absolutely essential, that the medical school should control a hospital of its own. There should be such an organization of the hospital staff as I have indicated, providing the requisite opportunities for the prolonged and thorough training of those preparing for the higher careers in medicine and surgery, and permitting the establishment of close and mutually stimulating relations between chief and assistants.

The professors of medicine and surgery occupy a peculiar position. They are teachers in the universities and at the same time teachers in the technical schools, the hospitals, which in this country are in only one or two instances, unfortunately, under the control of the university. As university instructors it is still a question just how much of the technical they shall teach, and as workers in the technical school, the hospital and in private practice, how much time they shall devote to laboratory investigation. It is doubtful if an ideal adjustment, if there were such a thing, could always be preserved, because in one individual there reigns a passion for laboratory pursuits, in another the love of the practical and the reward which practice may bring. Barker[8] has recently, in his memorable address, mooted this subject. Emphasizing the evils of the proprietary school and the inadequateness of what he designates as the "pseudo-university school," he proposes the name "semi-university school" for the "six or eight best medical schools in the United States," for the reason that only the subjects of the first two years are taught by men (university professors) "who do not engage in the private practice of medicine" and "who give their whole time and energies to the teaching and investigation of the sciences which they represent." It is to be noted that the true "university medical school," in the sense in which this designation is used by Barker, exists nowhere and probably never has existed.

The professors who teach in the departments of the last two years "are either not paid at all or are paid small sums, almost always less than the remuneration which pertains to a university chair, and almost always too little to provide the professor with a living income." "It is obvious," Barker continues, "that if those who teach the clinical subjects have to make their living from private practice, they will be compelled to direct their activities so as not to interfere with that practice." And further, he says, "I should like to see what the result would be if men with these capacities were bred to university careers, were placed in charge of hospitals especially constructed and endowed for university purposes and were sufficiently paid to permit them to give up private practice entirely and to devote their whole time and strength to teaching and investigating in such hospitals." Time permits only the very briefest consideration of this proposition, with which I am in the fullest sympathy, and which for a long time, perhaps for 20 years or more, I have seriously debated. Certain objections may nevertheless, I believe, with great propriety be urged against prohibiting the acceptance of fees by professors of surgery in universities.

---

8. Llewellys Franklin Barker (1867–1943) was a Canadian (M.D., University of Toronto) who joined the Hopkins staff in 1891. Although his primary interests were in anatomy and neurology, he was elected to succeed the great William Osler (1849–1919) as Hopkins's physician-in-chief in 1904. Barker was a proponent of medical school faculties that devoted full time to teaching rather than teaching on a part-time basis. The address that Halsted refers to appeared in *American Medicine*, July, 1902.

1. To be an impressive teacher of surgery, to attract important cases in large numbers, to exert an influence far and wide as a surgeon, to know his subject thoroughly, the surgeon must operate every day and always. A very considerable part of the surgeon's time must be spent in the operating room; more and more, it would seem, as time advances, for the number and variety of operations which a general surgeon performs each year is prodigiously increasing.

Professor von Mikulicz writes me from Breslau, "When I was a student in Vienna there were days, particularly in winter, when not a single operation occurred in the University clinic, so scarce was the operative material. Today the number of cases for operation is so great in the large German clinics that even when operations are conducted simultaneously on two tables we find that three or more hours of intense work is required almost every day." Through the kindness of friends in Boston and New York I am able to append the reports which testify to the great increase in the number of operations performed in a year in the Massachusetts General, the Boston City, the Roosevelt and the New York Hospitals. The statistics furnished by the venerable Massachusetts General Hospital are particularly instructive. In the entire decennium prior to the discovery of anaesthesia only 385 operations were performed in the hospital, an average of 38.5 operations a year. In the first decade subsequent to the employment of ether 1893 operations were performed, an average of 189 per year. In the decade preceding Lister's visit (1876) to this country, from 1868–1878, 7696 operations were performed. In the next decade only 10,119 operations were performed in this hospital; but from 1894–1904, 24,270 were performed; and in the year 1903, over three thousand operations were performed in the Massachusetts General Hospital.

The other hospitals mentioned show an increase in similar proportions. It may surprise some that the decade following the introduction of antiseptic surgery, from 1878 to 1888, should show such a slight increase. This may be taken as an indication of what is true, viz., that the majority of the operations which are done today were not only not attempted, but were not known fifteen years ago. Indeed many of them were unthinkable before the introduction of antiseptic surgery.

MASSACHUSETTS GENERAL HOSPITAL

Number of operations performed in decade previous to discovery of ether 385.

Number of operations performed in decade subsequent to discovery of ether 1893.

Number of operations performed in decade previous to use of antiseptics in this country (1878) 7696.

Number of operations performed in decade subsequent to use of antiseptics 10,119.

Number of operations performed during last ten years (1894–1904) 24,270.

Number of operations performed during year 1903 3109.

BOSTON CITY HOSPITAL
In 1878 316 operations were performed.
From 1878 to 1887, inclusive, 5882 operations were performed.
From 1893 to 1902, inclusive, 16,269 operations were performed.
In 1902 1923 operations were performed.

ROOSEVELT HOSPITAL, NEW YORK
In 1878 132 operations were performed.
From 1878 to 1887, inclusive, 4060 operations were performed.
From 1894 to 1903, inclusive, 18,181 operations were performed.
In 1903 2719 operations were performed.
Operations in the Gynaecological division are included.

NEW YORK HOSPITAL
In 1878 142 operations were performed.
From 1878 to 1887, inclusive, 2706 operations were performed.
From 1894 to 1903, inclusive, 13,002 operations were performed.
In 1903 1680 operations were performed.

2. With a fixed salary the surgeon may devote himself to the work of his choice, whatever that may be. If his tendencies are in the direction of research, he will neglect his operative work; if he is a natural operator, he will chafe under the restrictions which prohibit the acceptance of fees so easily within his reach.

I know of one or two men today occupying important chairs of surgery in Germany, to whom operating is less agreeable than teaching, and whose clinics, in consequence, suffer greatly from want of surgical material. Billroth had comparatively and actually little operating to do when in the days of sepsis he was most earnestly engaged in his microscopic studies and laboratory pursuits; and Thiersch, although one of the greatest names in surgery, was not a great operator and had small operative material even for his day.

3. An able and successful surgeon probably would not for the sake of fame merely and the usual professor's or any feasible salary be content to operate so constantly and to incur the anxieties attendant upon a large surgical practice. Indeed, he probably could not relinquish all fees if he would, for the exigencies of his family and his tastes would prohibit his doing so. Young and comparatively untried men could, of course, be induced to take the position, and some of these would undoubtedly regret the compact.

4. Barker proposes, if necessary, to give the professors of the practical branches (technical professors we may call them) a larger salary than the others; but this would at once place the purely scientific men in

an awkward position; it would pave the way for discontent among the chemists and physicists and others, who might with propriety claim that their salaries should be increased because they, too, might make a fortune if they were allowed to turn their ideas or discoveries to commercial account. As a matter of fact, professors of chemistry and physics accept fees, and all professors are at liberty to do so.

5. After all, the hospital, the operating room and the wards should be laboratories, laboratories of the highest order, and we know from experience that where this conception prevails not only is the cause of higher education and of medical science best served, but also the welfare of the patient is best promoted. It remains with the teachers of medicine and surgery to make them so. The surgeon and the physician should be equipped and should be expected to carry on work of research; they hold positions which should make them fertile in suggesting lines of investigation to their assistants and associates; they should not only be productive themselves, but should serve as a constant stimulus to others.

I should like to see the plan which Dr. Barker advocates carried out to the letter, and if it should succeed no one would rejoice more than I. But I would not advocate giving the surgeon or physician a larger salary than the others. The salaries of all must eventually be increased at least two or three-fold. There is, however, a compromise which even at present is altogether feasible. Let the surgeon be permitted to accept remuneration for services to certain patients operated upon in the hospital which the university provides or controls. His consultation and operations should all take place at the hospital. He might under only very exceptional circumstances be permitted to visit a patient in his town or state. Under special circumstances he might well be permitted to visit a patient in another state, if it were impossible for that patient to come to him. Private patients in a hospital need consume little or no more of the chief surgeon's time than the patients in the public wards.

While it has been my main purpose in this address to call attention to certain defects in the existing methods of medical education, especially in the opportunities for the advanced training of surgeons in this country, I would not be understood to minimize or to decry the great achievements of American surgery. Courage, ingenuity, dexterity, resourcefulness are such prominent characteristics of our countrymen that it would have been surprising if from the labors of her many earnest and devoted teachers and practitioners there had not resulted contributions to the science and art of surgery which have carried the fame of American surgery throughout the civilized world. The names of your own Nathan Smith[9] and Jonathan Knight[10] will always be treasured not only by this university, but wherever the history of surgery is cultivated. There is barely time for even the briefest reference to the recent contributions of America's surgeons to their art and science, but I should do my countrymen scant justice did I fail to emphasize the importance of at least one monumental contribution, which, I believe, redounds more to the glory of American surgery than any achievement of the past. It is hardly possible to overestimate the value of the modern work on the subject of appendicitis nor to attribute to it too great a share in stimulating and clearing the way for the great strides made in the entire field of abdominal surgery in the past 12 or 14 years. It is convincing testimony to the advanced character of this epochal work that continental surgeons were for several years unable fully to comprehend and accept the teachings of their co-workers in the new country. As operators some of our surgeons are not surpassed by any I have seen; there are, I believe, few operations in surgery which cannot be performed as well in this country as anywhere in the world, and not a few operations are best performed by the surgeons of America.

---

9. Nathan Smith (1762–1829); see page 104.

10. Jonathan Knight (1789–1864) held a Yale professorship for 51 years. He was appointed professor of anatomy and physiology at the school's founding in 1813 and became professor of surgery in 1838. He became Connecticut's leading surgeon and was twice elected president of the American Medical Association.

Bibliography

This bibliography includes only source and reference material. Other works mentioned in the text or in the footnotes have been indexed; see "Medical and surgical works" and "Medical journals" as well as individual entries in the Index.

Adams, G. W.
Doctors in Blue
Henry Schumann, New York, 1952

Austin, R. B.
Early American Medical Imprints, 1668–1820
U.S. Government Printing Office, Washington, D.C., 1961

Bell, J. W.
The Colonial Physician and Other Essays
Science History, New York, 1975

Billings, J. S.
"History of Surgery" in Frederic S. Dennis's *System of Surgery*
Lea Brothers, Philadelphia, 1895

Brieger, G. H.
"American Surgery and the Germ Theory of Disease"
Bulletin of the History of Medicine 40:135, 1966

Brieger, G. H.
Medical America in the Nineteenth Century: Readings from the Literature
Johns Hopkins Press, Baltimore, 1972

Churchill, E. D.
To Work in the Vineyard of Surgery: The Reminiscences of J. Collins Warren
Harvard University Press, Cambridge, 1958

Cohn, I.
Rudolph Matas
Doubleday, New York, 1960

Concise Dictionary of American Biography
Charles Scribner's Sons, New York, 1964

Concise Dictionary of American History
Charles Scribner's Sons, New York, 1962

Crowe, S. J.
Halsted of Johns Hopkins
Charles C. Thomas, Springfield, Ill., 1957

Cunningham, H. H.
Doctors in Gray, 2d Edition
Louisiana State University Press, Baton Rouge, La. 1960

Davis, L.
J. B. Murphy: Stormy Petrel of Surgery
G. P. Putnam's Sons, New York, 1938

Dictionary of American Biography
Charles Scribner's Sons, New York

Donaldson, G. A.
"The First All-New-England Surgeon"
American Journal of Surgery 135:471, 1978

Earle, A. S.
"The Germ Theory in America: Antisepsis and Asepsis (1867–1900)"
Surgery 65:508, 1969

Earle, A. S.
"Nathan Smith and his Contributions to Surgery"
Surgery 54:41, 1963

Fishbein, M.
A History of the American Medical Association, 1847–1947
W. B. Saunders, Philadelphia, 1947

Francis, S. W.
Biographical Sketches of New York Surgeons
John Bradburn, New York, 1866

From the Surgeon's Library
Reprinted from *Surgery, Gynecology and Obstetrics*
Franklin H. Martin Memorial Foundation
Chicago, Illinois, 1959

Garrison, F. H.
History of Medicine, 4th Edition
W. B. Saunders, Philadelphia, 1929
Reprinted 1960

Gordon, M. B.
Aesculapius Comes to the Colonies
Ventnor, Ventnor, N. J. 1949

Gross, S. D.
"A Century of American Medicine, 1776–1876: Surgery"
American Journal of the Medical Sciences 7:431, 1876
Reprinted by Old Hickory Bookshop, Brinklow, Md., 1962

Gross, S. D.
Lives of Eminent American Physicians and Surgeons
Lindsay & Blakiston, Philadelphia, 1861

Guerra, F.
American Medical Bibliography: 1639–1783
Lathrop C. Harper, New York, 1962

Guthrie, D.
A History of Medicine
Nelson and Sons, London, 1945

Hall, R. J.
"Suppurative peritonitis due to ulceration and suppuration of the

vermiform appendix"
New York Medical Journal 43:662–63, 1886

Harris, S.
Woman's Surgeon: J. Marion Sims
MacMillan, New York, 1950

Heuer, G. W.
"Dr. Halsted"
Supplement to *Bulletin of Johns Hopkins Hospital*, No. 90, February, 1952

Holloway, L. M.
Medical Obituaries: American Physicians Biographical Notices in Selected Medical Journals before 1907
Garland, New York, 1981

Horner, W. E.
Necrological Notice of Dr. Philip Syng Physick
Haswell, Barrington and Haswell, Philadelphia, 1838

Kelly, E. C.
Encyclopedia of Medical Sources
Williams & Wilkins, Baltimore, 1948

Kelly, H. A.
Cyclopedia of American Medical Biography
W. B. Saunders, Philadelphia, 1912

Kelly, H. A. and Burrage, W. L.
American Medical Biographies
Norman, Remington, Baltimore, 1920

Keys, T. E.
The History of Surgical Anesthesia
Henry Schumann, New York, 1945
Reprinted by Dover Publications, New York, 1963

Langstaff, J. B.
Dr. Bard of Hyde Park
E. P. Dutton, New York, 1942

Leonardo, R. A.
History of Surgery
Froben Press, New York, 1943

Major, R. H.
A History of Medicine
Charles C. Thomas, Springfield, Illinois, 1954

Marti-Ibanez, F.
History of American Medicine: A Symposium
M. D. Publications, New York, 1958

Meade, R. H.
An Introduction to the History of General Surgery
W. B. Saunders, Philadelphia, 1968

Mease, J.
"A Short Account of the Life of Doctor John Jones," in *The Surgical Works of the Late John Jones*
Wrigley and Berriman, Philadelphia, 1795

Medicine in Colonial Massachusetts, 1620–1820
The Colonial Society of Massachusetts, Boston, 1980
Distributed by the University Press of Virginia

Morton, L. T.
Garrison and Morton's Medical Bibliography
Argosy Book Stores, New York, 1961

Mumford, J. G.
A Narrative of Medicine in America
J. B. Lippincott, Philadelphia, 1903

Myer, J. S.
Life and Letters of Dr. Beaumont
C. V. Mosby, St. Louis, 1912

New York Times Obituaries Index, 1858–1968
The New York *Times*, New York, 1970

"Obituary: Samuel White"
New York Journal of Medicine 4:425, 1845

Olch, P. D.
"William S. Halsted and Local Anesthesia"
Anesthesiology 42:479, 1975

Olch, P. D.
"William Halsted's New York Period, 1874–1886"
Bulletin of the History of Medicine 40:495, 1966

Osler, W.
"The Inner History of the Johns Hopkins Hospital"
Johns Hopkins Medical Journal 125:184, 1969

Packard, F. R.
History of Medicine in the United States
Paul B. Hoeber, New York, 1931
Reprinted by Hafner Publishing, New York, 1963

Penfield, W.
"Halsted of John Hopkins"
Journal of the American Medical Association 210:2214–18, 1969

Pool, E. H. and McGowan, F. J.
Surgery at the New York Hospital One Hundred Years Ago
Paul B. Hoeber, Inc., New York, 1930

Randolph, J.
A Memoir of Philip Syng Physick
Collins, Philadelphia, 1839

Ravitch, M. M.
A Century of Surgery: The History of the American Surgical Association
J.B. Lippincott, Philadelphia, 1981

Richmond, P. A.
"American Attitudes toward the Germ Theory of Disease"
Journal of the History of Medicine 9:428, 1954

Ridenbaugh, M. Y.
The Biography of Ephraim McDowell
Charles L. Webster, New York, 1890

Rutkow, I. M.
"William Stewart Halsted and the Germanic Influence on Education and Training Programs in Surgery"
Surgery, Gynecology and Obstetrics 147:602, 1978

Schachner, A.
Ephraim McDowell
J. B. Lippincott, Philadelphia, 1921

Shryock, R. H.
Medicine in America: Historical Essays
Johns Hopkins Press, Baltimore, 1966

Sigerist, H. E.
American Medicine
W. W. Norton, New York, 1962

Singer, C. and Underwood, F. A.
A Short History of Medicine
Oxford University Press, New York, 1962

Smith, E. A.
The Life and Letters of Nathan Smith
Yale University Press, New Haven, 1914

Smith, H. H.
"History of Surgery, and Bibliographic Index of American Writers in
A System of Operative Surgery
Lippincott, Grambo, Philadelphia, 1852

Stone, R. F.
Biography of Eminent American Physicians and Surgeons
Carlon & Hollenbeck, Indianapolis, Ind., 1894

Thacher, J.
American Medical Biography
Cotton and Barnard, Boston, 1828

Truax, R.
The Doctors Warren of Boston
Houghton Mifflin, Boston, 1968

Viets, H. R.
"James Thacher and his Influence on American Medicine"
Virginia Medical Monthly 76:384, 1949

Wangensteen, O. H. and Wangensteen, S. D.
The Rise of Surgery
University of Minnesota Press, Minneapolis, 1978

Warren, E.
The Life of John Collins Warren, M.D.
Ticknor and Fields, Boston, 1860

Warren, J. C.
Surgical Observations on Tumors
Crocker and Brewster, Boston, 1837

Williams, S. W.
American Medical Biography
L. Merriam, Greenfield, Mass., 1845

Winthrop, J.
The History of New England from 1630 to 1649
Phelps and Farnham, Boston, 1825,
Reprinted by the Arno Press, New York, 1972

Index

About the Editor

A. SCOTT EARLE grew up in historic Lexington, Massachusetts. He served during World War II with the army's Tenth Mountain Division and then attended Harvard College, where under the influence of George Sarton, Professor of the History of Science, he developed an interest in medical history. After his graduation, Dr. Earle taught biology at Boston University and then entered Harvard Medical School; he received his M.D. degree in 1953.

Dr. Earle completed his surgical training at Boston's Peter Bent Brigham Hospital in 1959 and then practiced surgery in rural Idaho until 1970. During this time he wrote a number of articles on the history of surgery in America and edited the first edition of this anthology.

From 1970 to 1972 Dr. Earle received further training in plastic surgery at Cleveland's University Hospitals and then was appointed Director of the Division of Plastic Surgery at the Cleveland Metropolitan General Hospital. He is a Diplomate of both the American Board of Surgery and the American Board of Plastic Surgery and is Associate Professor of Plastic Surgery at Case Western Reserve University School of Medicine. He resides in Shaker Heights, Ohio, with his wife Barbara and their family. In addition to his interest in the history of surgery, Dr. Earle is an enthusiastic photographer.

WITHDRAWN

5/92⁷   9· 8/⁰⁴   ①⁴⁶7 – ¹¹/⁰⁸